IP2009

Milestones in Drug Therapy
MDT

Inhibitors of Monoamine Oxidase B

Pharmacology and Clinical Use in Neurodegenerative Disorders

Edited by I. Szelenyi

Birkhäuser Verlag
Basel · Boston · Berlin

Editor's Address:

Prof. I. Szelenyi
ASTA Medica AG
Dept. of Pharmacology
Weismüllerstrasse 45
D-6000 Frankfurt/Main 1

Library of Congress Cataloging-in-Publication Data

Inhibitors of monoamine oxidase B: pharmacology and clinical use in
  neurodegenerative disorders/edited by I. Szelenyi.
    Includes bibliographical references and index.
    ISBN 3-7643-2782-0 (acid-free paper)—ISBN 0-8176-2782-0 (acid-free paper)
    1. Nervous system—Degeneration—Chemotherapy. 2. Monoamine oxidase—
Inhibitors—therapeutic use. 3. Selegiline. 4. Parkinsonism—Chemotherapy.
I. Szelenyi, I. (Istvan), 1941–   .
    [DNLM: 1. Monoamine Oxidase Inhibitors—pharmacology. 2. Monoamine
Oxidase Inhibitors—therapeutic use. 3. Nerve Degeneration—drug effects.
4. Nervous System Diseases—drug therapy. QV 77.5 I56]
II. Series: Milestones in Drug Therapy.
RC365.I54 1993
616.8'0461—dc20

Deutsche Bibliothek Cataloging-in-Publication Data

Inhibitors of monoamine oxidase B: pharmacology and clinical
use in neurodegenerative disorders/ed. by I Szelenyi. – Basel;
Boston; Berlin: Birkhäuser, 1993
  (Milestones in drug therapy)
  ISBN 3-7643-2782-0 (Basel . . .)
  ISBN 0-8176-2782-0 (Boston . . .)
NE: Szelenyi, Istvan [Hrsg.]

© 1993 Birkhäuser Verlag Basel
    P.O. Box 133
    CH-4010 Basel
    Switzerland

Printed in Germany on acid-free paper

ISBN 3-7643-2782-0
ISBN 0-8176-2782-0

To my son, Stefan

Contents

Preface   ix
List of Contributors   xi
List of Abbreviations   xiii
Introduction   xv

Parkinson's Disease: A Brief Introduction

1. Anatomy of the Human Basal Ganglia
   H. Braak and E. Braak   3
2. The Pathophysiological Basis of Parkinson's Disease
   M. Gerlach and P. Riederer   25
3. Parkinson's Disease and Its Existing Therapy
   P.-A. Fischer   51

Chemistry and Pharmacology of Monoamine Oxidase B Inhibitors

4. Medicinal Chemistry of Present and Future MAO-B
   Inhibitors
   J. Gaál and I. Hermecz   75
5. *l*-Deprenyl: A Unique MAO-B Inhibitor
   E. E. Polymeropoulos   109
6. Pharmacology of Monoamine Oxidase Type B Inhibitors
   K. Magyar   125
7. The Pharmacological Basis of the Therapeutic Effect of
   (−)-Deprenyl in Age-Related Neurological Diseases
   J. Knoll   145
8. Neurotoxins and Monoamine Oxidase B Inhibitors: Possible
   Mechanisms for the Neuroprotective Effect of (−)-Deprenyl
   V. Glover and M. Sandler   169
9. The Mode of Action of MAO-B Inhibitors
   M. Gerlach, P. Riederer and M. B. H. Youdim   183
10. Pharmacokinetics and Clinical Pharmacology of Selegiline
    E. H. Heinonen, M. I. Anttila and R. A. S. Lammintausta . . .   201
11. Preclinical Evaluation of *l*-Deprenyl: Lack of
    Amphetamine-Like Abuse Potential
    *S. Yasar, G. Winger, B. Nickel, G. Schulze and
    S. R. Goldberg*   215

Clinical Experience with Monoamine Oxidase B Inhibitors

12. The History of *l*-Deprenyl
    M. J. Parnham 237
13. MAO-B Inhibitors in Neurological Disorders with Special
    Reference to Selegiline
    K. Wessel 253
14. (−)-Deprenyl Combined with L-Dopa in the Treatment of
    Parkinson's Disease
    T. S. Elizan. 277
15. Neuroprotective Effects of MAO-B Inhibition: Clinical
    Studies in Parkinson's Disease
    P. A. LeWitt. 289
16. Alzheimer's Disease and *l*-Deprenyl: Rationales and
    Findings
    P. N. Tariot, L. S. Schneider, S. V. Patel and B. Goldstein .. 301
17. Do MAO-B Inhibitors Have Any Role in the Treatment of
    Depression?
    G. Laux. 319
18. The Therapeutic Place and Value of Present and Future
    MAO-B Inhibitors – *l*-Deprenyl as the Gold Standard
    P. Riederer and M. B. H. Youdim 327

Appendix I

Chemical Structures and Pharmacological Features of MAO-B
Inhibitors
W. Paul and I. Szelenyi 339

Appendix II

Explanation of the Nomenclature for Optical Isomers
E. E. Polymeropoulos 359

Subject Index 361

Preface

Drug development is one of the most exciting, yet sometimes frustrating enterprises in the world. Inter alia, it requires intuitiveness, attention to detail and the ability to interpret preclinical data in terms of their clinical practicability, even if the clinical efficacy decides their definite fate.

Monoamine oxidase inhibitors are typical examples of such an exciting development with the inherent "ups" and "downs". About 40 years ago, monoamine oxidase (MAO) inhibitors were recognized as therapeutic agents for the treatment of depression. Despite promising results with the first generation of MAO inhibitors, their benefit was overshadowed by serious side-effects. The relatively young MAO research sustained severe set-backs. In fact, in the late 1960s very little was heard about MAO research.

In 1965, a young Hungarian scientist, J. Knoll, described the pharmacological profile of a compound, E-250. Perhaps influenced by Kline's exacting and provocative paper (1958), they considered the compound to be a "psycho-energizer". Since that time, MAO research has recovered from its initial stalemate. Isoenzymes were discovered and basic research proceeded rapidly. E-250, now under the new name "deprenyl" was recognized as a specific MAO-B inhibitor. During that same period, the treatment of Parkinson's disease underwent remarkable and sustained progress, although that progress raised other pros and cons.

Although the old "Danube-Monarchy" had decayed by 1918, and the "iron curtain" descended in 1948, the well-known intellectual contacts apparently remained intact between the nations along the blue Danube.

From the therapeutical point of view it was obvious that inhibition of MAO type-B, the major dopamine metabolizing enzyme in the nigro-striatal system, could lead to an enhancement of the attenuated supply. The idea that such a compound could have another, probably more important indication was then recognized by P. Riederer and M. Youdim upriver in Vienna.

The introduction of *l*-deprenyl (now called selegiline) revolutionized the treatment of Parkinson's disease. *l*-Deprenyl was the first selective MAO-B inhibitor to be used in clinical practice, and it has remained the sole such agent until the present.

Meanwhile, several other selective MAO-B inhibitors have been developed. Some of them are still in the preclinical phase, others are already in different stages of clinical development. However, *l*-deprenyl appears to remain in the centre of attention; to date more than 1700 papers have been published on this fascinating compound. Besides its enzyme inhibitory activity, additional properties have been discovered which might be advantageous in the therapy of Parkinson's disease, and are probably also beneficial in the treatment of other diseases, e.g. Alzheimer's disease. The broad pharmacological profile of *l*-deprenyl may result in new therapeutic entities. The drug's high therapeutic value in the treatment of Parkinson's disease and future applications emerging from recent clinical studies received appropriate recognition in the form of the "Claudius Galenus Prize", awarded in Berlin in 1991.

The generic name of *l*-deprenyl, or $(-)$-deprenyl, was recently changed to selegiline. However, the authors of this volume were free to use either name; the "old" name, *l*-deprenyl, is somewhat more known from the literature and it indicates the stereospecifically active form.

The amount of information in the field of medical research is growing rapidly. This necessitates fast publication of the very latest results in order to present the most current state of a given compound. Against this background it seemed most appropriate to start a new series of monographs on recently marketed, promising drugs, an idea put forward by my friend and colleague, Kay Brune, Professor of Pharmacology at the University Erlangen-Nürnberg. I am happy that Birkhäuser Publishers were ready to take up and develop Brune's idea and thus to provide scientists with a series of highly topical monographs.

I am much indebted to Peter Riederer for his advice and assistance in working out the final structure. Special thanks are also due to Birkhäuser editor Johann C. F. Habicht for his help during the publication process. I also thank my colleagues, Hans Heinrich Homeier, Bernd Nickel, Fritz Stroman, and Ulrich Werner, for their help in preparing the subject index, and I gratefully acknowledge the technical assistance of my secretaries, Heidemarie Schnitzler and Uta Kolb. Finally, I thank my family and, especially, my young son, for their understanding in having to do without me so often.

My intent as editor and the aim of this book have, I believe, both been fulfilled. I hope that everyone with even a passing interest in inhibitors of MAO-B, particularly in *l*-deprenyl, will find this book to be informative. May the work contain some ideas worth developing and may it intensify the research on MAO-B inhibitors.

Schwaig, July 1992   Istvan Szelenyi

List of Contributors

Anttila, M. I., M.Sc. Orion Corporation Farmos, Research and Development, P.O. Box 425, 20101 Turku, Finland

Braak, E., Prof. Dr. rer. nat. habil., J. W. Goethe University, Department of Anatomy, Theodor Stern Kai 7, 6000 Frankfurt/Main, Germany

*Braak, H., Prof. Dr. med., J. W. Goethe University, Department of Anatomy, Theodor Stern Kai 7, 6000 Frankfurt/Main, Germany

*Elizan, T. S., M.D., Professor, Department of Neurology, Box 1137, The Mount Sinai Medical Center of the City University of New York, 1 Gustave L. Levy Place, New York, NY 10029, USA

Fischer, P.-A., M.D., Professor and Head, Department of Neurology, ZNN, Schleusenweg 2-16, 6000 Frankfurt 71, Germany

*Gaál, J., Ph.D., Biological Research, Chinoin Pharmaceutical and Chemical Works Ltd., To u. 1-5, 1045 Budapest, Hungary

Gerlach, M., M.D., Clinical Neurochemistry, Department of Psychiatry, University of Würzburg, Füchsleinstr. 15, 8700 Würzburg, Germany

Glover, V., D.Sc., Department of Chemical Pathology, Queen Charlotte's and Chelsea Hospital, Goldhawk Road, London W6 OXG, United Kingdom

*Goldberg, S. R., Ph.D., Head of Preclinical Pharmacology Laboratory, NIDA Addiction Research Center, P.O. Box 5180, Baltimore, MD 21224, USA

Goldstein, B., M.S., R.N.C., Monroe Community Hospital, 435 E. Henrietta Road, Rochester, NY 14620, USA

*Heinonen, E. H., M.D., Orion Corporation Farmos, Research and Development, P.O. Box 425, 20101 Turku, Finland

Hermecz, I., Ph.D., D.Sc., Chemical Research, Chinoin Pharmaceutical and Chemical Works Ltd., To u. 1-5, 1045 Budapest, Hungary

*Knoll, J., M.D., D.Sc., Professor and Head, Department of Pharmacology, Semmelweis University of Medicine, P.O. Box 370, 1445 Budapest, Hungary

Lammintausta, R. A. S., M.D., Ph.D., Orion Corporation Farmos, Research and Development, P.O. Box 425, 20101 Turku, Finland

*Laux, G., M.D., Associate Professor, Department of Psychiatry, University of Bonn, Sigmund-Freud-Str. 25, 5300 Bonn, Germany

*LeWitt, P. A., M.D., Professor of Neurology, Wayne State
University, School of Medicine, Clinical Neuroscience Program,
14800 West McNichols, Suite 001, Detroit, MI 48235, USA

*Magyar, K., M.D., D.Sc., Professor and Head, Department of
Pharmacodynamics, Semmelweis University of Medicine,
Nagyvarad ter 4, 1089 Budapest, Hungary

Nickel, B., Ph.D., Department of Pharmacology, ASTA Medica AG,
P.O. Box 100105, 6000 Frankfurt am Main 1, Germany

*Parnham, M. J., Ph.D. Associate Professor, Director, Parnham
Advisory Services, Hankelstr. 43, 5300 Bonn 1, Germany

Patel, S. V., M.R.C. Psych., Monroe Community Hospital, 435 E.
Henrietta Road, Rochester, NY 14620, USA

*Paul, W., B.Sc., Department of Scientific Information, ASTA
Medica AG, P.O. Box 100105, 6000 Frankfurt am Main 1,
Germany

*Polymeropoulos, E. E., Ph.D., Department of Scientific Information,
ASTA Medica AG, P.O. Box 100105, 6000 Frankfurt am Main 1

*Riederer, P., Ph.D., Professor, Clinical Neurochemistry, Department
of Psychiatry, University of Würzburg, Füchsleinstr. 15, 8700
Würzburg, Germany

*Sandler, M., M.D., Professor, Department of Chemical Pathology,
Queen Charlotte's and Chelsea Hospital, Goldhawk Road, London
W6 OXG, United Kingdom

Schneider, L., M.D., University of Southern California, School of
Medicine Tower Hall, 1171 Griffin Avenue, Los Angeles, CA
90033, USA

Schulze, G., M.D., Department of Neuropsychopharmacology, Free
University of Berlin, Spandauer Damm 130, 1000 Berlin 19,
Germany

*Tariot, P. N., M.D., Director, Psychiatry Unit, Monroe Community
Hospital, 435 E. Henrietta Road, Rochester, NY 14620, USA

*Wessel, K., Ph.D., Medical Department, ASTA Medica AG, P.O.
Box 100105, 6000 Frankfurt am Main, Germany

Winger, G., Ph.D., Department of Pharmacology, University of
Michigan Medical School, Medical Science Building, Ann Arbor,
MI 48104, USA

Yasar, S., M.D., Preclinical Pharmacology Laboratory, NIDA
Addiction Research Center, P.O. Box 5180, Baltimore, MD 21224,
USA

Youdim, M. B. H., Ph.D., Professor and Chairman, Department of
Pharmacology, Bruce Rappaport Faculty of Medicine, Technion,
Haifa, Israel

*to whom correspondence should be addressed.

List of Abbreviations

A	amphetamine
AAAD	aromatic L-amino acid decarboxylase
AD	Alzheimer's disease
BA	benzylamine
cAMP	3′,5′-cyclic adenosine monophosphate
CCK-8	cholecystokinin-8
COMT	catechol-O-methyltransferase
CSF	cerebrospinal fluid
DA	dopamine
DAT	dementia of Alzheimer type
DDC	dopa decarboxylase
L-dopa	3-hydroxy-L-tyrosine; levodopa
DOPAC	3,4-dihydroxyphenylacetic acid
DSP-4	N-(2-chloroethyl)-N-ethyl-2-bromo-benzylamine
FAD	flavin adenosine dinucleotide
GABA	γ-aminobutyric acid
GAD	glutamic acid decarboxylase
Glu	glutamic acid
GSH	L-glutathione
GSSG	oxidized glutathione
5-HIAA	5-hydroxyindoleacetic acid
5-HT	5-hydroxytryptamine (serotonin)
5-HTP	5-hydroxytryptophan
HVA	homovanillic acid
LD	levodopa
LGP	lateral segment of the globus pallidus
leu-enk	leucine-enkephalin
MA	methamphetamine
MAO	monoamine oxidase
MAOI	monoamine oxidase inhibitor(s)
MCTP	1-methyl-4-cyclohexyl-1,2,3,6-tetrahydropyridine
met-enk	methionine-enkephalin
MGP	medial globus pallidus
MHPG	3-methoxy-4-hydroxyphenylglycol
MPP$^+$	1-methyl-4-phenylpyridinium cation
MPTP	1-methyl-4-phenyl-1,2,3,6-tetrahydropyridine
NA	noradrenaline (norepinephrine)

NMDA	N-methyl-D-aspartate
6-OHDA	6-hydroxydopamine
PD	Parkinson's disease
PEA	β-phenylethylamine, or 2-phenylethylamine
PET	positron emission tomography
ROS	reactive oxygen species
SN	substantia nigra
SOD	superoxide dismutase
SSAO	semicarbazide sensitive amine oxidase
STN	subthalamic nucleus
TA	tyramine
VTA	ventral tegmental area

Introduction

This introduction presents a short summary of each chapter, by which I hope to focus the reader's interest on particular topics.

Braak and Braak (Chapter 1) describe the neuroanatomy of the basal ganglia. This excellent anatomical introduction is followed by a description of the pathophysiology of Parkinson's Disease (PD). Gerlach and Riederer (Chapter 2) focus their attention on underlying biochemical changes responsible for the impairment of nigrostriatal dopaminergic neurotransmission. Their chapter provides a detailed presentation of the biochemical parameters and, in addition, gives new insights into the pathophysiological function of the "motor-loop" in the pathogenesis of the motor disturbances in PD. The role of glia is also discussed. Fischer's contribution (Chapter 3) deals with the clinical signs of PD and summarizes existing therapy. An old proverb says: "the bad doctor treats symptoms, the good doctor treats ailments, but it is the rare doctor who treats patients". Fischer, a "rare doctor", emphasizes that symptoms and stages in PD should be treated on an individualized basis, since an adequate improvement can be achieved in a variety of ways.

Chapter 4 by Gaál and Hermecz summarizes the medicinal chemistry of MAO-B inhibitors up to the present. In addition, valuable explanations of the different kinds of enzyme inhibition are presented. Polymeropoulos (Chapter 5) discusses the differences in MAO-B inhibitory potency of the optical isomers of deprenyl from a structural point of view. Moreover, a series of selective, reversible, and irreversible MAO-B inhibitors is compared with the structure of *l*-deprenyl*. Using semiempirical quantum mechanical methods, the interaction between MAO-B inhibitors and the flavin adenosine nucleotide enzyme cofactor is also described.

The introduction to the chemistry of MAO-B inhibitors is followed by chapters dealing with their pharmacology. Magyar (Chapter 6), who has been working with these drugs for many years, reviews the action of several MAO-B inhibitors. He points out that certain MAO-B inhibitors have an intrinsic pharmacological activity which is not related to the enzyme inhibition. The mechanism of the "cheese reaction" and

---

*Synonyms: (−)-deprenyl, selegiline; see also Appendix II.

its absence after administration of certain MAO-B inhibitors is also discussed. Knoll (Chapter 7) focuses on selegiline; he divides the pharmacological actions of selegiline (l-deprenyl) into two types: single- and multiple-dose effects. Besides the highly potent and selective inhibition of MAO-B (a single-dose effect), selegiline administered repeatedly facilitates the activity of the nigrostriatal dopaminergic neurons, enhances superoxide dismutase and catalase activity in the striatum, and prevents age-related changes in the morphological features of neuromelanin granules within the neurocytes of the substantia nigra. Based on his experimental results, it seems likely that selegiline is able to protect the striatal dopaminergic system from natural aging. Glover and Sandler (Chapter 8) discuss possible mechanisms by which selegiline manifests its neuroprotective effects. They include prevention of protoxin activation and inhibition of substrate oxidation by MAO-B, enhancement of dopaminergic tone, and induction of superoxide dismutase. They point out that the latter is of particular interest and may correlate with longevity in different strains and species. Gerlach, Riederer and Youdim (Chapter 9) have evaluated all relevant aspects of the mode of action of selective MAO-B inhibitors and make special reference to the possible mechanisms responsible for the observed neuroprotective effects, i.e., the inhibition of oxidative stress and an indirect influence on the N-methyl-D-aspartate (NMDA) receptor by MAO-B inhibitors. Heinonen, Anttila and Lammintausta (Chapter 10) give an excellent overview of the pharmacokinetics and clinical pharmacology of selegiline (l-deprenyl). They clearly point out that the stereoisomeric configuration is maintained in the metabolism of the drug; no transformation into the (+)-form takes place, a finding which is supported by Yasar, Winger, Nickel, Schulze and Goldberg (Chapter 11). As I began editing this book, the question arose as to whether selegiline has abuse potential or whether this was a myth rooted in ignorance about its metabolism to (−)-amphetamine or the lack of clinical experience. Even if there is no clinical evidence for an addiction potential, this point, probably based on the often simplified representation of selegiline's metabolism has only been discussed sporadically. Goldberg's preclinical results now clearly confirm the clinical experience that with therapeutically relevant doses of selegiline there is no danger of abuse.

The clinical section of this book starts with an enjoyable contribution (Chapter 12) by Parnham who describes the fascinating journey of selegiline from "psychoenergizer" to milestone in parkinsonian therapy. This selective MAO-B inhibitor possesses a high degree of clinical usefulness in the treatment of PD. By preventing the breakdown of dopamine, l-deprenyl can prolong the efficacy of a particular dose of the dopamine precursor, L-dopa. l-Deprenyl, in combination with L-dopa and peripheral decarboxylase inhibitors, may prolong the life of parkinsonian patients. Wessel (Chapter 13) gives an overview of the

MAO-B-related and MAO-B-unrelated effects of selegiline. Besides demonstrating the clinical efficacy of selegiline by presenting valuable tables summarizing several clinical studies, he describes the undesired effects of the drug, both in monotherapy and in combination with L-dopa. Elizan (Chapter 14) reviews the combined selegiline/L-dopa therapy in PD. Her conclusion is that selegiline's anti-parkinsonian efficacy is not as dramatic as that of L-dopa, a statement that could be discussed controversially. However, the addition of selegiline to L-dopa early in PD allows for a smoother titration of the L-dopa dose and an easier maintenance of the latter drug at low optimal levels for as long as possible than would otherwise be the case. Her proposal, which may be of interest, is a "triple" combination of MAO-B inhibitor, dopamine agonist and L-dopa as initial therapy in *de novo* cases. In the preclinical section, Glover and Sandler discuss how deprenyl can act neuroprotectively. In Chapter 15, LeWitt collects all clinical results in order to demonstrate the clinical relevance of a possible neuroprotective effect of MAO-B inhibitors. Besides results from the well-known DATATOP study, he has included data from the new French Selegiline Multicenter Trial. Chapter 16, by Tariot, Schneider, Patel and Goldstein, summarizes all studies performed with selegiline in Alzheimer's disease (AD) up to the present. These authors clearly state that a rationale exists for the administration of selegiline to patients suffering from dementia of the Alzheimer type (DAT). There is some encouraging but no convincing evidence of the clinical benefit of selegiline in such cases. Large, well-controlled clinical studies are necessary before we can establish the putative effect of selegiline in AD. Laux (Chapter 17) evaluated the role of selegiline alone and in combination with phenylalanine and *l*-5-hydroxytryptophan in the treatment of depression; in the studies performed so far, higher doses were used than in the treatment of PD. Based on the multifaceted pharmacological profile of selegiline, Laux proposes to carry out controlled studies in patients with certain subtypes/subgroups of affective disorders in order to establish the therapeutic value of selegiline in the treatment of depression. Riederer and Youdim (Chapter 18) consider the possible future therapeutic uses of new MAO-B inhibitors. Of course, they had to base their projection on *l*-deprenyl, the only currently available MAO-B inhibitor used in the treatment of parkinsonism. From this point of view, they give an excellent short review of the pharmacological and biochemical profile of this compound and include some remarks on therapy. Based on our present experience with the interesting therapeutic uses of selegiline, the efficacy of new MAO-B inhibitors will presumably be judged using the drug as "gold standard".

Appendix I is intended for the cursory reader, the more specialized pharmacologist, the treating clinician, and the general practitioner; it summarizes chemical, pharmacological, and clinical data on the most important MAO-B inhibitors and lists their originators, drug development stage, and for marketed drugs, their brand or trade names and distributors.

Finally, Appendix II explains the correct nomenclature of enantiomers.

I. Szelenyi, Frankfurt, July 1992

Parkinson's Disease: A Brief Introduction

Inhibitors of Monoamine Oxidase B
Pharmacology and Clinical Use in Neurodegenerative Disorders
ed. by I. Szelenyi
© 1993 Birkhäuser Verlag Basel/Switzerland

CHAPTER 1
Anatomy of the Human Basal Ganglia

H. Braak and E. Braak

1 Introduction
2 Ventral and Dorsal Striatum
3 Ventral Pallidum, External and Internal Pallidal Segments
4 Subthalamic Nucleus
5 Substantia Nigra
6 Paranigral Nucleus and Pigmented Parabrachial Nucleus
7 Cortex Related Thalamic Nuclei and Reticular Nucleus of the Thalamus
8 Centromediano-Parafascicular Complex
9 Locus Coeruleus, Anterior Raphe Nuclei, Tuberomamillary Nucleus and
  Magnocellular Nuclei of the Basal Forebrain
  Summary
  References

1. Introduction

The limbic system exerts considerable influence on cortical areas and subcortical nuclei involved in the initiation, execution, and control of movements. Particularly dense projections to the accumbens nucleus and ventral striatum arise from the entorhinal region, hippocampal formation, and amygdala. The limbic data is transferred via the ventral pallidum and the mediodorsal thalamic nuclei to association areas of the frontal isocortex. This part of the frontal lobe is thought to initiate movements by influencing the dorsal striatum. From here, the information is transferred to both the external and internal segments of the pallidum. Eventually, the pallidal output reaches the anterior ventrolateral thalamic nuclei which relay data back to the cortex. The final loop includes the pons, cerebellum, and lower brain stem nuclei. Again, the thalamus integrates input and projects to cortical areas that contribute to the formation of corticonuclear and corticospinal fibers projecting down to the motor neurons of the lower brain stem and spinal cord (Figure 1).

This review concentrates on the topography, internal organization, neuronal types, and connectivity of the "basal ganglia" which provide the substrate for a parallel arrangement of numerous channels from the cortex to the motor thalamus [1–4]. Unfortunately, the frequently used term "basal ganglia" lacks precision. In this text, the term is used to

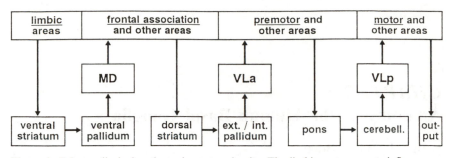

Figure 1. Scheme displaying the main motor circuits. The limbic system exerts influence on the ventral striatum. Via ventral pallidum and mediodorsal thalamus (MD) data is transported to the frontal association cortex which, in turn, projects to the dorsal striatum. From here, information is transferred via the external (ext.) and internal (int.) segments of the pallidum and anterior nuclei of the ventrolateral thalamus (VLa) to premotor areas. These project to the pontine gray and via cerebellum and the posterior nuclei of the ventrolateral thalamus (VLp) the data are relayed back to cortical areas generating the corticospinal tract (output).

include the telencephalic striatum and magnocellular nuclei of the basal forebrain, the diencephalic pallidum, the tuberomamillary and subthalamic nuclei, the mesencephalic substantia nigra, and the paranigral and pigmented parabrachial nuclei.

2. Ventral and Dorsal Striatum

The term "striatum" refers to closely related subcortical nuclei in basal portions of the telencephalon comprising the accumbens nucleus and ventral striatum, the caudate nucleus and the putamen. All these types of gray matter disclose a principally uniform composition of a small number of neuronal types. Bundles of myelinated fibers traverse the nuclei and give them a striated appearance.

The accumbens nucleus appears as the genuine center of the striatum (fundus striati, [5]). It forms the anteromedial striatal extremity and generates a superior (caudate nucleus), lateral (putamen), and inferior extension (ventral striatum). The ventral striatum fills much of the space below the anterior commissure extending down to the basal surface of the brain (Figure 2b). The ventral striatum and large parts of the accumbens nucleus are tightly interconnected with cortical areas and subcortical nuclei of the limbic system; these are combined in Figure 4 under the term "ventral striatum" [6–8].

The thick head of the caudate nucleus emerges from the accumbens nucleus. Posteriorly, it narrows into the body and gradually tapers off, diminishing to the tail. Putamen and caudate nucleus are incompletely separated by the fiber bundles of the internal capsule. The putamen spans from the external capsule to the external medullary lamina of the pallidum (Figure 2). The caudate nucleus and the putamen are grouped under the term "dorsal striatum" (Figures 4 and 5).

The striatum is composed of a few neuronal types. Predominating among these are the medium-sized spiny type-I neurons ([9, 10], spiny type-I: [11], spiny neuron: [12]). These cells exhibit a polygonal cell body which gives off a moderate number of dendrites radiating in all directions. The extensively branching dendrites show a spine-free proximal stem, while the more distal portions are densely covered with spines. The axon gives off extensive local collaterals that branch profusely within the reaches of the parent neuron. The collaterals preferentially terminate on proximal dendrites of neighboring type-I neurons and may thus link together local clusters of these cells. The terminal twig of the axon is very thin, sparsely myelinated, and leaves the striatum to terminate within the pallidum with small band-like arborizations oriented parallel to the medullary lamina. Part of the axons also reach the pars reticulata of the substantia nigra. The medium-sized spiny type-I neuron contains sparse basophilic material within the cell body. Lipofuscin granules are usually located at one pole of the cell body, with a tendency to extend into one of the proximal dendrites. The globular and pallid nucleus is centrally located (Figure 3; [10, 12, 13]).

Most type-I neurons are inhibitory GABAergic (gamma-amino-butyric acid) projection cells. Two subtypes exist, the first being characterized by an opiate peptide (mostly an enkephalin-like peptide), the second by substance P [7, 14]. Type-I neurons receive excitatory glutamatergic afferents from the cerebral cortex and a second excitatory projection from the thalamus, both terminating with asymmetrical contacts on the tips of their dendritic spines [15–17]. The dopaminergic projection fibers from the substantia nigra form symmetric contacts and impinge chiefly upon the stalk of the spines, while the intrinsic cholinergic terminals are usually found on proximal portions of the dendrites. Dopaminergic and cholinergic boutons are hence well positioned to regulate the excitatory input from cortical areas and thalamic nuclei. In contrast to the relatively well-known function of fast-acting neurotransmitters (glutamate opening an excitatory Na^+ channel, and GABA opening an inhibitory Cl^- channel), many questions remain as yet unanswered regarding the role of dopamine and acetylcholine in the striatum. Dopamine and acetylcholine work much slower than glutamate and GABA, as the former work through the stimulation of second messengers. Acetylcholine most likely exerts an excitatory effect on the GABA/enkephalin projection neurons, while dopamine appears to stimulate the GABA/substance P neurons and to inhibit the GABA/enkephalin cells. The cholinergic input, therefore, appears to serve as an antagonist to the dopaminergic input [6, 18]. The main function of both subtypes of type-I neurons appears to exert a controlled inhibitory influence on the tonically active projection cells of both the pallidum and the nigral pars reticulata.

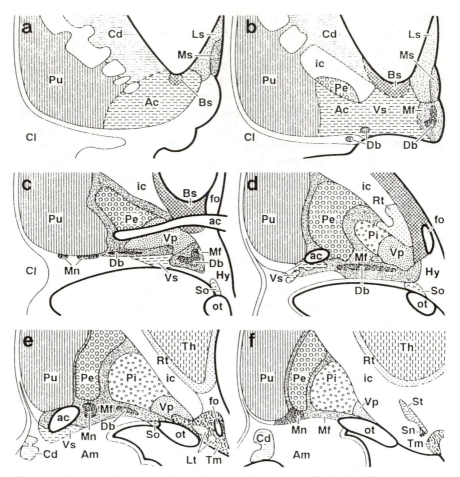

Figure 2. Diagram of coronal sections through the human basal forebrain. The series runs in an anterior posterior direction with each of the sections spaced apart by 3200 μm (800-μm thick pigment preparations). *Ac* accumbens nucleus, *Am* amygdala, *Bs* bed nucleus of the stria terminalis, *Cd* caudate nucleus, *Cl* claustrum, *Db* nucleus of the diagonal band, *Hy* hypothalamus, *Ls* lateral septal nucleus, *Lt* lateral tuberal nucleus, *Mf* magnocellular nuclei of the basal forebrain, *Mn* basal nucleus of Meynert, *Ms* medial septal nucleus, *Pe* external pallidal segment, *Pi* internal pallidal segment, *Pu* putamen, *Rt* reticular thalamic nucleus, *So* supraoptic nucleus, *Sn* substantia nigra, *St* subthalamic nucleus, *Th* thalamus, *Tm* tuberomamillary nucleus, *Vp* ventral pallidum, *Vs* ventral striatum; *ac* anterior commissure, *fo* fornix, *ic* internal capsule, *ot* optic tract.

Much less is known about the remaining striatal cell types; quite a number of them appear to function as local circuit neurons. The sources of input received by these cells are largely unknown and there is also little knowledge as to their efferent connections [7, 10].

The slender type-II neurons give rise to a few long, intertwining dendrites. Frequently, the main processes emerge from opposite poles of

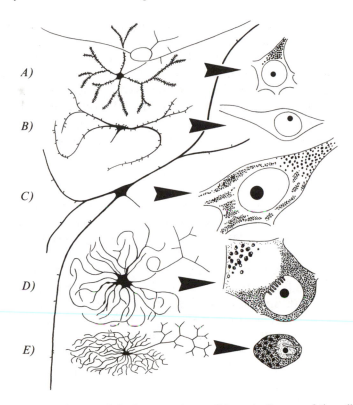

Figure 3. Neuronal types of the human striatum. Schematic diagram of the cells as seen in Golgi preparations (left side) are compared with pigment-Nissl characteristics of the same neurons (right side). *A*) Medium-sized spiny type-I neurons are predominately found in the human striatum. *B*) Slender type-II neurons with long dendrites and somatic spines. *C*) Large type-III neurons resembling nerve cells of the pallidum. *D*) Large aspiny type-IV neurons with dense spherical dendritic arbor and local axon. *E*) Small type-V cells with local axon and dark cell body (with permission from [10]).

the soma. The dendrites and also, especially, the soma possess a few spines (spiny type II: [11]). These cells receive only a small number of synaptic contacts. The pattern of axonal arborization and the target of the terminal axon are as yet unknown. The elongated cell body is devoid of lipofuscin pigment or it harbors a few tiny granules (Figure 3). Many of the type-II cells are GABAergic and contain, in addition, somatostatin and neuropeptide Y ([14]; personal observations).

The large multipolar type-III cells generate a small number of thick and extended dendrites with a few spines. The cell body contains finely granulated and widely dispersed lipofuscin pigment (leptodendritic neuron: [12]). These cells have many features in common with the principal cells of the pallidum and may represent displaced pallidum neurons (Figure 3; [10]).

The voluminous aspiny type-IV cells (aspiny neuron: [19]; aspiny type II: [11]; spidery neuron: [12]) display a polygonal rounded soma and emit numerous thin dendrites. The winding dendrites are relatively short and frequently branch off into secondary twigs. Typically, a spherical dendritic domain results. The axon branches extensively into terminal twigs close to the parent soma. The cell body contains a small nucleus in an off-center position opposite a tightly packed agglomeration of lipofuscin granules. The nuclear membrane facing the pallid center of the cell body exhibits numerous deep enfolds. The Nissl material accumulates in irregular masses and is located in the peripheral cytoplasm (Figure 3). Type-IV cells contain choline acetyltransferase, and many of the excitatory cholinergic fibers within the striatum probably derive from the large aspiny nerve cells [14]. The fibers exert excitatory effects on GABA/enkephalin type-I neurons [6].

The small to medium-sized aspiny type-V cells ([11]; aspiny type I: [20], microneuron: [12]) appear as dwarfed versions of the type-IV cells. The dendrites break up into a swirling mass of thin branches and more than one axon may project from these cells. The axons branch profusely in the vicinity of the cell body. Type-V neurons contain unusually large and well stained lipofuscin granules and the cell body is rich in diffusely distributed Nissl material. Also, type-V neurons contain parvalbumin (personal observation).

Many authors differentiate a further cell type with very small soma, a few moderately branching dendrites and a thin axon (aspiny type III: [13]).

The dorsal striatum is composed of two compartments, patches (=striosomes) and matrix. This division is less obvious or absent in the ventral striatum [21]. The irregularly outlined patches are lacking in acetylcholinesterase (striosomes, constituting 10–20% of the striatal volume [22, 23, 24], but are surrounded by an acetylcholinesterase-rich matrix. Patches and matrix are also distinguishable on the basis of differences in their content of various neuromodulators or neurotransmitters. Furthermore, afferent and efferent connections are divided with respect to these compartments. Patches tend to receive inputs from limbic structures and frontal association cortex, while the matrix receives, predominantly, afferents from the central region of the cortex related to sensorimotor processing. Isocortical layer-V pyramidal cells preferentially project to the patches, while deep layer-III pyramidal cells target the matrix [25].

Dopaminergic fibers apparently exert their influence within patches via D2 receptors and within the matrix via D1 receptors. During early development, initial dopamine-containing terminals form islands corresponding to the future patches (proto-striosomes). Later, they expand and fill the matrix [26, 27]. Matrix type-I neurons preferentially project to the pallidum and nigral pars reticulata, thereby establishing the main output system, whereas patch type-I neurons generate a relatively small projection directed to the pars compacta of the substantia nigra, a system which is likely to be involved in the feedback modulation of the striatum [28]. Somatostatin-containing type-II cells occur in both matrix and patches. Their long dendrites are capable of spanning the boundaries of both compartments and may thus serve as a link from matrix to patches [18].

Inferior portions of the accumbens nucleus and the ventral striatum receive significant projections from olfactory areas, the basolateral nuclei of the amygdala, the subiculum of the hippocampal formation, the entorhinal region, and adjoining orbitofrontal temporopolar isocortical associations areas. They also receive input from the retrosplenial region and anterior cingulate areas. The limbic-dominated ventral striatum projects to the ventral pallidum and a few other limbic areas of the upper brain stem (Figure 4; [4, 6−8, 29]).

The dorsal striatum receives topographically organized projections from virtually all areas of the isocortex. Association areas project to the caudate nucleus while the sensorimotor cortex of the central region projects mostly to the putamen and has a somatotopic representation of the body in the form of obliquely oriented strips [30−32]. The topographically organized thalamostriatal projection originates in intralaminar thalamic nuclei and the centromediano-parafascicular complex. The neurotransmitter used by the excitatory thalamo-striatal projection is not yet known.

The next major source of input is from the dopaminergic neurons of substantia nigra. In the adult brain, the dopamine terminals are homogeneously distributed throughout the striatum. Less dense projections to the striatum stem from GABAergic histamine-containing nerve cells of the hypothalamic tuberomamillary nucleus, from serotonergic and dopaminergic nerve cells of the anterior raphe nuclei, and possibly also from noradrenergic neurons of the locus coeruleus (Figure 5).

Projection fibers from the dorsal striatum approximate a rough topography and terminate within the pallidum and the substantia nigra. Each of the targets receives input from independent homogeneous clusters of striatal type-I neurons. The projection to the external pallidal segment derives from the GABA/enkephalin cells, while the projection to the internal pallidal segment and the adjoining nigral pars reticulata stems from GABA/substance P neurons [33]. Patch neurons of the accumbens nucleus and adjoining portions of the caudate nucleus aim toward the dopamine neurons of the substantia nigra and midbrain tegmentum (Figure 5, [34]).

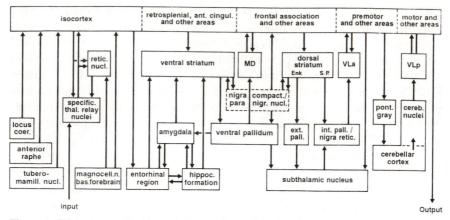

Figure 4. Diagram showing the main connections of the basal ganglia in more detail than in Figure 1. For details see text.

3. Ventral Pallidum, External and Internal Pallidal Segments

The diencephalic pallidum is the most anterior part of the hypothalamus; its internal organization differs considerably from that of the striatum. Therefore, it seems obsolete to continue to use the term "lentiform nucleus" which combines the telencephalic putamen andthe diencephalic pallidum. The "pallidum" derives its name from the pallid gray of fresh material, which is due to the high content of myelinated fibers. Its external segment is separated from the convex putamen by the external medullary lamina. The corresponding internal lamina separates the internal pallidum from the external

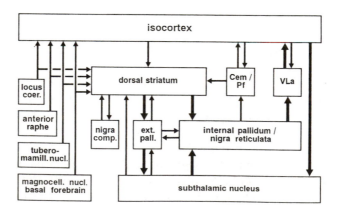

Figure 5. Circuits of the dorsal striatum show in more detail than in Figure 4. See text for explanations.

segment. The posterior extremity of the pallidum is continuous with the closely related pars reticulata of the substantia nigra [36]. The internal pallidum is equivalent to the entopenduncular nucleus of nonprimate mammalian species. The boundaries of the ventral pallidum are less clearly defined [7, 36]. Anteromedially, it is in close contact to the bed nucleus of the stria terminalis and the reticular nucleus of the thalamus. Inferiorly, it abuts the nucleus of the diagonal band and the tuberomamillary nucleus. The ventral pallidum joins the lateral hypothalamus and stretches beneath the anterior commissure (Figure 2; [7]).

The pallidum is largely populated by large, elongated nerve cells that are spaced widely apart from each other. Golgi studies do not show significant differences between the nerve cells populating the three compartments of the pallidum. The cell bodies generate thick and far-reaching dendrites which are sparsely spined and branch only occasionally. The dendrites are preferentially oriented parallel to the medullary laminae and perpendicular to the incoming striatal axons. They are densely covered by synaptic boutons [36]. The incoming axons of the striatal type-I neurons form a dense plexus around the dendrites and, in doing so, retain topographical segregations of the striatal input. Fine axon-like processes arise from the thick dendrites. The main axon leaves the pallidum and terminates within nuclei of the thalamus or the subthalamic nucleus. The large GABAergic nerve cells contain few lipofuscin granules and strongly basophilic Nissl bodies. Small nerve cells with short, thin dendrites and, possibly, a local axon have also been observed [37]. The pallidum as well as the related nigral pars reticulata harbor a large amount of endogenous iron within both glial cells and neurons [7].

The ventral pallidum receives a mixture of GABA/substance P and GABA/enkephalin projections from the ventral striatum and dopaminergic fibers from the substantia nigra and midbrain tegmentum. It projects mainly to the mediodorsal nuclei of the thalamus and relays data to the frontal association areas of the isocortex. The ventral pallidum also projects to the subthalamic nucleus and the amygdala (Figure 4).

The external and internal segments of the pallidum and the nigral pars reticulata receive topographically arranged projections from the dorsal striatum. GABA/enkephalin terminals appear as densely placed punctae along the dendrites of the principal cells in the external segment while the internal segment is filled with GABA/substance P fibers (Figures 4 and 5; [38–40]).

The external pallidum provides a dense GABAergic projection to the subthalamic nucleus and sparser projections to the striatum, internal pallidal segment, and nigral pars reticulata. The main feature of the external pallidum is that it establishes – via the subthalamic nucleus – an "indirect" pathway to the main pallidal output structure, the internal segment (Figures 4 and 5). Activation of the inhibitory projection from the striatum suppresses nerve cells within the external pallidal segment and thereby disinhibits (stimulates) the subthalamic nucleus which, in turn, activates the internal pallidum. The inhibitory action of the internal pallidum eventually leads to suppression of thalamic activity and, accordingly, provides a negative feedback to the cortex (Figures 5 and 6).

The internal pallidum issues a "direct" pathway to a number of thalamic nuclei. Activation of inhibitory striatal projection neurons suppresses part of the activity in the internal pallidum and thus results in the stimulation of related thalamic nuclei, i.e., it results in a positive feedback to the cortex. It appears important to note that the two populations of striatal projection neurons with their different pallidal targets have opposing effects on cortical motor activity. It should be recalled that dopamine appears to exert an opposing influence on the two striatal pathways with inhibition of the indirect pathway (via GABA/enkephalin neurons) and excitation of the direct pathway (via GABA/substance P neurons). By promoting the direct pathway and delaying the indirect one, dopamine guides the mainstream of data passing through the cortico-striato-thalamo-cortical circuit [6]. Clear separation of the two pathways in the limbic basal ganglia circuit is missing (Figure 4).

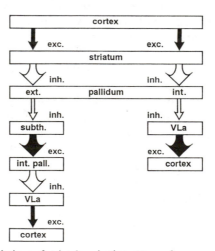

Figure 6. The two populations of striatal projection neurons have opposing effects on cortical motor activity. The indirect pathway via GABA/enkephalin neurons, external pallidum, subthalamic nucleus, and internal pallidum eventually leads to suppression of thalamic and cortical activity (left side), while the direct pathway via GABA/substance P neurons and internal pallidum results in an activation of cortical motor activity (right side). Excitatory influence is indicated by black arrows while inhibitory projections are displayed by open arrows. Broad arrows indicate a strong input, thin arrows a weak input.

4. Subthalamic Nucleus

The subthalamic nucleus (body of Luys) is well developed in primates and appears as lens-shaped gray matter with sharp boundaries. It is situated above the internal capsule or cerebral peduncle and, posteriorly, superimposes part of the substantia nigra (Figures 2f, 7a–d).

The grey matter appears to be formed of a single nerve cell type [41]. The medium-sized spindle-shaped nerve cells generate relatively long dendrites. Thin branches of these dendrites may be endowed with irregularly spaced spines. The axon gives off numerous local collaterals, while the main trunk leaves the nucleus and terminates in the internal pallidal segment and nigral pars reticulata. Rafols and Fox [42] identified small local circuit neurons in the monkey. Whether such cells are present in the human brain is unknown at present.

One of the main features of the subthalamic nucleus is that it receives a remarkably dense and topographically organized input from the cerebral cortex; especially the primary motor area and premotor frontal fields project to this gray matter (Figures 4 and 5; [7]). Furthermore, it receives input from the ventral pallidum and external pallidal segment and sends, in a topographical fashion, a particularly powerful excitatory, glutamatergic projection to the internal segment of the pallidum and nigral pars reticulata. The subthalamic nucleus can, therefore, be considered to be one of the driving forces in the system of the basal ganglia. Only sparse projections reach the external pallidum and the striatum (Figure 5).

5. Substantia Nigra

The substantia nigra is a heteromorphic gray matter located in the inferior tegmentum where is borders on the cerebral peduncles. It extends throughout the midbrain from the posterior tip of the mamillary bodies to the level of the oculomotor nucleus [43–46]. The nuclear gray matter can be divided into three territories: a cell-dense pars compacta (equivalent to the rodent "A9" cell group), a cell-sparse pars diffusa, and the pars reticulata [47].

The pars compacta is formed by an anterior group of subnuclei which are located close to the superior border of the nucleus, while the posterior group occupies a deeper position. Cell-sparse zones above the posterior portion are denoted as "pars diffusa". Seven well-defined subnuclei that are constant in location form the pars compacta. The anterior portion comprises three subnuclei (anteromedial, anterointer-

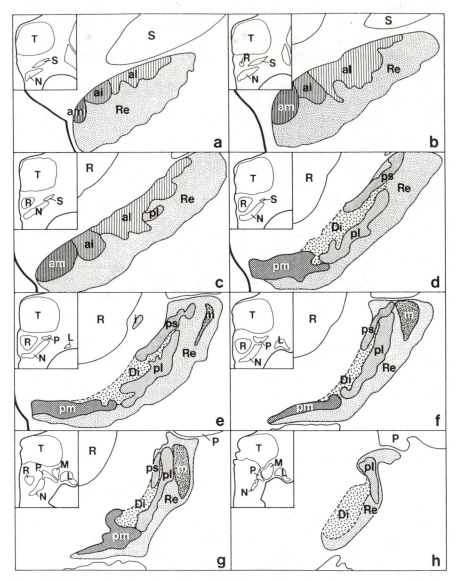

Figure 7. Series of frontal sections through the human substantia nigra, cut perpendicular to the intercommissural axis (Forel's axis). The series runs in an anterior posterior direction with each of the sections spaced 1600 μm apart. The line drawings show the boundaries of the various subnuclei. *Di* pars diffusa, *L* lateral geniculate body, *M* medial geniculate body, *N* nucleus niger, *P* peripeduncular nucleus, *R* nucleus ruber, *Re* nigra pars reticulata, *S* subthalamic nucleus, *T* thalamus, *ai* anterointermediate subnucleus, *al* anterolateral subnucleus, *am* anteromedial subnucleus, *i* islands of melanin-containing nerve cells in the perirubral formation – perirubral subnucleus, *m* magnocellular subnucleus, *pl* posterolateral subnucleus, *pm* posteromedial subnucleus, *ps* posterosuperior subnucleus (with permission from [47]).

mediate, and anterolateral subnucleus). The posterior portion consists of two cell plates bent at a blunt angle (posteromedial and posterolateral subnucleus), a hook-like formation (posterosuperior subnucleus), and a wedgeshaped cell assembly deeply penetrating into the pars reticulata (magnocellular subnucleus: [47]). Small groups of melanin-containing nerve cells are also found in the perirubral area. These groups are partly contiguous with pars compacta. The cells are here referred to as the perirubral subnucleus (Figure 7e; equivalent to the rodent "A8" group). Compartments either rich or poor in acetyl-cholinesterase have been delineated in the nigra pars compacta [48].

The pars reticulata occupies the inferolateral portion of the substantia nigra. To a large extent, it contains the dendrites of the pars compacta neurons [49]. Scattered among this dendritic network are relatively few nerve cells which remain devoid of neuromelanin granules. Glial cells and many of the large nerve cells of the pars reticulata contain a remarkable amount of iron.

Three basic neuronal types are found within the substantia nigra (Figure 8). Large melanin-laden type-I nerve cells constitute the predominating cell type of the pars compacta subnuclei. Isolated cells of this type may also occur in the pars diffusa and pars reticulata. The dark appearance of the substantia nigra is due to the presence of the type-I cells. Their large and fusiform cell bodies give off a few remarkably thick, sparsely branching dendrites [47, 50]. Dendritic processes of many type-I cells are arranged in bundles and extend into the pars diffusa and pars reticulata. The dendrites of the substantia nigra neurons generally do not extend beyond the boundaries of the nuclear complex. Some type-I neurons have dendrites profusely covered with spines, while others remain virtually devoid of them. The axon arises with a thick, cone-shaped initial segment. The cells are well endowed with peripherally located and sharply outlined elongated Nissl bodies extending into the proximal dendrites. The central portion of the perikaryon is lightly stained in Nissl preparations. The spherical nucleus is eccentrically located and contains a large nucleolus. One pole of the cell body is filled with tightly packed neuromelanin granules. The amount of neuromelanin varies within individual cells. Like the Nissl material, the pigment granules tend to extend into the dendrites (Figure 8). Neuromelanin is formed as an oxidative byproduct of the biosynthesis of dopamine. In the adult human brain, the presence of neuromelanin pigment marks the catecholamine-synthesizing nerve cells [45]. Relatively little is known about the possible colocalization of neuropeptides in dopaminergic nerve cells. Cell groups projecting to the ventral striatum may also contain cholecystokinin and neurotensin [14]. There are some toxins known to destroy selectively the dopaminergic nerve cells in primates (MPTP: 1-methyl-4-phenyl-1,2,3,6-tetrahydropyridine).

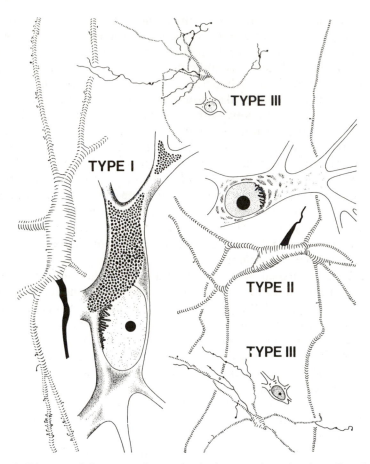

Figure 8. Diagram of the neuronal types in the human substantia nigra. Type-I neurons exhibit an eccentrically located nucleus, elongated patches of Nissl material, and neuromelanin granules extending into the proximal dendrites. Type-II neurons have a small and centrally located nucleus and Nissl bodies arranged around the nucleus. Type-III neurons are small and contain a dark nucleus and pallid cytoplasm with intensely stained lipofuscin granules. The three neuronal types can easily be recognized in pigment Nissl preparations (with permission from [47]).

Nerve cells devoid of melanin constitute the medium-sized to large type-II cells that form the bulk of the reticulata neurons, but these may also occur in other portions of the nucleus. Type-II cells vary in size and shape and generate sparsely branching dendrites. Their cell bodies frequently show well-defined Nissl bodies concentrically arranged around the centrally placed nucleus. Type-II cells accumulate variable amounts of lipofuscin granules (Figure 8). These cells are GABAergic; it is unknown at present whether they contain additional neuropeptides.

Type-III cells are small, local circuit neurons which occur in all subdivisions of the nuclear complex [47, 51]. Their spindle-shaped cell body gives rise to very thin and spineless dendrites. The pale cytoplasm contains characteristic lipofuscin granules which allow recognition of type-III cells in Nissl preparations counterstained for lipofuscin pigment. Type-III cells may generate more than one local axon (Figure 8). The density of type-III cells varies considerably within the different subnuclei of the pars compacta.

All subdivisions of the substantia nigra receive considerable input from both the ventral striatum and GABA/substance P neurons of the dorsal striatum. Even projections terminating within the pars reticulata mainly contact the dendrites of pars compacta neurons. Caudatonigral fibers appear to terminate within anterior portions of the nuclear gray, while putaminonigral fibers reach more posterior parts. Projections from the accumbens nucleus seem to concentrate on anteromedial cell groups. The dopaminergic cells of the substantia nigra generate the predominantly ipsilateral and topographically organized nigrostriatal projection, the comb bundle (Figure 5, [52]). Anteromedial subnuclei and the adjoining paranigral nucleus mainly project to the ventral striatum. Anterolateral subnuclei and perirubral cells project to the head of the caudate nucleus while posteromedial subnuclei target the putamen. The GABAergic type-II neurons project to the thalamus (VL) and superior colliculus and provide a tonic inhibition of its intermediate and deep layers [53].

6. Paranigral Nucleus and Pigmented Parabrachial Nucleus

The paranigral nucleus is contiguous with the anteromedial subnucleus of the nigral pars compacta. The nuclei of both sides form an arch that covers the interpeduncular nucleus. Superiorly, the paranigral nucleus continues into the pigmented parabrachial nucleus, a leaf-like and sagittally oriented structure that accompanies the linear nucleus of the oral raphe system. The linear raphe nucleus and the pigmented parabrachial nucleus are embedded within the masses of decussating myelinated fibers of the superior cerebellar peduncle [44]. The paranigral nucleus and the pigmented parabrachial nucleus (both equivalent to the rodent "A10" group) are easily distinguishable from the linear raphe nucleus on account of the neuromelanin deposits within their constituent nerve cells. Little is known concerning the afferent connections of these nuclei which provide the major dopaminergic projections to the amygdala, the hippocampal formation, and entorhinal region. Additionally, the isocortical motor areas, anterior cingulate fields, and frontal association areas of the isocortex receive a dense projection.

7. Cortex-Related Thalamic Nuclei and Reticular Nucleus of the Thalamus

Relay nuclei of the thalamus provide specific input to the isocortex with richly myelinated fibers forming columnar terminal arborizations in layers II–V of defined cortical areas. Intralaminar nuclei inclusive of the centromediano-parafascicular complex generate an additional set of poorly myelinated and diffusely arranged fibers which are less specific. These spread throughout more than one cortical area and terminate in layers I and VI [54, 55].

The reticular nucleus incompletely covers the lateral portions of the thalamus and is thus well placed to receive collaterals from both thalamocortical and corticothalamic fibers. In addition, the reticular nucleus receives a dense cholinergic input from the magnocellular nuclei of the basal forebrain (Figure 4) and is – in rodents and cats – also reached by a strong GABAergic projection from the external segment of the pallidum [56]. It remains however to be elucidated whether such a pallidal input exists in primates and in man [6]. The GABAergic principal cells of the thalamic reticular nucleus do not project to the cortex, but send their axons exclusively to other nuclei of the thalamus. This kind of arrangement suggests that some part of modulation of the basal ganglia may occur at the level of the reticular thalamic nucleus.

8. Centromediano-Parafascicular Complex

The centromediano-parafascicular complex is well developed in primates. It receives input from the internal segment of the pallidum and a number of other sources, including limbic areas and cerebellum (Figure 5, [57]). Anterior intralaminar nuclei and the centromediano-parafascicular complex are the main sources of a powerful thalamic projection to the matrix compartment of the dorsal striatum. Projection cells of the centromedian nucleus preferably target the putamen, while those of the parafascicular nucleus project to the caudate nucleus. Inferior portions of the parafascicular nucleus and the subjacent sub-parafascicular nucleus project to the ventral striatum.

9. Locus Coeruleus, Anterior Raphe Nuclei, Tuberomamillary Nucleus, and Magnocellular Nuclei of the Basal Forebrain

The locus coeruleus is located close to the lateral angle of the fourth ventricle in the pontine tegmentum. The column-like nucleus commences at the level of the motor trigeminal nucleus and extends anteriorly up to the posterior border of the inferior colliculus. The chief cell of this nucleus is a melanin-laden neuron with a rounded, medium-sized to large cell body which is easily distinguishable from neuronal types of neigh-boring nuclear grays. The locus coeruleus projects to the entire cerebral cortex, cerebellum, lower brain stem, and spinal cord. It also sends a small projection to the dorsal striatum (Figure 5). It is unclear at present, how-ever, whether this connection is constantly established in the human brain.

Serotonin-containing nerve cells are encountered within the complex of raphe nuclei which, in the human brain, are separated into an anterior group with ascending projections and a posterior group with descending projections. The anterior raphe complex comprises a dorsal, a central, and a linear raphe nucleus. Predominant among the neuronal types forming these nuclei are large lipofuscin pigment-laden cells which are likely to represent the serotonin-producing neurons [58]. It should be noted, however, that the raphe nuclei also contain a number of non-serotonergic cells. The anterior raphe nuclei do not only project to cortical targets, but also send serotonergic fibers to all subdivisions of the striatum (Figure 5, [59]). However, a substantial proportion of the raphe projection is dopaminergic [14].

The tuberomamillary nucleus extends throughout the lateral tuberal and mamillary region of the hypothalamus and is closely associated with fibers of the median forebrain bundle (Figure 2e). Large, lipofuscin-laden nerve cells predominate within the gray matter [60]. Most tuberomamil-lary neurons synthesize GABA and contain a variety of additional substances including histamine, adenosine and galanin [61]. Tubero-mamillary neurons generate widespread projections to the cerebral cortex in approximately the same magnitude as those of the magnocellular basal forebrain nuclei [62]. In this context, it appears important to note that they also send projections to the striatum (Figure 5).

Clusters of large, multipolar nerve cells located in the basal forebrain form three major nuclei, i.e., the medial septal nucleus, the nucleus of the diagonal band, and the basal nucleus of Meynert. All these nuclei are incompletely surrounded by the small-celled substantia innominata (Fig. 2; [63]). Leaf-like extensions of the magnocellular nuclear complex pene-trate extensively into the external and internal medullary laminae of the pallidum and form the peripallidal subnucleus. The magnocellular nuclei contain different neuronal types. Most of the large neurons synthesize acetylcholine. Another type of large neuron is GABAergic and contains, in addition, a variety of neuropeptides [62]. The basal forebrain nuclei receive major input from cortical areas and subcortical nuclei of the limbic system and provide a massive cholinergic projection to the mediodorsal thalamic nuclei (MD, transferring limbic data from ventral pallidum to frontal association cortex, Figure 1, [64]), the reticular nucleus of the thalamus, the amygdala, and the entire cerebral cortex (Figure 4). Thus far, peripallidal cholinergic nerve cells have received little attention, but cortical afferents and a direct input from the striatum have been reported [65]. The targets of the peripallidal cholinergic nerve cells have not yet been identified.

Summary

In this brief review we have provided data on the topography, neuronal types, and connections of the human basal ganglia. We have concentrated on striatum, pallidum, subthalamic nucleus, substantia nigra, and related structures. The description of basal ganglia circuits is incomplete without taking notice of the important input from limbic structures. However, many details concerning the morphology and connectivity of the inconspicuous limbic compartment of the basal ganglia are as yet unknown. The isocortex-dominated dorsal striatum, in contrast, has received particular attention during the past decades. Each of the two subtypes of striatal projection cells establishes a major pathway to the thalamus. The GABA/enkephalin cells of the striatum furnish a long way via external pallidum, subthalamic nucleus and internal pallidum to the motor thalamus while the GABA/substance P cells directly project to the internal segment of the pallidum. The two pathways have opposing effects on cortical motor activity.

Acknowledgements

This study was supported by the Deutsche Forschungsgemeinschaft. The skillful assistance of Ms. Szasz in preparing the drawings is gratefully acknowledged.

References

[1] Nauta HJW. A proposed conceptual reorganization of the basal ganglia and telencephalon. Neuroscience 1979; 4: 1875–1881.
[2] Mehler WR. The basal ganglia – circa 1982. A review and commentary. Appl Neurophysiol 1981; 44: 261–290.
[3] Nauta WJH, Domesick VB. Afferent and efferent relationships of the basal ganglia. In: Evered D, O'Connor M, editors. Functions of the basal ganglia. CIBA foundation symposium, vol. 107. London: Pitman, 1984: 3–29.
[4] Rolls ET. Information processing and basal ganglia function. In: Kennard C, Swash M, editors. Hierarchies in neurology. A reappraisal of a Jacksonian concept. London: Springer, 1989: 123–142.
[5] Brockhaus H. Zur feineren Anatomie des Septum und des Striatum. J Psychol Neurol 1942; 51: 1–56.
[6] Alexander GE, Crutcher MD, DeLong MR. Basal ganglia-thalamocortical circuits: Parallel substrates for motor, oculomotor, "prefrontal" and "limbic" functions. Progr Brain Res 1990; 85: 119–146.
[7] Alheid GF, Heimer L, Switzer RC. Basal ganglia. In: Paxinos G, editor. The human nervous system. New York: Academic Press, 1990: 483–582.
[8] Groenewegen HJ, Berendse HW, Meredith GE, Haber SN, Voorn P, Wolters JG, Lohman AHM. Functional anatomy of the ventral, limbic system-innervated striatum. In: Willner P, Scheel-Krüger J, editors. The mesolimbic dopamine system: From motivation to action. Chichester: Wiley & Sons, 1991: 19–59.
[9] Fox CA, Andrade AN, Hilman DE, Schwyn RC. The spiny neurons in the primate striatum: A Golgi and electron microscopic study. J Hirnforsch 1971; 13: 181–201.

[10] Braak H, Braak E. Neuronal types in the striatum of man. Cell Tiss Res 1982; 227: 319–342.

[11] Graveland GA, Williams RS, DiFiglia M. A Golgi study of the human neostriatum: Neurons and afferent fibers. J Comp Neurol 1985; 234: 317–333.

[12] Yelnik J, Francois C, Percheron G, Tande D. Morphological taxonomy of the neurons of the primate striatum. J Comp Neurol 1991; 313: 273–294.

[13] DiFiglia M, Pasik P, Pasik T. A Golgi study of neuronal types in the neostriatum of monkeys. Brain Res 1976; 114: 245–256.

[14] Semba K, Fibiger HC, Vincent SR. Neurotransmitters in the mammalian striatum: Neuronal circuits and heterogeneity. Can J Neurol Sci 1987; 14: 386–394.

[15] Groves PM. A theory of the functional organization of the neostriatum and the neostriatal control of voluntary movement. Brain Res Rev 1983; 5: 109–132.

[16] Bolam JP. Synapses of identified neurons in the neostriatum. In: Evered D, O'Connor M, editors. Functions of the basal ganglia. CIBA foundation symposium, vol. 107. London: Pitman, 1984: 30–47.

[17] Smith AD, Bolam JP. The neural network of the basal ganglia as revealed by the study of synaptic connections of identified neurones. Trends Neurosci 1990; 13: 259–265.

[18] Gerfen CR. Synaptic organization of the striatum. J Electr Micr Techn 1988; 10: 265–81.

[19] Fox CA, Andrade AN, Schwyn RC, Rafols JA. The aspiny neurons and the glia in the primate striatum: A Golgi and electron microscopic study. J Hirnforsch 1971; 13: 341–362.

[20] Pasik P, Pasik T, DiFiglia M. The internal organization of the neostriatum in mammals. In: Divac I, Berg RE, editors. The Neostriatum. Oxford: Pergamon Press 1979: 5–36.

[21] Martin LJ, Hadfield MG, Dellovade TL, Price DL. The striatal mosaic in primates: Patterns of neuropeptide immunoreactivity differentiate the ventral striatum from the dorsal striatum. Neuroscience 1991; 43: 397–417.

[22] Graybiel AM. Neurotransmitters and neuromodulators in the basal ganglia. Trends Neurosci 1990; 13: 244–254.

[23] Graybiel AM, Ragsdale CW. Biochemical anatomy of the striatum. In: Emson PC, editor. Chemical Neuroanatomy. New York: Raven Press, 1983: 427–504.

[24] Johnston JG, Gerfen CR, Haber SN, van der Kooy D. Mechanisms of striatal pattern formation: Conservation of mammalian compartmentalization. Developm Brain Res 1990; 57: 93–102.

[25] Parent A. Extrinsic connections of the basal ganglia. Trends Neurosci 1990; 13: 254–258.

[26] Graybiel AM. Correspondence between the dopamine islands and striosomes of the mammalian striatum. Neuroscience 1984; 13: 1157–1187.

[27] Graybiel AM. Neurochemically specified subsystems in the basal ganglia. In: Evered D, O'Connor M, editors. Functions of the basal ganglia. CIBA foundation symposium, vol. 107. London: Pitman, 1984: 114–149.

[28] Giménez-Amaya JM, Graybiel AM. Compartmental origins of the striatopallidal projection in the primate. Neuroscience 1990; 34: 111–126.

[29] Haber SN, Lynd E, Klein C, Groenewegen HJ. Topographic organization of the ventral striatal efferent projections in the rhesus monkey: An anterograde tracing study. J Comp Neurol 1990; 293: 282–298.

[30] Alexander GE, DeLong MR, Strick PL. Parallel organization of functionally segregated circuits linking basal ganglia and cortex. Annual Rev Neurosci 1986; 9: 367–381.

[31] Goldman-Rakic PS, Selemon LD. Topography of corticostriatal projections in nonhuman primates and implications for functional parcellation of the neostriatum. In: Jones EG, Peters A, editors. Cerebral Cortex. Sensory-motor areas and aspects of cortical connectivity, vol. 5, New York: Plenum, 1986: 447–466.

[32] Nauta WJH. Circuitous connections linking cerebral cortex, limbic system, and corpus striatum. In: Doane BK, Livingston KE, editors. The limbic system. New York: Raven Press, 1986: 43–54.

[33] Reiner A, Anderson KD. The patterns of neurotransmitter and neuropeptide co-occurrence among striatal projection neurons: Conclusions based on recent findings. Brain Res Rev 1990; 15: 251–265.

[34] Hedreen JC, DeLong MR. Organization of striatopallidal, striatonigral, and nigrostriatal projections in the macaque. J Comp Neurol 1991; 304: 569–595.

[35] Fox CA, Andrade AN, LuQui IJ, Rafols JA. The primate globus pallidus: A Golgi and electron microscopic study. J Hirnforsch 1974; 15: 75–93.

[36] Heimer L, Switzer RC, Van Hoesen GW. Ventral striatum and ventral pallidum. Components of the motor system? Trends Neurosci 1982; 5: 83–87.

[37] Francois C, Percheron G, Yelnik J, Heyner S. A Golgi analysis of the primate globus pallidus. I. Inconstant processes of larger neurons, other neuronal types and afferent axons. J Comp Neurol 1984; 227: 182–199.

[38] Beach TG, McGeer EG. The distribution of substance P in the primate basal ganglia: An immunohistochemical study of baboon and human brain. Neuroscience 1984; 13: 29–52.

[39] Haber SN, Watson SJ. The comparative distribution of enkephalin, dynorphin and substance P in the human globus pallidus and basal forebrain. Neuroscience 1985; 14: 1011–1024.

[40] Mai JK, Stephens PH, Hopf A, Cuello AC. Substance P in the human brain. Neuroscience 1986; 17: 709–739.

[41] Yelnik J, Percheron G. Subthalamic neurons in primates. A quantitative and comparative analysis. Neuroscience 1979; 4: 1717–1743.

[42] Rafols JA, Fox CA. The neurons in the primate subthalamic nucleus: A Golgi and electron microscopic study. J Comp Neurol 1976; 168: 75–112.

[43] Hassler R. Zur Normalanatomie der Substantia nigra. Versuch einer architektonischen Gliederung. J Psychol Neurol 1937; 48: 1–55.

[44] Olszewski J, Baxter D. Cytoarchitecture of the human brain stem. Basel, New York: Karger, 1954.

[45] Saper CB, Petito CK. Correspondence of melanin-pigmented neurons in the human brain with A1–A14 catecholamine cell groups. Brain 1982; 105: 87–102.

[46] Van Domburg PHMF, ten Donkelaar HJ. The human substantia nigra and ventral tegmental area. In: Beck F, Hild W, Kriz W, Pauly JE, Sano Y, Sano Y, Schiebler TH., editors. Advances in Anatomy, Embryology and Cell Biology, vol. 121. Berlin: Springer, 1991: 1–132.

[47] Braak H, Braak E. Nuclear configuration and neuronal types of the nucleus niger in the brain of the human adult. Human Neurobiol 1986; 5: 71–82.

[48] Jiminez-Castellanos J, Graybiel AM. Subdivisions of the primate substantia nigra pars compacta detected by acetylcholinesterase histochemistry. Brain Res 1987; 437: 349–354.

[49] Schwyn RC, Fox CA. The primate substantia nigra: A Golgi and electron microscopic study. J Hirnforsch 1974; 15: 95–126.

[50] Yelnik J, Francois C, Percheron G, Heyner S. Golgi study of the primate substantia nigra. I. Quantitative morphology and typology of nigral neurons. J Comp Neurol 1987; 265: 455–472.

[51] Francois C, Percheron G, Yelnik J, Heyner S. Demonstration of the existence of small local circuit neurons in the Golgi-stained primate substantia nigra. Brain Res 1979; 172: 160–164.

[52] Percheron G, Francois C, Yelnik J. Spatial organization and information processing in the core of the basal ganglia. In: Carpenter MB, Jayaraman A, editors. The basal ganglia II. New York: Plenum Publ. Corp., 1987: 205–226.

[53] Hikosaka O. Motor programming in basal ganglia. In: Ito M, editor. Neural programming. Basel: Karger, 1990: 101–109.

[54] Jones EG. The thalamus. New York: Plenum Press, 1985.

[55] Strick PL. How do the basal ganglia and cerebellum gain access to the cortical motor areas? Behav Brain Res 1985; 18: 107–123.

[56] Haber SN. Neurotransmitters in the human and non-human primate basal ganglia. Human Neurobiol 1986; 5: 159–168.

[57] Fénelon G, Francois C, Percheron G, Yelnik J. Topographic distribution of pallidal neurons projecting to the thalamus in macaques. Brain Res 1990; 520: 27–35.

[58] Ohm TG, Heilmann R, Braak H. The human oral raphe system. Architectonics and neuronal types in pigment-Nissl preparations. Anat Embryol 1989; 180: 37–43.

[59] Saper CB. Diffuse cortical projection systems: Anatomical organization and role in cortical function. In: Plum F, editor. Handbook of physiology. The nervous system, vol. V. Bethesda: American Physiological Society, 1987: 169–210.

[60] Braak H, Braak E. Anatomy of the human hypothalamus (chiasmatic and tuberal region). Progr Brain Res. 1992; 93: in press.

[61] Panula P, Airaksinen MS, Pirvola U, Kotilainen E. A histamine-containing neuronal system in human brain. Neuroscience 1990; 34: 127–132.

[62] Saper CB. Cholinergic system. In: Paxinos G, editor. The human nervous system. New York: Academic Press, 1990: 1095–1113.
[63] Ulfig N. Configuration of the magnocellular nuclei in the basal forebrain of the human adult. Acta anat 1989; 134: 100–105.
[64] Hreib KK, Rosene DL, Moss MB. Basal forebrain efferents to the medial dorsal thalamic nucleus in the rhesus monkey. J Comp Neurol 1988; 277: 365–390.
[65] Mesulam MM, Mufson EJ. Neural inputs into the nucleus basalis of the substantia innominata (Ch4) in the rhesus monkey. Brain 1984; 107: 253–274.

Inhibitors of Monoamine Oxidase B
Pharmacology and Clinical Use in Neurodegenerative Disorders
ed. by I. Szelenyi
© 1993 Birkhäuser Verlag Basel/Switzerland

CHAPTER 2
The Pathophysiological Basis of Parkinson's Disease

M. Gerlach and P. Riederer

1   Introduction
2   Presynaptic Changes in Dopaminergic Neurons of the Nigro-Striatal System
3   The Functional State of Postsynaptic Dopaminergic Receptors
3.1 Classification of Dopamine Receptors
3.2 Specific Roles of the Dopamine Receptor Subtypes in Motor Control
3.3 The Postsynaptic Dopamine Receptor Retains its Functional Activity
4   Changes in the Motor-Loop
5   The Extrastriatal Dopaminergic Pathobiochemistry
6   Dysfunction of Non-Dopaminergic Systems in Parkinson's Disease
6.1 Degeneration of Noradrenergic System
6.2 The Degeneration of Serotonergic Systems
6.3 The Degeneration of Cholinergic Systems
6.4 Preservation of GABAergic Systems?
6.5 The Dysfunction of Peptidergic Systems
7   The Role of the Glia
8   Research Strategies for the Future
     Summary
     References

1. Introduction

Parkinson's syndrome, or parkinsonism, involving the clinical symptoms first described in 1817 by James Parkinson [1], occurs in a variety of disorders of the central nervous system (CNS), and is basically characterized by dysfunction of the dopaminergic nigro-striatal system. It may, or in rare cases it may not, be associated with distinct anatomical damage to melanin-containing neurons of the substantia nigra (SN), changes in the neuronal cytoskeleton including the presence of Lewy bodies, and pathological changes in other neuronal systems, often as part of a more widespread process [2]. The term Parkinson's disease (PD) is properly restricted to paralysis agitans, the idiopathic form of parkinsonism, associated with the formation of Lewy bodies and the loss of neurons in the pars compacta of the SN (SNC), which has been known since the time of Tretiakoff [3] as the system principally at risk in this disorder. It can be accompanied by nonspecific or age-related brain pathology, and a variety of other coincidental lesions elsewhere in the CNS.

Biochemically, the salient feature of the illness is the selective degeneration of the dopaminergic nigro-striatal system, and this profoundly disturbs neurotransmission of signals throughout the basal ganglia. In 1960, Ehringer and Hornykiewicz [4] reported for the first time that the principal biochemical manifestation of this damage is a pronounced deficiency of dopamine (DA) in the striatum (caudate nucleus and putamen) of patients with PD. Subsequent to this remarkable finding, the disease has been treated with L-dopa (L-3,4-dihydroxyphenylalanine) as a way of restoring striatal DA levels [5, 6]. The reversal of the clinical signs by treatment with L-dopa, and the finding that the degree of striatal DA deficiency correlates significantly with the extent of cell loss in the SNC and the severity of parkinsonian disability, especially akinesia [7], have consistently pointed to the nigro-striatal dopaminergic impairment as the lesion primarily responsible for the motor deficits in PD.

These insights stimulated many scientists to investigate the physiological function of DA. In recent years, DA has been recognized as a neurotransmitter, and a wealth of information has been discoverd about almost every aspect of the normal dopaminergic function in the mammalian brain. The identification of further neurotransmitters such as adrenaline (A), acetylcholine (ACh), γ-aminobutyric acid (GABA), glutamic acid (Glu) or noradrenaline (NA) has permitted the mapping of several neuronal systems within the brain. Measurement of the concentrations of these neurotransmitters and of the activity of their specific synthesizing enzymes in human autopsy material has allowed us to make certain assumptions concerning the nature and the number of these biochemically distinct neuronal systems. Taken together with conventional clinico-pathological correlations, such assays may give an indication of which neuronal systems have been affected by the disease.

For these reasons, neurotransmitter concentrations may serve as indices of the extent of the neuronal destruction. The levels of their principal metabolites and the characteristics of their receptor sites give an idea of presynaptic neuronal activity (the ratio of the concentration of the metabolites to the corresponding neurotransmitter) and of the functional state of the target neurons (increased or decreased sensitivity of the receptors).

This paper will review some of the neurochemical findings which were obtained at autopsy from analysis of the brains from patients with PD. Special attention will be paid to clarifying the possible clinical implications of the observed changes, and to the relevance of the glia in the pathogenesis of PD. In addition, future research strategies will be discussed.

2. Presynaptic Changes in Dopaminergic Neurons of the Nigro-Striatal System

In PD, DA concentrations are profoundly reduced in all structures belonging to the nigro-striatal system, such as the SNC, the putamen,

Table 1. Concentrations of dopamine in various brain regions of patients with Parkinson's disease.

Brain region	Decrease in % of control
Basal ganglia	
Caudate nucleus	90[a]
Putamen	96[a]
Substantia nigra	83[a]
Globus pallidus	90[a]
Subcortical regions	
Nucleus accumbens	58[b]
Medial olfactory area	22[c]
Lateral olfactory area (olfactory tubercle; substantia innominata; anterior perforate substance)	0.0[c]
Lateral hypothalamic area	90[b]
Amygdaloid nucleus	45[d]
Ventral tegmental area (VTA)	50[d]
Cortical regions	
Parolfactory cortex (Brodmann area 25)	90[c]
Frontal cortex	61[d]
Entorhinal cortex	68[d]
Cingulate cortex	52[d]
Hippocampus	68[d]

[a]Birkmayer and Riederer, 1975 (ref. [8]); [b]Price et al., 1978 (ref. [9]); [c]Farley et al., 1977 (ref. [10]); [d]Scatton et al., 1984 ref. [11]).

the caudate nucleus, and the globus pallidus (Table 1). In principle, striatal DA loss is characteristic of parkinsonian syndromes of whatever etiology [7]. The degree of striatal DA deficiency is significantly correlated with the degree of cell loss in the SNC and the severity of parkinsonian disability, especially akinesia [7]. The studies of Riederer and Wuketich [12] have shown that striatal DA content must be reduced by 70% or more before clinical symptoms become apparent.

In addition to the loss of DA, the DA metabolites 3,4-dihydroxy-phenylacetic acid (DOPAC) and homovanillic acid (HVA) are markedly reduced; while the amounts of DOPAC were reduced to a greater extent than those of DA, the fall in HVA levels was less pronounced (Table 2). Since DOPAC levels are most probably representative of the metabolism of DA in nerve terminals [14], and the oxidation of DA to DOPAC is catalyzed by intraneuronal monoamine oxidase (MAO), it can be assumed that DOPAC is a more sensitive marker for the degenerative process than HVA. The production of HVA requires both MAO and catechol-O-methyl transferase (COMT), but is probably the result of extraneuronal metabolism of DA, 3-methoxytyramine and/or DOPAC (the latter diffusing out of the nerve terminals for subsequent metabolism by COMT). The less pronounced reduction of HVA could therefore reflect an increase of extraneuronal

Table 2. Concentrations of dopamine and metabolites in the brain of patients with Parkinson's disease (according to Riederer et al. [13]).

Brain region	DA	DOPAC	HVA
		in % of the control	
Putamen	4	10	29
Substantia nigra	7	2	48
Hippocampus	47	68	106
Frontal cortex	66	38	66

DA, dopamine; DOPAC, 3,4-dihydroxyphenylacetic acid; HVA, homovanillic acid.

DA-turnover due to an increased presynaptic release of DA on the part of surviving dopaminergic neurons.

The impairment of dopaminergic neurotransmission in the nigro-striatal system is also characterized by the diminished activity of the DA-synthesizing enzymes tyrosine hydroxylase (TH) and dopa decarboxylase (DDC) (Table 3). TH catalyzes the rate-limiting reaction in the synthesis of catecholamines [22]. It is likely that TH protein decreases due to denervation of dopaminergic neurons, so that reduced activities are observed. In harmony with this assumption, levels of L-erythro-biopterin, the natural cofactor for TH, were diminished in the striatum of parkinsonian patients [23]. *In vitro*, however, the response of the residual TH enzyme under stimulating conditions shows no differences between controls and patients with PD (Table 3; see also [17]). Thus, it may be concluded that, in such patients, the functional state of TH in surviving neurons is likewise unaltered compared to controls. Indeed, calculations of TH activity on the basis of TH protein have given normal values in the SN, and a significant fourfold increase of homospecific TH activity in the caudate nucleus (Table 3; see also [18]). Although the activity of DDC is profoundly reduced, there is obviously enough enzyme activity present to account for any increased DA formation in the striatum of patients receiving therapeutic doses of L-dopa [19].

In contrast to the DA-synthesizing enzymes TH and DDC, the activity of the DA-catabolyzing enzymes MAO-B and COMT seem to be unchanged (Table 3), reflecting the fact that these enzymes are not preferentially localized in the nigro-striatal dopaminergic nerve terminals.

The cause of the reduced activities of mitochondrial respiratory-chain enzymes (Table 3) and their relationship to the pathogenesis and progression of PD are unknown. Of all the respiratory-chain complexes Complex I is the largest and probably most vulnerable to disturbances of the structural and functional integrity of membranes. A non-specific reduction of mitochondrial respiratory-chain enzyme activities in

Table 3. Pathobiochemistry of the nigro-striatal system in Parkinson's disease.

	Brain region	in % of controls
Activities of dopamine-metabolizing enzymes		
Dopa decarboxylase	Putamen	4[a]
	Caudate nucleus	9[a]
Tyrosine hydroxylase	Substantia nigra	46[b]
	Putamen	16[b]
	Caudate nucleus	60[c]
after Fe^{2+}-stimulation	Caudate nucleus	50[c]
homospecific activity	Caudate nucleus	396[d]
Catechol-O-methyl	Substantia nigra	82[e]
transferase	Putamen	78[e]
	Caudate nucleus	70[e]
Monoaminoxidase-B	Substantia nigra	125[f]
Activities of mitochondrial respiratory-chain enzymes		
NADH cytochrome c reductase (Complex I)	Substantia nigra	66[g]
Succinate cytochrome c reductase	Substantia nigra	62[g]

[a]Lloyd and Hornykiewicz, 1970 (ref. [15]); [b]Riederer et al., 1978 (ref. [16]); [c]Rausch et al., 1988 (ref. [17]); [d]Mogi et al., 1988 (ref. [18]); [e]Lloyd et al., 1975 (ref. [19]); [f]Riederer et al., 1989 (ref. [20]); [g]Reichmann and Riederer, 1989 (ref. [21]).

response to some other metabolic disturbances or drug treatment in parkinsonian patients cannot be excluded, particularly because L-dopa, through its conversion to quinones, may produce "oxidative stress" (a cellular state in which an imbalance arises between the processes that generate cellular oxidants and cellular antioxidant defenses).

3. The Functional State of Postsynaptic Dopaminergic Receptors

3.1. Classification of Dopamine Receptors

Based on radioreceptor analysis, the existence of multiple DA receptor subtypes ($D_1 - D_5$) has been proposed [24, 25]. However, only D_1 and D_2 DA receptors seem to fulfill all the criteria for a receptor site. Molecular cloning has corroborated the presence of at least two DA receptor subtypes [26, 27]. Recently, a D_3 receptor, which shows an extensive similarity in its amino acid sequence of the D_2 receptor, but differs from the latter by the apparent lack of adenylate cyclase coupling, has been isolated and characterized pharmacologically [28].

The classification of central DA receptors into D_1 and D_2 subtypes, originally based on biochemical criteria, has gained further support by the identification of selective agonists and antagonists for both receptor types (for a review, see [29]). The biochemical, pharmacological, and

Table 4. Classification of dopamine receptors (modified according to Markstein and Vigouret [30]).

	D$_1$	D$_2$
Stimulation of adenylate cyclase	Yes	No
Dopamine	Agonist (in µmol/l)	Agonist (in nmol/l)
Apomorphine	Partial agonist or antagonist	Agonist (in nmol/l)
Selective agonists	SKF 38393 CY 208-243	Bromocriptine LY 171555 RU 24-213
Selective antagonist	SCH 23390	Sulpiride
Prolactin secretion	No	Inhibition
Parathormone release	Stimulation	No
Induction of emesis	No	Yes
Behavioral effect	Non-stereotyped sniffing	Stereotyped sniffing, gnawing

behavioral characteristics of these subtypes are shown in Table 4. The principal difference between the two types is the manner of their linkage to adenylate cyclase. Stimulation of the D$_1$ receptor increases cyclic AMP (cAMP) formation, while stimulation of the D$_2$ receptor either inhibits production of cAMP or else has no effect.

3.2. Specific Roles of the Dopamine Receptor Subtypes in Motor Control

The D$_2$ receptor seems to be responsible for most of the behavioral effects of DA agonists, such as stereotypy, locomotion, and vomiting, as well as for their psychomimetic activity, whereas any important physiological role for the D$_1$ receptor has been questioned. However, recent studies with newly available D$_1$-selective agonists and antagonists strongly suggest that the D$_1$ receptor also participates in motor control (for a review, see [30]). Evidence is now accumulating that D$_1$ and D$_2$ receptors do not regulate motor behavior independently, but are functionally linked. In experimental animals (rats and mice) doses of D$_1$ agonists and of D$_2$ agonists, which when given alone failed to change motor activity, when given together produced marked behavioral activation (for a review, see [30]). Furthermore, clinical experience [31, 32] suggests that agonists (pergolide, CQ-32084 and the aeorphine SDZ-201-678) with D$_1$- and D$_2$-stimulatory activity are therapeutically more effective than pure D$_2$ agonists such as bromocriptine and lisuride. The most likely explanation for these observations is that D$_1$ and D$_2$ receptors interact in a synergistic manner and that D$_2$ receptor-mediated behavioral responses are only expressed

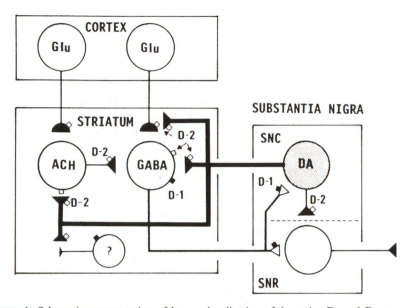

Figure 1. Schematic representation of known localization of dopamine D_1 and D_2 receptor subtypes in the nigro-striatal system. GLU, glutaminergic neurons; ACH, cholinergic neurons; GABA, γ-aminobutyric acidergic neurons; SNC, the pars compacta of the substantia nigra; SNR, the pars reticulata of the substantia nigra. D_1-receptors occur only on post-synaptic elements. D_2-receptors occur on pre- and postsynaptic elements (from [30], with permission).

when D_1 receptors are also activated. This hypothesis implies that the effects of selective D_2 agonists depend in some way on the presence of endogenous DA which can provide the necessary tonic D_1 receptor-threshold.

At the cellular level, D_1 and D_2 receptors have been shown to produce opposing biochemical effects. For instance, in striatal preparations activation of the D_1 receptor enhances the formation of cAMP and the neuronal release of GABA, whereas stimulation of the D_2 receptor produces the opposite effect [33, 34]. Robertson and Robertson [35] proposed that the synergistic effect of D_1 and D_2 agonists is mediated by actions in anatomically separate regions.

Figure 1 depicts a schematic representation of the known localization of D_1 and D_2 receptors in the nigro-striatal system. In the striatum D_1 receptors are exclusively of postsynaptic location, whereas D_2 receptors occur on both post- and presynaptic neuronal elements. Presynaptic D_2 receptors (the so-called DA autoreceptors) form part of a negative feedback system by which the synthesis and release of DA is regulated in an inhibitory fashion. D_1 receptors seem to occur on terminals of the GABAergic neurons in the SN, whereas D_2 receptors occur presynaptically on dendrites and the soma of dopaminergic neurons.

3.3. The Postsynaptic Dopamine Receptor Retains Its Functional Activity

Although the disturbances in presynaptic dopaminergic neurons in the nigro-striatal system of patients with PD are very pronounced, radioligand-binding studies in autopsy brain tissue from PD patients [36–50] suggest that there is usually no dramatic loss of D_1 and D_2 receptors. The investigation of the D_2 receptor binding have given contradictory results. Table 5 summarizes the results of these investigations; it shows that increased, unchanged, and decreased binding of various dopaminergic ligands to D_2 receptors has been reported. Most of these discrepant data are probably due to the variety of drug treatment strategies that have been used, and to the heterogeneity of the patient populations. The most detailed studies up to the present [39, 50] show that, in untreated patients, the extent of binding is only slightly altered. However, since these studies have hitherto only been done on total brain tissue, the presence of increased receptor binding in certain localized areas of the striatum cannot be excluded. Studies using positron emission tomography (PET), which permits *in vivo* investigation of DA receptors, do in fact show (at least in untreated PD patients in the early stages of the disease) that there is a slightly increased degree of binding for the DA antagonist spiroperidol [51, 52]. It may be that this early supersensitivity of D_2 receptors is lost during the course of PD, either because of the dopaminergic treatment (L-dopa, DA agonists) or because of the progression of the disease, and thus, in the final phases of the disease, one may even observe reduced binding, as has been reported in several studies (Table 5).

Table 5. The binding of dopaminergic ligands to the D_2-receptor in Parkinson's disease.

Reference	Caudate nucleus	Putamen	Effect of L-dopa therapy
Reisine et al., 1977 [40]	−	0	−
Lee et al., 1978 [41]	+	+	0
Rinne et al., 1979 [42]	+	+	0
Quik et al., 1979 [43]	0	n.i.	0
Winkler et al., 1980 [44]	−	n.i.	n.i.
Rinne et al., 1981 [45]	−	−	−
Riederer and Jellinger, 1982 [46]	n.i.	−	−
Bokobza et al., 1984 [47]	0	+	+
Guttman and Seeman, 1985 [48]	+	+	0
Guttman et al., 1986 [49]	0	+	0
Seeman et al., 1987 [50]	+	+	0
Rinne et al., 1991 [39]	−	0	0

−, decreased density of D_2-binding sites or negative effect of L-dopa therapy; +, increased density of D_2-binding sites or positive effect of L-dopa; 0, no change in the density of D_2-binding sites or no effect of L-dopa; L-dopa, L-3,4-dihydroxyphenylalanine; n.i., not investigated.

However, "normal" binding of a ligand to the DA receptor, derived from a Scatchard plot from which B_{max} and K_d values have been calculated, is merely evidence that the receptor protein recognizes the receptor ligand; it gives no indication about the functioning of receptor. Therefore, receptor-binding techniques, unless coupled with functional tests, are of only limited value in the quest for insights into the function of the receptor amplification and effector systems. So far no studies of this kind have been made in PD. However, the clinical efficacy of DA agonists such as bromocriptine and lisuride shows that, in about 75% of patients with PD, the postsynaptic receptor response remains effective until the end-stage of the disease is reached. However, in about 25% of cases the binding of [^{3}H]spiroperidol (a D_2 receptor antagonist) to D_2 receptors in the putamen of patients with PD is not changed, although the patients had been non-responders to anti-Parkinson drugs during the final stage of the illness. In such cases, early studies have shown that adenylate cyclase exhibits insufficient response to stimulation by DA [53]. These observations suggest disturbances in receptor-effector coupling and/or a greater than 90% loss of presynaptic neurons.

4. Changes in the Motor-Loop

Our conception of the organization of basal ganglia has changed markedly over the past decade, due to significant advances in our understanding of the anatomy, physiology, and pharmacology of these structures. Independent evidence from each of these fields has reinforced a growing perception that the functional architecture of the basal ganglia is essentially parallel in nature, regardless of the perspective from which these structures are viewed. Current evidence suggests that the basal ganglia are organized into several structurally and functionally distinct "circuits" that link the cortex, the basal ganglia and the thalamus (for a review, see [54, 55]). A simplified scheme of the "motor-loop" is shown in Figure 2. In brief, this circuit, like other basal ganglia-thalamo-cortical circuits, represents a re-entrant pathway through which influences emanating from specific areas of the cortex are returned to certain of those same areas after intermediate processing within the basal ganglia and the thalamus. In primates, the inputs to the basal ganglia portion of the motor circuit are focused principally on the putamen. This part of the striatum receives topographic projections from the primary motor cortex and from at least two premotor areas, including the arcuate premotor area and the supplementary motor area (for a review, see [55]). Within the circuit are two projection systems that arise from separate sub-populations of neurons of the putamen, and which terminate within the medial segment of the globus pallidus

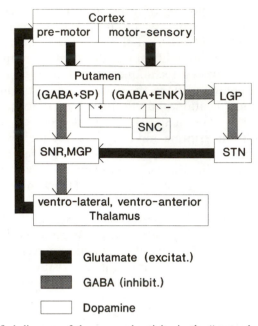

Figure 2. Simplified diagram of the neuronal activity in the "motor loop" (modified from Albin et al. [54]). GABA, γ-aminobutyric acid; ENK, enkephaline: LGP, the lateral segment of the globus pallidus; MGP, medial segment of the globus pallidus; SNC, the pars compacta of the substantia nigra; SNR, the pars reticulata of the substantia nigra; SP, substance P; STN, subthalamic nucleus.

(MGP) and the pars reticulata of the SN (SNR). The "direct" pathway arises from neurons of the putamen that contain both GABA and substance P, and which project directly to the motor portions of MGP and SNR (Figure 2). The "indirect" pathway, on the other hand, arises from neurons of the putamen that contain both GABA and enkephalin, and whose influences are conveyed to the basal ganglia output nuclei only indirectly, through a sequence of connections involving the lateral segment of the globus pallidus (LGP) and the subthalamic nucleus (STN) (Figure 2).

The role of DA within the basal ganglia appears to be a complex one, with many aspects still undefined. There are, however, indications that nigro-striatal dopaminergic projections may exert opposing effects on the "direct" and "indirect" pathways (for a review, see [55]) (Figure 2). Thus, the nigro-striatal innervation exerts an overall excitatory influence on the GABA/substance P-containing neuronal systems (which affect the output-regions of the basal ganglia via the "direct" pathway), and an overall inhibitory influence on the GABA/enkephalin-containing neuronal systems (which affect the nuclear regions of the LGP via the "indirect" pathway). Ultimately, therefore, this dopaminergic modulation of the striatum reinforces the cortically initiated activation either through an accelerated transmission of impulses via the "direct" pathway (which exerts an overall excitatory effect on the thalamus) or through a slowing down of impulse transmission via the "indirect" pathway (which in the end exerts an inhibitory effect on the thalamus).

The most recent animal experiments using the primate MPTP (1-methyl-4-phenyl-1,2,3,6-tetrahydropyridine) model of PD [56], in which the regional glucose utilization and thus the presynaptic activity was determined with the aid of the 2-deoxyglucose-uptake method [57–59], point to the fact that a reduction of nigro-striatal dopaminergic function leads to an increase in the activity of the striatal neurons projecting to the LGP and to a decrease in the activity of the striatal neurons projecting to the MGP and SNR. Figure 3 schematically represents the pathophysiological consequences of this differential effect on the striatal GABAergic projecting neurones in PD. In the final analysis this effect leads to a disinhibition of the output-regions of the basal ganglia and, thus, to an enhanced inhibition of the thalamo-cortical projection. The complex nature of these GABAergic under- and over-activities within the "motor-loop" may be the reason why GABA-mimetic drugs do not play any role in the treatment of the disease. In fact, progabide failed to

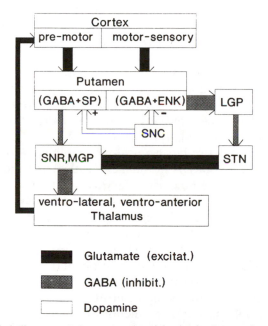

Figure 3. Simplified diagram of the neuronal activity in the "motor loop" in Parkinson's disease (modified from Albin et al. [54]). GABA, γ-aminobutyric acid; ENK, enkephaline; LGP, the lateral segment of the globus pallidus; MGP, the medial segment of the globus pallidus; SNC, the pars compacta of the substantia nigra; SNR, the pars reticulata of the substantia nigra; SP, substance P; STN, subthalamic nucleus.

show antiparkinson activity, and the benzodiazepines may at best only work by improving rigidity [60].

This hypothetical formulation of the pathophysiology of the motor symptomatology in PD is reinforced by the results of further animal experiments (for a review, see [54, 61]): for example, in rats the administration of DA receptor antagonists diminishes the concentration of substance P in the striatum and in the SNR; rats with brain lesions produced with 6-hydroxydopamine show an increase in the extent of GABA receptor binding in the LGP and a decrease in the SNC. Admittedly, however, there are few data and not a single systematic investigation of the biochemical parameters relevant in this connection has been carried out on brain tissue of patients who have died with PD.

5. The Extrastriatal Dopaminergic Pathobiochemistry

Reductions in the concentration of DA are not, however, restricted to the basal ganglia of patients with PD, but also occur to a variable extent in the mesocortical (cingulate gyrus, hippocampus, frontal cortex) and mesolimbic (nucleus accumbens, area olfactoria, lateral hypothalamus) projection areas of the area tegmenti ventralis (VTA) (Table 1). Early investigations by Riederer et al. [16], in which a sustantially decreased activity of TH (-70%) was found in the adrenal cortex tissues of patients who had died with PD, already pointed to a generalized involvement of the whole dopaminergic system in this disease. In studies on adrenal cortical tissue taken from PD patients for the purpose of autologous transplantation of this tissue to the caudate nucleus, a pronounced loss of DA (-80%) was in fact discovered [62, 63]. Decreased levels of DA were recently even demonstrated in the retina of deceased patients with PD [64].

Although no correlative biochemical-morphological studies are available, the observed loss of DA in the mesocortical and mesolimbic brain areas is most likely due to the neuronal degeneration of the dopaminergic cell bodies in the VTA which project to the frontal cortex and also to a variety of limbic forebrain regions. Due to the present lack of any biochemical-clinical correlations, it is difficult to evaluate the pathophysiological significance of the changes in DA concentrations in extrastriatal forebrain regions. What experimental evidence is available (for a review, see [65]) indicates that mesolimbic dopaminergic neurons (new nomenclature: ventral component of the mesostriatal dopaminergic system) not only have motor functions (for example, manipulations of the dopaminergic neurons in the nucleus accumbens produce marked changes in locomotor activity), but may also play a role in the regulation of emotional behavior. Anatomically, the ventral striatum is innervated by prefrontal and limbic cortical areas [65] and, therefore, the dopaminergic nerve terminal networks in the ventral striatum play an important part in the integrative mechanisms involving limbic and prefrontal cortex microcircuits ("complex loop"). Hence, any disturbance of dopaminergic neurotransmission in some cortical and, particularly, limbic areas, may play a role in the pathophysiology of affective changes seen in patients with PD. In addition, it may be assumed that the imbalanced mesolimbic dopaminergic system in the advanced stages of PD will favor the development of pharmacotoxic (L-dopa) psychosis. However, bearing in mind the glutamate hypothesis of schizophrenia [66], a functional imbalance between DA and Glu in the "complex loop" could also be involved in eliciting a pharmacotoxic psychosis [67].

6. Dysfunction of Non-Dopaminergic Systems in Parkinson's Disease

PD is not only a DA-deficiency syndrome, it additionally shows disturbances in other neurotransmitter and neuropeptide systems that interact with the basal ganglia dopaminergic system. The role of these non-dopaminergic changes seems to be indirect, and to be largely determined by two factors: a) the extent to which the corresponding neuronal systems influence the dopaminergic function of the basal ganglia, and b) the extent of the changes themselves.

6.1. Degeneration of Noradrenergic Systems

Cell loss in the locus ceruleus is also a characteristic change in PD [2]. For this reason the concentrations of NA and of 3-methoxy-4-hydroxy-phenylglycol (MHPG, the main metabolite of NA) as well as the activity of DA β-hydroxylase (the enzyme specific for the synthesis of NA) are reduced to a variable degree in many brain regions in PD, including the basal ganglia and associated brain stem areas, as well as extrastriatal regions [4, 68, 69]. This widespread NA deficiency suggests that both the locus ceruleus noradrenergic systems and the lateral tegmental noradrenergic systems are affected in PD.

6.2. The Degeneration of Serotonergic Systems

The moderate decrease of serotonin (5-HT) and its metabolite 5-hydroxy indoleacetic acid (5-HIAA) in several regions of the parkinsonian brain, including the basal ganglia, hypothalamus, hippocampus, and frontal cortex, as well as in some raphe nuclei and the lumbar spinal cord [69, 70] seems to be reflected by a substantial loss of neurons in the dorsal raphe [2] which gives rise to ascending serotonergic pathways. No gross changes in the characteristics of the serotonergic receptors are associated with altered serotonergic neurotransmission in the striatum of patients with PD [71].

6.3. The Degeneration of Cholinergic Systems

Studies of the enzymes associated with cholinergic neurotransmission (acetyl cholinesterase, choline acetyltransferase) indicate that the cholinergic neurons in the extrapyramidal nuclei are relatively well preserved in PD [72–74]. From the pathophysiological viewpoint, the sparing (even though it is only partial) of striatal cholinergic interneurons, in contrast with the profound dopaminergic deficiency, might explain the effectiveness of anticholinergic medication on motor symptoms of the disease. It is usually accepted that the loss of dopaminergic inhibition on cholinergic neurons causes cholinergic hyperactivity in the striatum (for a review, see [75, 76]). Hence, the rationale behind the treatment of PD is based upon the reduction of striatal cholinergic activity, either by enhancing dopaminergic inhibition through the administration of L-dopa or dopaminergic agonists, or via the administration of cholinergic receptor antagonists.

In contrast to non-demented patients with PD, choline acetyltransferase activity has been found to be significantly reduced in several cortical regions of demented patients with PD [77, 78]. Most likely, the reduction in cortical and hippocampal choline acetyltransferase activity is related to the cell loss in the nucleus basalis of Meynert, since most of the cholinergic innervation of the cerebral cortex arises from the nucleus basalis of Meynert, the median septum, and the nucleus of the diagonal band of Broca, and cholinergic cells of the nucleus basalis of Meynert degenerate in proportion to the degree of dementia [2]. Damage to the cholinergic innominato-cortical pathway also occurs in other degenerative conditions associated with intellectual deterioration, and particularly in Alzheimer's disease (for a review, see [79]). There are several similarities in the dementia associated with these two groups of disorders: both diseases involve degeneration of cholinergic, noradrenergic and also somatostatinergic neurons (for a review, see [80]); and the characteristic histopathological features of Alzheimer's disease (neurofibrillary tangles, senile plaques, granuvacuolar degeneration) may also be seen in PD patients – particularly in those who show intellectual deterioration (for a review, see [79]). Hence, damage to the cholinergic innominato-cortical pathway might be implicated in the pathophysiology of dementia, a common terminal feature of PD.

6.4. Preservation of GABAergic Systems?

The results obtained from studies concerning the GABAergic system in PD are contradictory. It is, for this reason, difficult to draw firm conclusions about the state of GABAergic systems in PD. The activity of glutamic acid decarboxylase (GAD, a GABA-synthesizing enzyme) has been reported to be decreased in large parts of the brain, particularly in the basal ganglia and the cerebral cortex [74, 81, 82]. In contrast to this finding, the concentration of GABA has been found to be elevated in the striatum [83, 84]. The density of GABA receptors, measured with ^{3}H-GABA, the distribution of which differs from that of the neuronal GABA marker GAD, is not significantly affected in most areas of the parkinsonian brain [85]. The decreased GABA receptor binding observed in the SN [85] is probably due to the loss of dopaminergic neurons in this region, since GABA receptors are located on these neurons (see Figure 1). As the majority of parkinsonian patients die with such concomitant factors as bronchopneumonia, associated with anoxia, decreased GAD activity might well reflect the vulnerability of this enzmye to terminal conditions. Measurements of GABA levels, however, were also markedly influenced by autopsy conditions. For example, GABA concentrations doubled within a few minutes of death, but thereafter rose at a rate equivalent to a 35% increase between 1 and 24 h [86]. Furthermore, the proportion of the free GABA concentration that represents neurotransmitter is unclear, since GABA, aside from its neurotransmitter role, is a metabolic intermediate and is present in both neurons and glia [87].

6.5. The Dysfunction of Peptidergic Systems

Among the numerous neuronal markers that are abnormal in PD, the following five neuropeptides are of particular interest: cholecystokinin (CCK-8), methionine-enkephalin (met-enk), leucine-enkephalin (leu-enk), substance P, and somatostatin. Although diminished concentrations of these neuropeptides in several brain regions have been described, the majority of other neuropeptides (thyrotropin releasing hormone, vasopressin, neurotensin, bombesin, neuropeptide Y and vasoactive intestinal peptide) do not appear to show altered concentrations (for a review, see [88]).

Most of CCK-8-containing neurons appear to be preserved in PD, at least as far as can be deduced from brain concentrations, which are generally normal. A moderate decrease in CCK-8-like immunoreactivity in the SN (− 30%) might, however, reflect some degeneration of CCK-8-containing neurons [89]. Investigations in rats have shown that CCK-8 coexists with DA in certain neurons originating in the VTA and innervating the medial and posterior portions of the nucleus accumbens [90]. However, no changes in CCK-8-like immunoreactivity were observed in the areas of this projection in patients with PD.

Brain levels of met-enk and leu-enk are usually normal in most brain regions in PD, although a decrease in the concentrations of met-enk-like immunoreactivity of about −70% has been observed in the SN, of about the same extent in the VTA, and of about −30% in both the putamen and in the globus pallidus [91]. Leu-enk levels are also reduced by 60–70% in the putamen and globus pallidus. These findings rather tend to contradict the concept (developed in section 2.4 above) concerning the pathophysiological displacement in the "motor-loop" in PD, according to which one might expect an increased number of enkephalinergic neurons (see Figure 3). However, the methodological difficulties associated with the methods for the determination of neuropeptides (antibody specifity, gross-reactivity), and the hitherto small number of available data require further experimental verification. Interestingly, the concentration of none of these neuropeptides was significantly changed in the caudate nucleus and the nucleus accumbens.

The concentration of substance P-like immunoreactivity was found to be decreased to the extent of about 30–40% only in the globus pallidus and the SN [92, 93], which might correspond to dysfunction of striato-pallidal and striato-nigral neurons containing this peptide. On the basis of the pathophysiological displacement in the "motor-loop" (Figure 3), one might expect a decreased number of neurons to show immunoreactivity to substance P in the putamen of patients with PD.

Although somatostatin levels are unaltered in most cortical areas, a moderate decrease (30–50%) has been observed in the frontal cortex and hippocampus in patients in whom there was clinical evidence of intellectual deterioration [94]. Since somatostatin is contained in the interneurons in the cerebral cortex, decreases in cortical somatostatin concentrations might indicate that some cortical lesions are associated with intellectual deterioration in this disease. A similar decrease in cortical somatostatin levels has been observed in patients with Alzheimer's disease [95]. The concentrations of somatostatin-like immunoreactivity were also reported to be decreased in the cerebrospinal fluid of patients with senile dementia of Alzheimer type and PD [96]. Hence, it can be concluded that somatostatinergic dysfunction plays a role in the pathophysiology of dementia.

With the exception of the association between cortical somatostatin deficiency and intellectual deterioration [94, 95], the role of neuropeptides in the pathophysiology and clinical picture of PD is not yet fully understood. However, with regard to the changes localized in the basal ganglia and related brain areas there is a wealth of information indicating the existence of strong functional interactions between the dopaminergic neurons and several non-dopaminergic systems. This functional neurotransmitter interrelationship suggests that at least some of the non-dopaminergic changes observed in the basal ganglia of patients with PD may influence, in either a positive or a negative direction, the symptoms produced by the striatal loss of DA.

7. The Role of the Glia

Neurons and capillaries in the CNS are embedded in a network, i.e., a "syncytium" of glial cells (primarily astrocytes and oligodendrocytes). Although these cells constitute approximately half the volume of the brain, and form isolating elements around synapses as well as blood vessels, and cover the surface of the ventricles, we know very little about their functions. Nevertheless, during recent years our knowledge of astroglial cell characteristics and function during maturation and in the adult nervous system has increased appreciably (for a review, see [97]). The spatial position of astrocytes between the neurons and the vascular endothelium might allow the astrocytic syncytium to act as a pathway for diffusion or active transport of substances between the environment of the neurons and the cerebral blood vessels and ventricles. Furthermore, the intimate morphological arrangements between astrocytes and neurons might reflect biochemical cooperation between these cells. Astrocytes in the adult nervous system are in a unique position to regulate the environment of neurons and, thereby, their sensitivity.

The lack of knowledge concerning the physiological significance of the glia and, above all, the unavailability of uncontaminated glial tissue for experimental investigation (because of the difficulty of separating glia from neurons and other non-glial tissue) may well be the reason why involvement of the glia in the pathogenesis of PD has hitherto not been taken into consideration. One of the currently favored hypotheses of the pathogenesis of PD, the "oxidative stress hypothesis" (imbalance between the formation of cellular oxidants and the antioxidative processes), is based on the notion that an excess of oxygen-derived compounds such as hydrogen peroxide, as well a hydroxyl and superoxide radicals are essentially responsible for the destruction of dopaminergic neurons (for a review, see [98]).

The superoxide radical is formed *in vivo* in a variety of ways (for a review, see [99]). A major source of it is the activity of mitochondrial and microsomal electron transport chains. Whereas cytochrome oxidase keeps all the partially-reduced oxygen intermediates tightly bound to its active site, some other components of the mitochondrial electron-transport chain (e.g., ubiquinone) link electrons directly to molecular oxygen. Since O_2 accepts electrons one at a time, the superoxide radical is released. Hydrogen peroxide, which *per se* is not toxic to cells, is generated by several enzymes, such as L-amino acid oxidase and MAO.

However, damage is done when hydrogen peroxide comes into contact with the reduced forms of heavy metal ions, e.g., iron (II) or copper (I). These decompose the hydrogen peroxide to the highly reactive hydroxyl radical (the Fenton reaction). A recent finding that such a reaction can proceed in the brain of patients with PD comes from post-mortem investigations [100–102], in which a shift of the iron(II):iron(III) ratio in the SNC from almost 2:1 in the normal brain to 1:2 in the parkinsonian brain was found. *In vitro* experiments show (for a review, see [99]) that oxygen-radical-generating systems damage biological structures, for example, by oxidizing membrane lipids and by fragmenting DNA. Indirect evidence for an increased peroxidation of membrane lipids in PD comes from experiments in which a significant increase of malondialdehyde levels was found in the SN of patients with PD [103].

As already mentioned, the MAO-catalyzed oxidation of DA includes hydrogen peroxide among its products. It is assumed that the major proportion of DA is metabolized via this reaction, and it is conceivable that in certain unfavorable circumstances increased amounts of cytotoxic radicals may be formed within the brain. Table 6 summarizes the essential reasons why the SN in particular exhibits an especially great sensitivity to such radicals. Most recently, however, immunocytochemical and immunohistochemical investigations [104–106] have re-examined the original assumption that high MAO activity is present in the SN. For example, Konradi et al. [104] were unable to demonstrate either MAO-A or MAO-B antibody reactions in the SN of deceased persons. On the other hand, the glia surrounding the SN contained high activity of MAO-B and showed a strong MAO-B antibody reaction. This would signify that the DA which is formed in the neurons of the SN is not broken down there, but rather in the surrounding glial cells. What this means is that the hydrogen peroxide formed in the glia would have to diffuse back into the neurons of the SN in order to exert a neurotoxic effect (which is apparently quite possible, as *in vitro* experiments in cultured cells indicate; for a review, see [99]), and there generate radicals via the Fenton reaction. This last step does not,

Table 6. Biochemical parameters that may contribute to the increased vulnerability of substantia nigra neurons to degeneration in Parkinson's disease.

1. High activity of Fe^{2+}-dependent tyrosine hydroxylase.
2. High concentration of reactive (free) iron.
3. Low or reduced enzymatic capacity (catalase, SOD) to detoxify free radicals (superoxide radical ion, hydroxyl radical) and hydrogen peroxide.
4. Low or reduced concentration of antioxidants (ascorbic acid, vitamin E).
5. High turnover of monoamines (hence a high synthesis of hydrogen peroxide).
6. Intraneuronal activity of MAO and aldehyde dehydrogenase.
7. High affinity of neurotoxins for uptake mechanism.
8. High rate of autoxidation and melaninization.

MAO, monoamine oxidase; SOD, superoxide dismutase.

however, take place within the neurons either, as the latest experiments suggest [107]. These semiquantitative histological investigations have shown increased iron (III) concentrations (which indirectly point to the occurrence of the Fenton reaction and, thus, to an increased formation of hydroxyl radicals) not in the pigmented neurons of the basal ganglia, but only in astrocytes, macrophages, reactive microglia, and non-pigmented neurons. These findings thus suggest the conclusion that processes which induce the formation of hydroxyl radicals are only occurring in the glia. On the basis of the extremely short biological half-lives of this radical it is, therefore, questionable whether this highly reactive species can even reach and let alone damage structures such as lipid membranes, DNA, or mitochondria which are esssential for the survival of the neurons.

8. Research Strategies for the Future

In spite of the incontrovertible success of L-dopa substitution therapy in PD, the treatment of the accompanying psychological and vegetative symptoms, and of the L-dopa-induced motor and psychic side-effects pose completely or at least very extensively unresolved problems [108–110]. Of particular clinical relevance is the problem that 20% of patients with PD do not respond to L-dopa treatment [111]. One must further consider that the currently used drug treatment strategies (new pharmaceutical formulations of L-dopa, MAO inhibition, the application of DA receptor agonists or DA uptake blockers) do not cure the underlying cause of the disease, but at best merely slow down its progression [112–114]. The strategies for designing future investigations therefore concentrate above all on these two essential aims:

1) The improvement of the symptomatic treatment, and
2) The development of a rational treatment aimed at the underlying pathomechanism of the disease.

To attain the first objective, bearing in mind the recent insights obtained into the pathophysiological displacements in the "motor-loop", systematic investigations are required in those regions which belong to this regulatory circuit. This will require that, in addition to DA, other relevant neurotransmitters, above all GABA and Glu, should be investigated in detail. Future investigations of the receptors for these neurotransmitters should, however, not be restricted to their binding-relationship for the appropriate ligands, but should also be combined with tests designed to assess their functioning.

   To attain the second of these objectives it is essential to clarify the underlying mechanisms responsible for the neurodegeneration. Although the partial elucidation of the pathogenic mechanisms responsible

for the toxic actions of neurotoxins such as MPTP and 6-hydroxydo-
pamine has provided some insights into how neurons may degenerate
(for a review, see [115]), and has been the basis of several hypotheses
concerning the pathogenesis of PD (for example, oxidative stress;
MPTP-like endogenous or environmental toxic substances); the causes
of the chronic nigral cell death and the underlying mechanisms remain
elusive. As already indicated in section 2.7, this might well be because
we first require knowledge of the biochemical cooperation that exists
between the neuronal and glial cells before we can check out the various
hypotheses of the pathogenesis of PD. If we accept that the glial
cells provide important metabolic substrates for the energy metabolism
of the neurons, and also serve to remove degradative products and,
to some extent, even toxic metabolites, then future investigations
must explain to what extent the glial anti-oxidant status (e.g., vitamins
C and E, reduced glutathione) or the activity of glial detoxifying
enzymes (catalase, superoxide dismutase) may be altered in patients
with PD.

Summary

The chronically progressive degeneration of the dopaminergic nigrostriatal neurons, and the consequent deficiency in dopamine in the
striatum of patients with Parkinson's disease is causally responsible for
the observed motor symptoms of the disease, and the basis of therapy
with L-dopa and dopamine agonists. Biochemically, the impairment of
nigro-striatal dopaminergic neurotransmission is characterized not only
by a strong reduction in the concentration of dopamine and of its
metabolites 3,4-dihydroxyphenylacetic acid and homovanillic acid, but
also by the loss of activity of the dopamine-synthesizing enzymes
tyrosine hydroxylase and dopa decarboxylase. In contrast, the activity
of the dopamine-metabolizing enzyme monoamine oxidase appears to
be unchanged. Equally unchanged, and functionally competent are
postsynaptic dopamine receptors in the striatum of patients with
Parkinson's disease. Biochemical findings in the late phase of the
disease, however, point to multiple disturbances in neurotransmission
and neuromodulation of various transmitter and modulator systems
(noradrenaline, serotonin, γ-aminobutyric acid, various neuropeptides)
in basal ganglia, but also additional disturbances in limbic and cortical
regions. This chapter provides a detailed presentation of the biochemical parameters, and in addition gives fresh insights into the pathophysiological function of the "motor-loop" in the pathogenesis of the motor
disturbances in Parkinson's disease. Additionally, the role of the glia in
this pathogenesis is considered, and future research strategies are put
forward.

Acknowledgements

Research carried out in the laboratories of the authors was generously supported by grants from the Bundesministerium für Forschung und Technologie (01 KL 9013).

References

[1] Parkinson J. An essay on the shaking palsy. London: Willingham and Rowland, 1817.

[2] Jellinger K. Pathology of Parkinson's syndrome. In: Calne DB, editor. Handbook of experimental pharmacology, Vol 88. Berlin Heidelberg: Springer-Verlag, 1989: 47–112.

[3] Tretiakoff C. Contribution a l'etude de l'anatomie pathologique du locus niger [dissertation]. Paris: Univ. of Paris, 1919.

[4] Ehringer H, Hornykiewicz O. Verteilung von Noradrenalin und Dopamin (3-Hydroxytyramin) im Gehirn des Menschen und ihr Verhalten bei Erkrankungen des extrapyramidalen Systems. Wien Klin Wschr 1960; 72: 1236–9.

[5] Birkmayer W, Hornykiewicz O. Der L-Dioxyphenylalanin (L-DOPA) Effekt bei der Parkinson-Akinese. Wien Klin Wschr 1961; 73: 787–8.

[6] Barbeau A, Murphy A, Sourkes GF. Excretion of dopamine in diseases of basal ganglia. Science 1961; 133: 1706–8.

[7] Bernheimer H, Birkmayer W, Hornykiewicz O, Jellinger K, Seitelberger F. Brain dopamine and the syndromes of Parkinson and Huntington. J Neurol Sci 1973; 20: 415–55.

[8] Birkmayer W, Riederer P. Responsibility of extrastriatal areas for the appearance of psychotic symptoms. J Neural Transm 1975; 37: 175–81.

[9] Price KS, Farley IJ, Hornykiewicz O. Neurochemistry of Parkinson's disease: relation between striatal and limbic dopamine. Adv Biochem Psychopharmacol 1978; 19: 293–300.

[10] Farley IJ, Price KS, Hornykiewicz O. Dopamine in the limbic regions of the human brain: normal and abnormal. Adv Biochem Psychopharmacol 1977; 16: 57–64.

[11] Scatton B, Javoy-Agid F, Montfort JC, Agid J. Neurochemistry of monoaminergic neurons in Parkinson's disease. In: Usdin E, Carlsson A, Dahlström A, Engel J, editors. Catecholamines: Neuropharmacology and central nervous system – therapeutic aspects. New York: Liss A, 1984: 43–52.

[12] Riederer P. Wuketich S. Time course of nigrostriatal degeneration in Parkinson's disease: a detailed study of influential factors in human brain amine analysis. J Neural Transm 1976; 38: 277–301.

[13] Riederer P, Sofic E, Konradi C. Neurobiochemische Aspekte zur Progression der Parkinson-Krankheit: Post-mortem-Befunde und MPTP-Modell. In: Fischer PA, editor. Spätsyndrome der Parkinson-Krankheit. Basel: Editiones (Roche), 1986: 37–49.

[14] Zetterström T, Sharp T, Collin AK, Ungerstedt U. *In vivo* measurement of extracellular DA and DOPAC in rat striatum after various DA-releasing drugs: implications for the origin of extracellular DOPAC. Eur J Pharmacol 1988; 148: 327–34.

[15] Lloyd K, Hornykiewicz O. Parkinson's disease: activity of L-dopa decarboxylase in discrete brain regions. Science 1970; 170: 1212–3.

[16] Riederer P, Rausch WD, Birkmayer W, Jellinger K, Seemann D. CNS modulation of adrenal tyrosine hydroxylase in Parkinson's disease and metabolic encephalopathies. J Neural Transm [Supplement] 1978; 14: 121–32.

[17] Rausch WD, Hirata Y, Nagatsu T, Riederer P, Jellinger K. Human brain tyrosine hydroxylase: *in vitro* effects of iron and phosphorylating agents in the CNS of controls, Parkinson's disease and schizophrenia. J Neurochem 1988; 50: 202–8.

[18] Mogi M, Harada M, Kiuchi K, Kojima K, Kondo T, Narabayashi H, Rausch D, Riederer P, Jellinger K, Nagatsu T. Homospecific activity (activity per enzyme protein) of tyrosine hydroxylase increases in Parkinsonian brain. J Neural Transm 1988; 72: 77–81.

[19] Lloyd KG, Davidson L, Hornykiewicz O. The neurochemistry of Parkinson's disease: effect of L-dopa therapy. J Pharmacol Exp Ther 1975; 195: 453–64.
[20] Riederer P, Sofic E, Rausch WD, Hebenstreit G, Bruinvels J. Pathobiochemistry of the extrapyramidal system: a "short note" review. In: Przuntek H, Riederer P, editors. Early diagnosis and preventive therapy in Parkinson's disease. Wien New York: Springer-Verlag, 1989: 139–49.
[21] Reichmann H, Riederer P. Biochemische Analyse der Atmungskettenkomplexe verschiedener Hirnregionen von Patienten mit Morbus Parkinson, Symposium des BMFT "Morbus Parkinson und andere Basalganglienerkrankungen", Bad Kissingen, 1989: 44.
[22] Nagatsu T, Levitt M, Udenfriend S. Tyrosine hydroxylase: the initial step in norepinephrine biosynthesis. J Biol Chem 1964; 239: 2910–7.
[23] Nagatsu T, Yamaguchi T, Kato T, Sugimoto T, Matsuura S, Akino M, Nagatsu I et al. Biopterin in human brain and urine from controls and parkinsonian patients: application of a new radioimmunoassay. Clin Chim Acta 1981; 109: 305–11.
[24] Kebabian JW, Calne DB. Multiple receptors for dopamine. Nature 1979; 277: 93–6.
[25] Seeman P. Brain dopamine receptors. Pharmacol Rev 1980; 32: 229–313.
[26] Zhou QY, Grandy D, Thambi L, Kushner J, Van Tol H, Cone R et al. Cloning and expression of human and rat D_1 dopamine receptors. Nature 1990; 347: 76–80.
[27] Bunzow J, Van Tol H, Grandy D, Albert P, Salon J, Christie M et al. Cloning and expression of a rat D_2 dopamine receptor cDNA. Nature 1988; 336: 783–7.
[28] Sokoloff P, Giros P, Martres MP, Bouthenet ML, Schwartz JC. Molecular cloning and characterization of a novel dopamine (D_3) receptor as a target for neuroleptics. Nature 1990; 347: 146–51.
[29] Wachtel H. Antiparkinsonian dopamine agonists: a review of the pharmacokinetics and neuropharmacology in animals and humans. J Neural Transm [P-D Sect] 1991; 3: 151–201.
[30] Markstein R, Vigouret JM. Is D-1 receptor stimulation important for the anti-parkinson activity of dopamine agonists? In: Przuntek H, Riederer P, editors. Early diagnosis and preventive therapy in Parkinson's disease. Wien New York: Springer-Verlag, 1989: 257–69.
[31] Ringwald E, Hirt D, Markstein R, Vigouret JM. Dopamin-Rezeptoren-Stimulation in der Behandlung der Parkinson-Krankheit. Nervenarzt 1982; 53: 67–71.
[32] Rinne UK. Brain neurotransmitter receptors in Parkinson's disease. In: Marsden CD, Fahn S, editors. Movement disorders. London: Butterworths, 1982: 59–74.
[33] Stoof JC, Kebabian JW. Opposing roles for D-1 and D-2 receptors in efflux of cyclic AMP from rat neostriatum. Nature 1981; 294: 366–8.
[34] Girault JA, Spampinato U, Glowinski J, Besson MJ. In vivo release of [^{3}H]gamma-aminobutyric acid in the rat neostriatum. II. Opposing effects of D-1 and D-2-dopamine receptor stimulation in the dorsal caudate putamen. Neuroscience 1986; 19: 1109–17.
[35] Robertson GS, Robertson HA. D-1 and D-2 dopamine agonist synergism: separate sites of action? Trends Pharmacol Sci 1987; 8: 295–9.
[36] Raisman R, Cash R, Ruberg M, Javoy-Agid F, Agid Y. Binding of [^{3}H]SCH 23390 to D_1 receptors in the putamen of control and parkinsonian subjects. Eur J Pharmacol 1985; 113: 467–8.
[37] Pimoule C, Schoemaker H, Reynolds GP, Langer SZ. [^{3}H]SCH 23390 labeled D_1 dopamine receptors are unchanged in schizophrenia and Parkinson's disease. Eur J Pharmacol 1985; 114: 235–7.
[38] Rinne JO, Rinne JK, Laakso K, Lönnberg P, Rinne UK. Dopamine D-1 receptors in the parkinsonian brain. Brain Res 1985; 359: 306–10.
[39] Rinne JO, Laihinen A, Lönnberg P, Marjamäki P, Rinne UK. A post-mortem study on striatal dopamine receptors in Parkinson's disease. Brain Res 1991; 556: 117–22.
[40] Reisine TD, Fields JZ, Yamamura HI, Bird ED, Spokes E, Schreiner PS et al. Neurotransmitter receptor alterations in Parkinson's disease. Life Sci 1977; 21: 335–44.
[41] Lee T, Seeman P, Rajput A, Farley IJ, Hornykiewicz O. Receptor basis for a dopaminergic supersensitivity in Parkinson's disease. Nature 1978; 273: 59–61.
[42] Rinne UK, Sonninen V, Laaksonen H. Responses of brain neurochemistry to levodopa treatment in Parkinson's disease. In: Poirier LJ, Sourkes TL, Bedard PJ, editors. Advances in neurology, Vol 24. New York: Raven Press, 1979: 259–74.

[43] Quik M, Spokes EG, Mackay AVP, Bannister R. Alterations in [³H]spiperone binding in human caudate nucleus, substantia nigra and frontal cortex in the Shy Drager syndrome and Parkinson's disease. J Neurol Sci 1979; 43: 429–37.

[44] Winkler MH, Berl S, Whetsell WO, Yahr MD. Spiroperidol binding in the human caudate nucleus. J Neural Transm 1980; 16: 45–51.

[45] Rinne UK, Lönnberg P, Koskinen V. Dopamine receptors in the parkinsonian brain. J Neural Transm 1981; 51: 97–109.

[46] Riederer P, Jellinger K. Dopaminerge (D₂) Rezeptorfunktion bei Parkinson-Krankheit, Morbus-Alzheimer, seniler Demenz und Schizophrenie. In: Fischer PA, editor. Psychopathologie des Parkinson-Syndroms. Basel: Editiones (Roches), 1982: 71–80.

[47] Bokobza B, Ruberg M, Scatton B, Javoy-Agid F, Agid Y. [³H]Spiperone binding, dopamine and HVA concentrations in Parkinson's disease and supranuclear palsy. Eur J Pharmacol 1984; 99: 167–75.

[48] Guttman M, Seeman P. L-dopa reverses the elevated density of D₂ dopamine receptors in Parkinson's diseased striatum. J Neural Transm 1985; 64: 93–103.

[49] Guttman M, Seeman P, Reynolds GP, Riederer P, Jellinger K, Tourtellotte WW. Dopamine D₂ receptor density remains constant in Parkinson's disease: no explanation for late-onset diminished response to L-dopa. Ann Neurol 1986; 19: 487–92.

[50] Seeman P, Bzowej NH, Guan HC, Bergeron C, Reynolds GP, Bird ED et al. Human brain D₁ and D₂ dopamine receptors in schizophrenia, Alzheimer's disease, Parkinson's, and Huntington's diseases. Neuropsychopharmacol 1987; 1: 5–15.

[51] Rinne UK, Laihinen A, Rinne JO, Någren K, Bergman J, Ruotsalainen U. Positron emission tomography (PET) demonstrates dopamine D-2 receptor supersensitivity in the striatum of patients with early Parkinson's disease. Movement Disorders 1990; 5: 55–9.

[52] Rinne JO, Laihinen A, Någren K, Bergman J, Ruotsalainen U, Solin O et al. PET demonstrates different behavior of striatal D₁ and D₂ receptors in early Parkinson's disease. J Neurosci Res 1990; 27: 494–9.

[53] Riederer P, Rausch WD, Birkmayer W, Jellinger K, Danielczyk W. Dopamine-sensitive adenylate cyclase activity in the caudate nucleus and adrenal medulla in Parkinson's disease and in liver cirrhosis. J Neural Trans [Supplement] 1978; 14: 153–61.

[54] Albin RL, Young AB, Penney JB. The functional anatomy of basal ganglia disorders. Trends Neurosci 1989; 12: 366–75.

[55] Alexander GE, Crutcher MD. Functional architecture of basal ganglia circuits: neural substrates of parallel processing. Trends Neurosci 1990; 13: 266–71.

[56] Mitchell IJ, Clarke CE, Boyce S, Robertson RG, Peggs D, Sambrook MA et al. Neural mechanisms underlying parkinsonian symptoms based upon regional uptake of 2-deoxyglucose in monkeys exposed to l-methyl-4-phenyl-1,2,3,6-tetrahydropyridine. Neurosci 1989; 32: 213–26.

[57] Schwartz WJ, Smith CB, Davidsen L, Savaki H, Sokoloff L. Metabolic mapping of functional activity in the hypothalamo-neurohypophysical system of the rat. Science 1979; 205: 723–5.

[58] DeLong MR, Alexander GE, Georgopoulos AP, Crutcher MD, Mitchel SJ, Richardson RT. Role of basal ganglia in limb movements. Human Neurobiol 1984; 2: 235–44.

[59] Filion M, Tremblay L, Bedard PJ. Abnormal influences of passive limb movement on the activity of globus pallidus neurons in parkinsonian monkeys. Brain Res 1988; 444: 165–76.

[60] Kapp W. Benzodiazepine bei Morbus Parkinson. In: Bergmann H, Fitzal S, Kapp W, Steinbereithner K, editors. Benzodiazepine: Klinische Bedeutung und Anwendung. Wien München Bern: Wilhelm Maudrich-Verlag, 1987: 129–35.

[61] DeLong MR. Primate models of movement disorders of basal ganglia origin. Trends Neurosci 1990; 13: 281–5.

[62] Carmichael SW, Wilson RJ, Brimijoin WS, Melton III LJ, Okazaki H, Yaksh TL et al. Decreased catecholamines in the adrenal medulla of patients with Parkinsonism. New Engl J Med 1988; 318: 254.

[63] Stoddard SL, Ahlskog JE, Kelly PJ, Tyce GM, van Heerden JA, Zinsmeister AR et al. Decreased adrenal medullary catecholamines in adrenal transplanted parkinsonian patients compared to nephrectomy patients. Exp. Neurol 1989; 104: 218–22.

[64] Harnois C, Dipaolo T. Decreased dopamine in the retinas of patients with Parkinson's disease. Investigative Opthalmol Visual Sci 1990; 31: 2473–5.

[65] Fuxe K, Agnati LF, Kalia M, Goldstein M, Andersson, K, Härfstrand. Dopaminergic systems in the brain and pituitary. In: Flückiger E, Müller EE, Thorner MO, editors. The role of brain dopamine: basic and clinical aspects of neuroscience, Vol 1. Berlin New York: Springer-Verlag, 1985: 11–25.

[66] Kim JS, Kornhuber HH, Schmid-Burgk W, Holzmüller B. Low cerebrospinal fluid glutamate in schizophrenic patients and a new hypothesis on schizophrenia. Neurosci Lett 1980; 20: 379–82.

[67] Riederer P, Kornhuber J, Gerlach M, Danielczyk W, Youdim MBH. Glutamatergic-dopaminergic imbalance in Parkinson's disease and paranoid hallucinatory psychosis. In: Rinne UK, Nagatsu T, Horowski R, editors. International Workshop Berlin Parkinson's Disease. Bussum: Medicom Europe, 1991: 10–23.

[68] Riederer P, Birkmayer W, Seemann D, Wuketich S. Brain-noradrenaline and 3-methoxy-4-hydroxyphenylglycol in Parkinson's syndrome. J Neural Transm 1977; 41: 241–51.

[69] Scatton B, Javoy-Agid F, Rouquier L, Dubois B, Agid Y. Reduction of cortical dopamine, noradrenaline, serotonin and their metabolites in Parkinson's disease. Brain Res 1983; 275: 321–8.

[70] Bernheimer H, Birkmayer W, Hornykiewicz O. Verteilung des 5-Hydroxytryptamins (Serotonin) im Gehirn des Menschen und sein Verhalten bei Patienten mit Parkinson-Syndrom. Wien Klin Wschr 1961; 39: 1056–9.

[71] Rinne UK, Lönnberg P, Koskinen V. Dopamine receptors in the parkinsonian brain. J Neural Transm 1981; 51: 97–106.

[72] Lloyd KG, Möhler H, Heitz P, Bartholini G. Distribution of choline acetyltransferase and glutamate decarboxylase within the substantia nigra and in other brain regions from control and parkinsonian patients. J Neurochem 1975; 25: 789–95.

[73] Rinne UK, Riekkinen P, Sonninen V, Laaksonen H. Brain acetylcholinesterase in Parkinson's disease. Acta Neurol Scand 1973; 49: 215–26.

[74] McGeer PL, McGeer EG. Enzyme associated with the metabolism of catecholamines, acetylcholine and GABA in human controls and patients with Parkinson's disease and Huntington's chorea. J Neurochem 1976; 26: 65–76.

[75] Tarsy D. Dopamine-acetylcholine interaction in the basal ganglia. In: Fields WS, editor. Neurotransmitter function: basic and clinical aspects. New York: Stratton International, 1977: 213–46.

[76] Lehmann J, Langer SZ. The striatal cholinergic interneuron: synaptic target of dopaminergic terminals? Neuroscience 1983; 10: 1105–20.

[77] Ruberg M, Ploska A, Javoy-Agid F, Agid Y. Muscarinic binding and choline acetyltransferase activity in parkinsonian subjects with reference to dementia. Brain Res 1982; 232: 129–39.

[78] Ruberg M, Rieger F, Villageois A, Bonnet AM, Agid Y. Acetylcholinesterase and butyrylcholinesterase in frontal cortex and cerebrospinal fluid of demented and non-demented patients with Parkinson's disease. Brain Res 1986; 362: 83–91.

[79] Jellinger K. Morphology of Alzheimer's disease and related disorders. In: Maurer K, Riederer P, Beckmann H, editors. Alzheimer's disease. Epidemiology, neuropathology, neurochemistry, and clinics. Vienna New York: Springer-Verlag, 1990: 61–77.

[80] Moll G, Gsell W, Wichart I, Jellinger K, Riederer P. Cholinergic and monoaminergic neuromediator systems in DAT. Neuropathological and neurochemical findings. In: Maurer K, Riederer P, Beckmann H, editors. Alzheimer's disease. Epidemiology, neuropathology, neurochemistry, and clinics. Vienna New York: Springer-Verlag, 1990: 235–43.

[81] Gaspar P, Javoy-Agid F, Ploska A, Agid Y. Regional distribution of neurotransmitter synthesizing enzymes in the basal ganglia of human brain. J Neurochem 1980; 34: 278–83.

[82] Lloyd KG, Hornykiewicz O. L-glutamic acid decarboxylase in Parkinson's disease: effect of L-dopa therapy. Nature 1973; 243: 521–3.

[83] Kish SJ, Chang LJ, Mirchandani L, Rajput A, Gilbert J, Rozdilsky B et al. GABA is elevated in striatal but not extrastriatal brain regions in Parkinson's disease: correlation with striatal dopamine loss. Ann Neurol 1986; 20: 26–31.

[84] Perry TL, Javoy-Agid F, Agid Y, Fibiger HC. Striatal GABAergic neuronal acitivity is not reduced in Parkinson's disease. J Neurochem 1983; 40: 1120–3.

[85] Rinne UK, Koskinen V, Laaksonen H, Lönnberg P, Sonninen V. GABA receptor binding in the parkinsonian brain. Life Sci 1978; 22: 2225–8.

[86] Perry TL, Hansen S, Gandham SS. Postmortem changes of amino compounds in human and rat brain. J Neurochem 1981; 36: 406–12.

[87] Hertz L. Functional interactions between neurons and astrocytes. 1. Turnover and metabolism of putative amino acid transmitters. Prog Neurobio 1979; 13: 277–323.

[88] Javoy-Agid F, Ruberg M, Hirsch E, Cash R, Raisman R, Taquet H et al. Recent progress in the neurochemistry of Parkinson's disease. In: Fahn S, Marsden CD, Jenner P, Teychenne P, editors. Recent developments in Parkinson's disease. New York: Raven Press, 1986: 67–83.

[89] Studler JM, Javoy-Agid F, Cesselin F, Legrand JC, Agid Y. CCK-immunoreactivity distribution in human brain: selective decrease in the substantia nigra from parkinsonian patients. Brain Res 1982; 243: 176–9.

[90] Skirboll LR, Grace AA, Hommer DW, Rehfield JG, Goldstein M, Hokfelt T et al. Peptide-monoamine coexistence: studies of the actions of cholecystokinin-like peptide on the electrical activity of mid-brain dopamine neurons. Neuroscience 1981; 6: 2111–24.

[91] Taquet H, Javoy-Agid F, Hamon M, Legrand JC, Agid Y, Cesselin F. Parkinson's disease affects differently Met5 and Leu5-enkephalin in the human brain. Brain Res 1983; 280: 379–82.

[92] Mauborgne A, Javoy-Agid F, Legrand JC, Agid Y, Cesselin F. Decrease of substance P-like immunoreactivity in the substantia nigra and pallidum of parkinsonian brains. Brain Res 1983; 268: 167–70.

[93] Rinne UK, Rinne JO, Rinne JK, Laaksonen K, Lönnberg P. Brain neurotransmitters and neuropeptides in Parkinson's disease. Acta Physiol Pharmacol Latinoam 1984; 34: 287–99.

[94] Epelbaum J, Ruberg M, Moyse E, Javoy-Agid F, Dubois B, Agid Y. Somatostatin and dementia in Parkinson's disease. Brain Res 1983; 278: 376–9.

[95] Davies P, Katzman R, Terry RD. Reduced somatostatin-like immunoreactivity in cerebral cortex from cases of Alzheimer disease and Alzheimer senile dementia. Nature 1980; 288: 279–80.

[96] Strittmater M, Cramer H, Reuner C, Strubel D, Kuntzmann F. Somatostatin-like immunoreactivity and neurotransmitter metabolites in the cerebrospinal fluid of patients with senile dementia of Alzheimer type and Parkinson's disease. In: Maurer K, Riederer P, Beckmann H, editors. Alzheimer's disease. Epidemiology, neuropathology, neurochemistry, and clinics. Vienna New York: Springer-Verlag, 1990: 313–21.

[97] Hansson E, Rönnbäck L. Astrocytes in neurotransmission. Cell Molec Biol 1990; 36: 487–96.

[98] Götz ME, Freyberger A, Riederer P. Oxidative stress: a role in the pathogenesis of Parkinson's disease. J Neural Transm [Supplement] 1990; 29: 241–9.

[99] Halliwell B, Gutteridge JMC. Oxygen radicals and the nervous system. Trends in Neurosciences 1985; 8: 22–6.

[100] Sofic E, Riederer P, Heinsen H, Beckmann H, Reynolds GP, Hebenstreit G. Increased Iron (III) and total iron content in post mortem substantia nigra of Parkinsonian brain. J Neural Transm 1988; 74: 199–205.

[101] Riederer P, Sofic E, Rausch WD, Schmidt B, Reynolds GP, Jellinger K et al. Transition metals, ferritin, glutathione and ascorbic acid in parkinsonian brains. J Neurochem 1989; 52: 515–21.

[102] Sofic E, Paulus W, Jellinger K, Riederer P, Youdim MBH. Selective increase of iron in substantia nigra zona compacta of parkinsonian brains. J Neurochem 1991; 56: 978–82.

[103] Dexter DT, Carter CJ, Wells FR, Javoy-Agid F, Agid F, Lees A et al. Basal lipid peroxidation in substantia nigra is increased in Parkinson's disease. J Neurochem 1989; 52: 381–9.

[104] Konradi C, Svoma E, Jellinger K, Riederer P, Denney RM, Thibault J. Topographic immunocytochemical mapping of monoamine oxidase-A, monoamine oxidase-B and tyrosine hydroxylase in human post mortem brain stem. Neuroscience 1988; 26: 791–802.

[105] Westlund KN, Denney RM, Rose RM, Abell CW. Localization of distinct monoamine oxidase A and monoamine oxidase B cell populations in human brain stem. Neuroscience 1988; 25: 439–56.

[106] Konradi C, Kornhuber J, Froelich L, Fritze J, Heinsen H, Beckmann H et al. Demonstration of monoamine oxidase-A and -B in the human brainstem by a histochemical technique. Neuroscience 1989; 33: 383–400.

[107] Jellinger K, Paulus W, Grundke-Iqbal I, Riederer P, Youdim MBH. Brain iron and ferritin in Parkinson's and Alzheimer's diseases. J Neural Transm [P-D Sect] 1990; 2: 327–40.

[108] Fischer PA, Schneider E, Jacobi P. Ergebnisse der medikamentösen Parkinson-Therapie. Modifizierende und limitierende Faktoren. In: Fischer PA, editor. Parkinson plus. Berlin New York: Springer-Verlag, 1984: 4–18.

[109] Rinne UK. Problems associated with long-term levodopa treatment of Parkinson's disease. Acta Neurol Scand [Supplement] 1983; 95: 9–17.

[110] Parkes JD. Variability in Parkinson's disease; clinical aspects, causes and treatment. Acta Neurol Scand [Supplement] 1983; 95: 27–37.

[111] Birkmayer W, Riederer P, editors. Die Parkinson-Krankheit: Biochemie, Klinik, Therapie. 2nd ed. Vienna New York: Springer-Verlag, 1985: 127–36.

[112] Birkmayer W, Knoll J, Riederer P, Youdim MBH, Hars V, Marton J. Increased life expectancy resulting from addition of L-deprenyl to Madopar^R treatment in Parkinson's disease: a longterm study. J Neural Transm 1985; 64: 113–27.

[113] Tetrud J, Langston W. The effect of deprenyl (selegiline) on the natural history of Parkinson's disease. Science 1989; 245: 519–22.

[114] Parkinson Study Group. Effect of deprenyl on the progression of disability in early Parkinson's disease. N Engl J Med 1989; 321: 1364–71.

[115] Gerlach M, Riederer P, Przuntek H, Youdim MBH. MPTP mechanisms of neurotoxicity and their implications for Parkinson's disease. Eur J Pharmacol [Mol Pharmacol Sect] 1991; 208: 273–86.

Inhibitors of Monoamine Oxidase B
Pharmacology and Clinical Use in Neurodegenerative Disorders
ed. by I. Szelenyi
© 1993 Birkhäuser Verlag Basel/Switzerland

CHAPTER 3
Parkinson's Disease and Its Existing Therapy

P.-A. Fischer

1   Parkinson's Disease
1.1 Motor Symptoms
1.2 Mental Disorders
1.3 Disorders of the Autonomic Nervous System
1.4 Course of Parkinson's Disease
2   Current Therapy of Parkinson's Disease
2.1 L-Dopa Therapy
2.2 Therapy with Dopamine Agonists
2.3 Amantadine Therapy
2.4 Anticholinergic Therapy
2.5 Treatment with Monoamine Oxidase B Inhibitors
2.6 Surgical Therapy
2.7 Physiotherapy
3   The Implementation of Long-Term Pharmacotherapy and Its Problems
     References

1. Parkinson's Disease

The parkinsonian syndrome is characterized clinically by the motor symptoms akinesia, rigor, and resting tremor. These may occur concomitantly with mental disturbances and disorders of the autonomic nervous system. The degree and combination of the symptoms vary from case to case and during the course of the disease. With consideration of the motor signs of the disease, an akinetic-rigid and a tremor-dominant progress type is differentiated. Equal occurrence of akinesia, rigor, and tremor in one patient is designated as the equivalence type of parkinsonism.

1.1. Motor Symptoms

The term "akinesia" goes back to Kleist [1, 2], who was the first researcher to draw attention to the loss of expressive and unintentional accompanying movement, as well as a general lack of movement as an independent symptom in paralysis agitans. Akinetic patients have great difficulties in starting a movement at all, and in later ending the movement sequence in the desired way. Difficulties in starting walking as well as the propulsions are thus explained. The akinetic patients are impeded in rapid innervation and in gradual slowing down of the movement. The akinesia leads to an impoverishment of expressive movements. Amimia and loss of gesticulatory movements result. Gait is transformed into small steps and the fluency of motor movements is lost. Unintentional accompanying movements are absent. The micrographia characteristic for many parkinsonian patients is a sign of akinesia. Movements against gravity, e.g., standing up from the supine position, are impeded by the akinesia. Altogether, the akinesia leads to multifarious motor impairments which are manifested especially in routine daily tasks.

The rigor is manifested as a waxing resistance in passive movements. This occurs to an equal extent in flexors and extensors, and does not depend on the position of the limbs, on the respective phase of the movement sequence, or on the position of the body. If the muscles do not yield smoothly, but rather abruptly in passive movements, this signals a characteristic of parkinsonian rigor: the cogwheel phenomenon. In contrast to spasticity, the myostatic reflexes and the polysynaptic reflexes are affected to a small extent by the rigor. Pathological reflexes are always lacking. In rigor, the patient is unable to relax musculature, and a posture which has been taken is fixed. A movement carried out against resistance which is suddenly released is immediately slowed down.

Typical parkinsonian tremor is a resting tremor which diminishes in action and intention. It can be stimulated by emotional-affective stimuli and stresses. This is a resting tremor with a frequency between 3 Hz and 7 Hz and a peak at 5 Hz. Parkinsonian tremor is an alternating agonist-antagonist tremor. It occurs most frequently as a resting tremor which is more pronounced distally. Parkinsonian tremor stops in sleep and in the absence of alpha waves in the EEG.

1.2. Mental Disorders

Among the mental disorders, bradyphrenia is regarded as a specific symptom of parkinsonism. The term "bradyphrenia" was coined by Naville in 1922 [3]. This is taken to mean a slowing down and a prolongation of all mental processes, resulting in impaired ability to grasp and reduced ability to concentrate, as well as a delayed reaction capacity. The bradyphrenia is identical with subcortical dementia, described in patients with progressive supranuclear palsy [4]. There are close correlations between the degree of bradyphrenia and the motor akinesia. It is therefore understandable that the discussion of the justification for the diagnosis bradyphrenia is also conditional on the method of investigation and the theoretical approach, and it presents difficulties in differentiating it from impairments of motor origin, effects of depressive symptoms, and incipient demential changes.

Parkinson's disease (PD) is frequently, but by no means always, accompanied by depression. As a rule, the depressions do not have the severity of psychotic depressions. In the long-term course of PD, depressions show independent characteristics. The question as to whether depressive moods occur more often in the premotor phase of PD cannot be definitively answered.

Parkinson's disease may be complicated by demential disorders. Parkinson himself pointed out that the patients he described did not show any intellectual impairments [5]. In later series of investigations, the frequency of demential changes in parkinsonian patients has been quantified very divergently. This results, in particular, from differences in the nomenclature of dementia, but also from differences in the recording of findings and in the sample populations investigated. Recent investigations specifically employing experimental psychological methods have disclosed various disorders of subfunctions. Parkinson's disease is not always accompanied by changes in intellect, and also does not automatically lead to dementia. Because of the importance of concomitant brain diseases in giving rise to demential changes, additional cerebral diagnostics including imaging methods are indicated in the presence of intellectual disorders in parkinsonian patients [6–8].

1.3. Disorders of the Autonomic Nervous System

Numerous disorders of the autonomic nervous system were registered in parkinsonian patients [9, 10]. However, there are not autonomic disorders specific to the parkinsonian syndrome. Alimentary symptoms such as salivation, disorders of deglutition and constipation (the significance of which, for the patient, was already pointed out by Parkinson in 1817) [5], are of practical importance. He attributed the salivation to a swallowing disorder. In recent investigations, this assumption could be confirmed and the assumption of a hypersialosis can be refuted [11, 12]. The disorders of the autonomic nervous system may occur as chronic symptoms or as disorders with increasing degree of the symptoms. The latter include outbreaks of profuse sweating and acute disorders of temperature regulation. The characteristic seborrhoic faces ("ointment face") of parkinsonian patients results from a hypersecretion of skin surface lipids, the formation and release of which are under dopaminergic control.

In disorders of the autonomic nervous system occurring in the course of PD, symptoms which may be a consequence of the motor disorders (salivation, respiratory disorders, sleep disorders) are to be differentiated from symptoms which are a direct result of the dysequilibrium of neurotransmitters and the consequent disorders of the central nervous system. Moreover, there are numerous autonomic disorders (which are already frequent in elderly patients) for which a multifactorial genesis is to be assumed.

1.4. Course of Parkinson's Disease

As a rule, the familiar full picture of PD in which the pronounced symptoms akinesia, rigor, tremor, and bradyphrenia are combined develops in a chronic, progressive course from discrete beginnings. The symptoms of the disease are initially present only in one limb or on one side in about two-thirds of the cases. This was already pointed out by Parkinson in 1817 [5]. He gave a description of the development of the disease up to the immobile terminal stage which is still valid today. The widely used classification of the disease stages according to Hoehn and Yahr (1967) [13] is also oriented to this typical course. Besides the usual case with chronic progression of the disease symptoms, however, there are also observations in which the symptoms remain stationary over a long time, whereas a rapid worsening occurs in other cases.

Depending on the degree of cardinal motor symptoms, a tremor-dominant, an akinetic-rigid progressive form, and an equivalence type are differentiated. The tremor-dominant progressive form has the most favorable long-term prognosis. The overall impairment of the patients is less, their psycho-organic efficiency is better, and the progression of the symptoms is generally slower. On the other hand, patients with an akinetic-rigid progressive form or an equivalence type show greater deficiencies, are more greatly impaired subjectively, and are more depressive [14, 15]. Terminal stages of the disease develop from a parkinsonian syndrome with advanced symptoms. These are characterized by an increasing inability to move, a bent-over posture, a general slowing down, apathy, and occurrence of disorders of the autonomic nervous system. In these stages, secondary complications such as bronchopneumonia, urinary tract infections, and decubital ulcers are frequent. Akinetic crises are only observed in advanced stages of the disease. These are characterized by sudden beginning, pronounced akinesia with disorders of deglutition, respiratory disorders, outbreaks of sweating, disorders of temperature regulation, and intellectual slowing. These states last for hours to days, and are reversible. However, akinetic crises can also lead to death. They are explained by an acute exhaustion of cerebral dopaminergic neurons [16]. Parkinson's disease reduces the life expectancy [13]; the mortality rate was 2.9 times higher than in an average population comparable in age, sex, and race before the introduction of modern anti-parkinsonism therapy with L-dopa, dopamine agonists, and MAO-B inhibitors. In the meantime, the average duration of the disease has been increased by 3 to 4 years under modern therapy, and the life expectancy has come closer to that of healthy persons of the same age.

Parkinson's disease is a disease of the second half of life. The age of manifestation is at present around the 60th year of life. When the disease occurs before the 40th year of life it is designated as juvenile parkinsonism. Insidious beginning, primarily bilateral symptoms, the predominance of akinetic rigid symptoms, very slow progression, the absence of mental disorders, and the detection of further cases of the disease in the family are typical for juvenile parkinsonism.

Senile parkinsonism occurs as the other extreme; it manifests after the 70th year of life. In these cases, parkinsonian symptoms are often observed soon after surgery or secondary diseases; bilateral symptoms with all cardinal motor symptoms, rapid progression, pronounced psycho-organic disorders, and the tendency to exogenous psychoses are observed [17].

The age factor is of great significance for the whole problem of parkinsonism. In diagnostic terms, incipient parkinsonism is to be distinguished from age-dependent alterations in motor functions. Vascular encephalopathy and atrophic lesions of the brain with extrapyramidal symptoms play an important role in the differential diagnosis of PD. Moreover, the multimorbidity typically present in PD is of very great practical importance in more elderly patients. In the elderly, cardiovascular conditions, metabolic disorders, respiratory disorders, and degenerative diseases of the skeleton may frequently modify PD in the most diverse ways and diminish the success of therapeutic measures.

2. Current Therapy of Parkinson's Disease

The causes of PD are unknown. It is therefore not possible to prevent the disease. Parkinson's disease is based on a progressive substantia nigra lesion with degeneration of nigrostriatal neurons which has already become extensive by the time at which the first symptoms of the disease are manifest. Reliable markers for the nigra lesion (which is already present, but not yet symptomatic) are not available. Curative treatment of the substantia nigra changes is not known, thus, there is no causal treatment of the symptoms which are manifested clinically as PD. Results of investigations which indicate that the progression of the disease is slowed down by administration of monoamine oxidase B inhibitors have therefore attracted great interest [18–21]. A confirmation of these results could mean that it would be possible for the first time to affect the basic process in the nigrostriatal system by medication. All the other therapeutic measures which are applied at present in parkinsonian patients are symptomatic treatments. The point of departure of therapeutic measures is striatal dopamine deficiency as well as the dysequilibria between cerebral neurotransmitter and functional systems induced by this. Medication and surgical methods for symptomatic treatment of PD are available. They can be supported by physiotherapeutic measures and sociotherapy. The therapy which is administered at present in PD can be categorized as drug therapy of the dopamine deficiency and cell-mediated therapy of the dopamine deficiency (transplantations), as well as drug therapy of functional dysequilibria and surgical therapy of functional dysequilibria (stereotactic operations). Among these possibilities of treatment, medication plays the decisive role. Agents for which the main indication is the treatment of PD, as reflected in its motor symptoms, are to be distinguished from drugs with other main indications and which have positive effects on individual motor, mental or autonomic parkinsonian symptoms.

2.1. L-Dopa Therapy

L-Dopa therapy is at present the most effective method for treatment of PD. This treatment was introduced by Birkmayer and Hornykiewicz [22], and Barbeau et al. [23], both in 1961 and independently of each other. It has a positive effect on all motor symptoms of parkinsonism. The data on the improvement of the overall symptoms of parkinsonism vary between 50% and 80% of the initial value. In historical terms, L-dopa was the first method of treatment with which the akinesia and the bradyphrenia could be positively affected. The therapeutic effectiveness of the L-dopa therapy is the standard against which other methods of treatment are measured. The life expectancy of parkinsonian patients has been increased substantially since the introduction of L-dopa therapy [24–27].

Pure L-dopa and L-dopa in combination with peripherally active decarboxylase inhibitors are available for L-dopa therapy. Equivalent doses of the pure form and L-dopa/decarboxylase inhibitor combinations lead to the same improvement of parkinsonian symptoms. However, the administration of pure L-dopa is accompanied by more side-effects, of which gastrointestinal symptoms are the most prominent. About 80% of the parkinsonian patients treated orally with pure L-dopa complain temporarily of persistent nausea and aversion to food. In addition, therapy with L-dopa is accompanied by various cardiovascular side-effects; these side-effects are dose-dependent. In the combination of L-dopa with a peripherally active decarboxylase inhibitor, the peripheral conversion of L-dopa into dopamine and noradrenaline is prevented, so that the occurrence of gastrointestinal and cardiovascular side-effects is largely avoided. The combination of L-dopa with the peripherally active decarboxylase inhibitor benserazide or carbidopa reduces the amounts of L-dopa necessary to attain therapeutically active levels in the blood. In administration of L-dopa in combination with a decarboxylase inhibitor, only about one-fifth of the dose of L-dopa is required to attain the same kinetic effect as the administration of pure

L-dopa. On the other hand, the symptoms of parkinsonism cannot be reduced to a greater extent by combination of L-dopa with the peripherally active decarboxylase inhibitor than in administration of pure L-dopa. Only a certain improvement (which cannot be optimized by increasing the dose) is possible with dopa therapy in any case of the disease [28–30].

Because of the better tolerance, L-dopa therapy is, as a rule, administered today as a combination of L-dopa/decarboxylase inhibitors (benserazide or carbidopa). With this modification of L-dopa therapy, peripheral side-effects play only a minor role. The dose of L-dopa required in any given case must be established individually. This is achieved with a slowly rising dose monitored against the parkinsonism symptoms.

During long-term treatment with L-dopa, side-effects – which may result in a serious change in the overall clinical picture – occur with increasing duration of treatment. Extrapyramidal dyskinesias and fluctuations of the symptoms are of very great practical importance. The most frequent side-effects of long-term L-dopa therapy are extrapyramidal dyskinesias which are manifested to various extents in almost 90% of patients after several years of treatment. In phenomenological terms, the hyperkinesias induced by L-dopa most frequently consist of choreatic movement sequences, and more rarely of dystonic movements [31]. The choreoathetotic hyperkinesias most frequently affect the limbs, with preferential involvement of the upper limbs and the shoulder girdle, as well as of the face and the mouth region. The dystonic dyskinesias consist of slow and sometimes painful cramps of the distal limb segments. Painful foot dystonias are particularly characteristic. Apart from choreatic and dystonic disorders of movement, other extrapyramidal dyskinesias such as tics, ballismus, or myoclonias are also very rarely observed under L-dopa therapy. Choreoathetotic dyskinesias occur, in particular, as the optimal clinical effect of an individual dose of L-dopa. They are therefore only rarely felt to be irksome by the patient when they are very pronounced. On the other hand, the choreatic movement disorders often have an alarming and disturbing effect in the social environment of the patient. These hyperkinesias (which are associated with times of particularly good mobility) can be reliably reduced or eliminated by reducing the dose. However, this is achieved at the cost of an intensification of the parkinsonian symptoms.

As a rule, the dystonic dyskinesias are linked to phases of immobility and times of relative underdosing with L-dopa. They respond well to an additional dopaminergic stimulation. Sustained-release L-dopa preparations or dopamine agonists can be successfully used to treat the most frequent and especially irksome dystonic dyskinesias, i.e., the foot cramps which mostly occur in the early morning [32].

Sustained-release L-dopa preparations are new developments in which there is a delayed release compared to the standard medications [33, 34].

Because of the reduced bioavailability, it is necessary to reduce the dose by about 50% in comparison to the standard preparations. A general switch from L-dopa/decarboxylase inhibitor standard preparations to sustained-release preparations has not proved effective. Most patients complain of a delayed onset of action and an incomplete effect on symptoms, and of an unpredictable efficacy when treated only with sustained-release preparations. However, the specific administration of sustained-release preparations has proved effective in combination with standard therapy. Such special indications are foot dystonias in the early morning or nocturnal immobilities with sleep disorders which can be eliminated by taking sustained-release dopa in the evening.

After treatment with L-dopa for several years, there are fluctuations of the symptoms in more than half of the parkinsonian patients. A distinction is made between two forms of fluctuations, depending on whether correlations with the intake of medication can be established or whether the akinetic symptoms occur unpredictably. A decline in the deterioration of mobility associated with a single dose is categorized under the generic term "wearing-off phenomena". These most frequently occur as end-of-dose akinesias. Akinetic states occurring independently of the intake of medication are paroxysmal on-off phenomena which are also designated as random oscillations. The consequences for patients with symptom fluctuations are periods of more pronounced immobility which become longer with increasing duration of treatment. It is possible to treat the predictable fluctuations of the wearing-off phenomenon type, whereas the paroxysmal on-off phenomena cannot be treated. The genesis of the response fluctuations has not been clarified and is probably not uniform. Both peripheral and central mechanisms are discussed as pathogenetic factors. Among the peripheral factors, the pharmacokinetics of L-dopa, the effect of metabolites of L-dopa administered in unphysiologically high doses, disorders of absorption in the gastrointestinal tract, and impairments of transport through the blood-brain barrier play a role. A decrease in presynaptic storage in the context of the progressive degenerative lesion, alterations of receptor sensitivities, and interactions between cerebral neurotransmitter systems are the central mechanisms held responsible [35–38].

The therapeutic approaches in fluctuations of the effect of L-dopa attempt to attain a continuous cerebral supply of L-dopa. This is achieved by stabilizing the levels of L-dopa in the plasma by more frequent administration of single doses, and by use of sustained-release preparations and dietary measures. The latter consist of avoiding competition between mechanisms of transport of L-dopa and the neutral amino acids ingested with food by abstinence from high-protein meals. In addition, methods of parenteral treatment are used. It has been shown that the long-term infusion of L-dopa can achieve a stable clinical effect. However, this approach is not practically feasible in terms of therapy, since the acidity of L-dopa solutions necessitates high dilutions and, thus, very large amounts of fluid. An attempt is therefore made to improve the fluctuations by secondary medications, in particular, by oral or parenteral administration of dopamine agonists.

Symptomatic psychoses may occur during long-term therapy. After more than 5 years of treatment, psychotic episodes are to be reckoned with in about 20–30% of patients. Symptomatic psychoses in parkinsonian patients are not only observed after administration of L-dopa, but also after all other anti-parkinsonism drugs. Analyses of individual cases show that there are multifactorial reasons for this, and that the anti-parkinsonian agent is only one link of the chain of causes. The designation "dopa psychosis" that is sometimes used should be avoided [39].

2.2. Therapy with Dopamine Agonists

Administration of dopaminergic agonists in PD improves the symptoms by stimulation of postsynaptic receptors. The dopamine agonists which can be used in therapy are readily able to pass the blood-brain barrier. The dopamine agonists administered up to now act, in particular, on D2 receptors. The specificity of this dopamine receptor stimulation has not yet been completely clarified and is probably also different for various dopamine agonists. The direct postsynaptic stimulation by dopamine agonists enables therapeutic effects, even in advanced degeneration. The anti-parkinsonian action of apomorphine has been known for a long time. Use of this agent was initially abandoned because the side-effects were too severe. In recent years, apomorphine has again been used for parenteral treatment of cases of advanced parkinsonism. Since 1974, various ergot derivatives have been used successfully in the treatment of parkinsonism. Experience with bromocriptine (which was introduced into parkinsonism therapy in 1974 by Calne et al.) [40] is the longest and most extensive. Large-scale treatment figures were also available for lisuride and pergolide [41, 42]. Long-term monotherapy is possible with dopamine agonists. However, high doses have to be administered and the rate of side-effects is high compared to L-dopa therapy. During long-term monotherapy with bromocriptine, a decline of the effect and worsening of the parkinsonian symptoms could be detected [43].

The most important side-effect of the dopamine agonists are gastrointestinal symptoms, orthostatic hypotension, and psychotic symptoms. Peripheral vascular effects are possible with ergot derivatives in the form of vasospasms of the fingers, edema, and erythromegaly. It was striking in the long-term administration of dopamine agonists that they gave rise to fewer end-of-dose fluctuations and hyperkinesias.

The dopamine agonists were initially used mainly in combination with L-dopa in advanced cases of the disease [44]. Additional positive effects compared to placebo could be attained in this way. A saving of L-dopa of 30–40% was possible without diminution of efficacy; at the same time, there was a reduction of the hyperkinesias [45]. On the basis of these observations, the early use of dopamine agonists is recommended at present. The early administration of L-dopa in combination with a dopamine agonist enables a lower dose of L-dopa to be administered with the same efficacy. Combination treatments with early administration of L-dopa in combination with various dopamine agonists revealed roughly the same efficacy compared to the effectiveness of L-dopa on its own, but with a smaller number of extrapyramidal hyperkinesias and a later and less pronounced occurrence of symptom fluctuations [46–48].

Monotherapy with dopamine agonists is no longer recommended. The main importance of dopamine agonists consists in their combined administration with L-dopa. There is an additional indication for parenterally administered dopamine agonists in advanced cases with very severe fluctuations. Improvements in fluctuating parkinsonian patients can be attained with subcutaneous or intravenous drips. The main risk of this form of treatment is the high rate of psychoses. Management of an intermittent subcutaneous therapy with apomorphine is more convenient in practical terms.

2.3. Amantadine Therapy

Amantadine treatment of PD is based on the observation that parkinsonian symptoms improved after administration of virustatically acting amantadine salts. Systematic investigations of Schwab et al. in 1969 [49] verified the positive effect. Amantadine hydrochloride and amantadine sulfate are used. Under experimental conditions, the compounds bring about an improvement of the release of dopamine by alteration of the fluidity of membranes in high concentrations [50]. However, in addition, the antiglutamatergic effect is relevant with regard to the results of therapy [51]. The improvement of the overall parkinsonian symptoms in monotherapy is between 20% and 30%. The amantadine therapy is suitable for mild and incipient cases of the disease; and it is easy to administer. In particular, hypotonic dysregulations, livedo reticularis, edema, vertigo, and nausea, as well as rare exogenous psychoses were observed as side-effects.

A special indication for amantadine is the intravenous administration in akinetic crises.

2.4. Anticholinergic Therapy

The anticholinergic therapy of parkinsonian syndrome is the oldest method of pharmacotherapy. Belladonna preparations were successfully introduced into the treatment of parkinsonism by the Charcot School in the late 1800s [52]. Initially, various belladonna extracts and pure alkaloids were used. The "Bulgarian cure" initially consisted of a weak acid extract of the Bulgarian root prepared with wine. Besides atropine, it contained a mixture of readily interconverted alkaloids. Since the development of synthetic anticholinergics in 1946, belladonna preparations have hardly been used.

With anticholinergic therapy on its own, the overall symptoms are improved by about 20% in parkinsonism patients. The individual symptoms rigor and tremor respond better. The effect of anticholinergics is primarily manifested in an elimination of the functional dysequilibrium between acetylcholine and dopamine in the striatum as a consequence of the dopamine deficiency due to the disease [53, 54]. This equilibrium is established on a level lower than the norm, since the effects of the slowly developing deficiency of dopamine in the striatum are counteracted before the occurrence of clinical symptoms by a counterregulation with reduction of cholinergic activity.

It is unclear whether anticholinergics act in other ways above and beyond their balancing effect on the cholinergic-dopaminergic equilibrium in the striatum. The effectiveness of the various anticholinergic preparations is very similar. According to the investigations available, it cannot be unequivocally stated whether the various anticholinergics have different effects on certain symptoms of parkinsonism. The anticholinergics lead to an inhibition of salivary secretion. This side-effect is used therapeutically in hypersialosis. Among the side-effects of anticholinergics, particular attention has been paid to the frequent occurrence of symptomatic psychoses during therapy. As a rule, however, the etiology is multifactorial. Therapy with anticholinergics is also restricted by the possibility of inducing demential changes [55]. This assumption is based on findings according to which a cerebral cholinergic insufficiency syndrome is significant for dementia of Alzheimer type. Cholinergic insufficiency might be caused by long-term anticholinergic therapy in parkinsonism patients. Further side effects of anticholinergics are disorders of accommodation and micturition, tachycardia, and vertigo.

Anticholinergics may be sufficient for treatment of mild parkinsonian syndromes. There are divergent views on the use of anticholinergics in combination therapies. It is particularly controversial whether additional positive effects can be attained by simultaneous administration of anticholinergics in patients who are adequately treated with L-dopa, and clinical omission studies have led to divergent results.

2.5. Treatment with Monoamine Oxidase B Inhibitors

After recognition of the pathogenic significance of striatal dopamine deficiency for parkinsonian symptoms, apart from dopamine substitution, attempts were made to attain therapeutic effects by intervening at other sites of dopaminergic transmission. One possibility is delayed dopamine degradation by administration of monoamine oxidase inhibitors. However, in the beginning this approach was abandoned, again because of overshoot noradrenergic activity and occurrence of the "cheese effect" after consumption of foods containing tyramine.

After differentiation of two different MAO types (types A and B), which can also be selectively inhibited, renewed attention was paid to this therapeutic principle [56, 57]. Birkmayer et al. (1975) found an intensification of the antiakinetic effect of L-dopa and an improvement of fluctuations during long-term L-dopa therapy using the selective MAO-B inhibitor *l*-deprenyl (selegiline) [58]. In subsequent studies, the positive effects of selegiline on motor parkinsonian symptoms were confirmed and MAO-B inhibition was introduced as a further means of treating parkinsonism. Monotherapy with selegiline was only administered in mild parkinsonism in its early phase, and it brought about slight changes in the principal neurological symptoms. The majority of reports on the results of treatment with selegiline concern combination treatments with L-dopa. Open studies and double-blind investigations with different trial designs consistently confirmed a positive effect of selegiline on motor parkinsonism symptoms. With doses between 5 mg and, at most, 15 mg, slight to pronounced motor improvements were registered. In long-term administration, the effectiveness of selegiline treatment declines. Investigations on the saving effect of L-dopa in combined administration consistently showed that the dose of L-dopa may be reduced, but there are divergent views as to the extent of the feasible dose reduction.

Different methods of measurement and different study designs have been involved. Deprenyl is administered in daily doses of 5–10 mg; 10 mg inhibit at least 80% of MAO-B. An increase of the dose does not improve the therapeutic effect. Deprenyl is well tolerated. In monotherapy with selegiline, insomnia or sleep disorders were registered as the most frequent side-effects. The more serious side-effects observed in combination therapy with L-dopa were exogenous psychotic episodes and accentuation of L-dopa-induced hyperkinesias.

Besides the administration of selegiline in practical therapy of parkinsonism to reduce the use of L-dopa and to treat fluctuations in the effect, an early use is discussed because of a possible protracting effect on the progression of PD. As discussed in detail elsewhere in this book (Chapters 2, 7, 8, 9, 13, 16), these applications are based on pathogenetic concepts which can be designated as a radical hypothesis and as a neurotoxin hypothesis. In the context of physiological dopamine metabolism, H_2O_2 and cytotoxic free radicals formed in oxidative processes are biotransformed by special enzyme systems. Assuming that endogenously formed free radicals have a pathogenetic role in the development and progression of the basic neurodegenerative lesion in the substantia nigra in disturbance of detoxication mechanisms (radical hypothesis), MAO-B inhibition might have a protective or protractive effect on the course of the disease.

The clarification of the mechanism of action of MPTP intoxications has raised the question as to whether other chemically similar and so far unknown exotoxins might be relevant for the development and course of Parkinson's disease (neurotoxin hypothesis). The toxic action of MPTP can be abolished by preventive inhibition of MAO-B. Their protective action is based on a blockade of conversion of MPTP in MPDP and also in their actually toxic metabolites MPP+. MAO-B inhibition might have positive effects even in the presence of exotoxins when monoamine oxidase activity is also important for their biotransformation.

2.6. Surgical Therapy

Surgical treatment methods played a major role for a short time before the introduction of L-dopa therapy. The unsatisfactory results of drug treatment prompted numerous attempts of surgical treatment including severance of various fiber connections and cortical resections. The use of stereotactic targeting devices by Spiegel and Wycis (1947) [59] also enabled the surgical method to become established. It is possible to carry out stereotactic operations with great precision, even in deep areas of the brain which are difficult to reach. Cases with dominant tremor and rigor can be improved by stereotactic operations in the thalamic nucleus and subthalamic afferent and efferent neuronal structures. The akinesia cannot be affected by stereotactic interventions. Despite continuous improvement of the techniques of operation, decline of the surgical mortality (which is at present about 0.4%), and avoidance of severe side-effects such as speech disorders and pareses (1.5% and 0.5%), the number of stereotactic operations has greatly diminished after the introduction of modern methods of drug treatment. Surgical treatment in Parkinson's disease is never the first-line therapy. With inadequate efficacy of drug treatment and/or serious intolerances, however, tremor-dominant cases of the disease still constitute an indication for stereotactic operation.

A good general condition, the absence of serious internal concomitant diseases, and more severe psycho-organic changes are a prerequisite for the operation. Immediate postoperative improvements in tremor and rigor are reported in 80% to 90% of cases [60]. The surgical successes diminish with aging. Since the risk of postoperative speech disorders increases substantially after bilateral operations, stereotactic operations should only be carried out unilaterally. They are therefore particularly indicated in hemilateral tremor-dominant cases. In the presence of bilateral symptoms the stereotaxis should be confined to an operation on the dominant side.

New attempts at surgical treatment entail the transplantation of catecholamine-producing tissues into the brain of parkinsonian patients. On the basis of animal experiments in which experimentally induced striatal dopamine deficiency syndromes could be eliminated by transplantation of various tissues synthesizing dopamine, transplantations have also been carried out in parkinsonian patients since 1985. The first transplantations were carried out with autologous adrenal medulla. In this procedure, the patient's own adrenal medulla is implanted into the striatum. In the meantime, at least 300 transplantations of adrenal medulla have been carried out in parkinsonian patients, utilizing various methods of surgery. The results were non-uniform and are not easy to interpret, since different methods of operation and of anesthesia, postoperative care, and concomitant pharmacotherapy were applied. Altogether, a sustained improvement of the neurological symptoms and definitive functioning of the transplant could not be demonstrated as a consequence of the transplantation.

Since fetal dopamine-synthesizing ventral midbrain cells already yielded better transplantation results in animal experiments, an attempt was also made to obtain positive results of therapy using homologous fetal midbrain tissue in parkinsonian patients. It is estimated that more than 100 patients have since been treated in this way. Data which can be evaluated are only available for a few patients operated on in Sweden and the USA. An increased storage of L-dopa could be demonstrated in the region of transplantation in one patient by means of positron emission tomography [61]. Altogether, the results obtained in two patients treated with fetal midbrain tissue indicate an improvement of their clinical picture [62]. However, the observation periods are still too short, even in these positive cases, for an overall appraisal compared to other methods of treatment. The transplantation of fetal midbrain tissue is associated with a large number of unsolved medical, legal, and ethical problems. At present, this is an experimental therapy of which the possible value for the treatment of selected parkinsonian patients cannot yet be evaluated [63, 64].

2.7. Physiotherapy

All methods of drug and surgical treatment improve the possibilities of movement (but not of individual movements) by reduction or elimination of motor disorders. These must be practiced within a training program. An individual physiotherapeutic treatment program must be worked out for each parkinsonian patient as an accompaniment to long-term pharmacotherapy. This must take into account his/her general performance capacity and specific symptoms. The objective is to counteract the lack of movement and to practice movements which have been lost. Besides coordination exercises, balance exercises, rhythmic gymnastics, postural and walking exercises, respiratory gymnastics are of great importance in severely ill patients. Although, active movement training has first priority; this can be supported by massaging tense muscles. Movement exercises in moderately warm water are considered comfortable by most patients. Group gymnastics are beneficial after individual dose adjustment and initial therapy because of the multifarious external stimuli they provide to parkinsonian patients. In addition to group exercise, communication with other parkinsonian patients and their families may also be important aids in coping with the symptoms of the disease, as they counteract the tendency to self-isolation by parkinsonian patients as a consequence of their disease.

The speech disorders in parkinsonian patients constitute a particular problem. These can only be alleviated to a small extent by medication. Early logopedic treatment is indicated in these cases.

3. The Implementation of Long-Term Pharmacotherapy and Its Problems

The various anti-parkinsonian agents improve symptoms to varying extents in monotherapy. Since Parkinson's disease cannot be causally cured at present, the long-term effectiveness of therapy is a further important criterion to be considered in its practical application. Progression of the underlying substantia nigra lesion and an increase of the disease symptoms are to be expected during treatment of a parkinsonian patient over a period of several years. Since there are various effective methods available for treatment of parkinsonism, a choice must be made on an individual patient basis and it must be decided whether monotherapy of combination therapy is to be given. The establishment of the most favorable combinations of medication presupposes several years of analyses or comparable patient populations with different treatments. The time and effort required as well as the difficulties of such studies are obvious. The establishment of the most favorable combination of drugs and the most suitable use of time for the various principles of therapy is therefore the subject of a continuous scientific controversy. There are special difficulties when recommendations made for treatment of incipient disease cases are inferred from problems in the long-term administration of individual anti-parkinsonian agents or certain combinations of drugs [65–69].

Presently, a new increase of parkinsonian symptoms is evident for all methods of drug and surgical treatment in follow-up investigations conducted over several years. The decline in effect in the long-term course is not a specific phenomenon of a certain therapy. The situation is complicated in that different progressive forms of Parkinson's disease could be characterized by long-term analyses of clinical populations [14, 17]. With comparable initial symptoms, patients with only a brief response to the therapy are to be found as often as patients who continue to show a good improvement over long periods without an alteration of the drug dose [70]. The severity of the symptoms of parkinsonism before the beginning of treatment does not allow a prognosis with regard to the treatment result. On the other hand, the rapid development of symptoms and the response of the parkinsonian symptoms during the dose adjustment phase have proved to be good indicators for the later result of treatment. Moreover, the prognostic relevance of the reaction to parenterally administered L-dopa or the injection of dopamine agonists such as apomorphine is being tested in de-novo patients. Besides the indications for the rapidity and severity of the underlined substantia nigra lesion which can be inferred from these observations, the presence or absence of symptoms of additive brain diseases or a multisystemic spreading of the lesion is of prognostic significance.

It could already be shown during the introduction of L-dopa therapy that it often failed, particularly in patients with severe organic brain disorders and states of confusion as recorded in the prior history [24]. After the introduction of cranial computer tomography into clinical diagnostics, systematic investigations in parkinsonian patients revealed extranigral cerebral changes in an unexpectedly high percentage of cases [71, 72]. These mostly comprised brain atrophy or vascular encephalopathy. In therapy studies, it could be demonstrated that patients with pathological CT findings respond more poorly to treatment and have a more favorable long-term progress [74, 75]. A significant correlation of secondary cerebral diseases for the prospects of treatment in Parkinson's disease could be clearly shown in follow-up observations over many years. Cerebral polypathia evidently brings about a destabilization of the respective clinical picture via its effect on compensation mechanisms. Additive cerebral conditions may already be present in the occurrence of parkinsonian symptoms or may only supervene in the course of PD.

The presence of parkinsonian symptoms together with cerebral symptoms which do not belong to PD and are the manifestation of either or both a secondary cerebral disease or a multisystemic degeneration is designated as "Parkinson plus". The definition Parkinson plus is based on cases with primary parkinsonian symptoms and refers to the combination of Parkinson's disease with vascular encephalopathies or neuronal degenerative degradation lesions which are becoming ever more important in practice. The definition Parkinson plus includes the cases of multisystem degenerations which develop from initial parkinsonian symptoms. All the disease states mentioned have in common that signs of cerebral disease which do not belong to Parkinson's disease can be detected clinically or with additional diagnostic measures in these cases. The prognostic significance of these "non-Parkinson" symptoms increases with their number. In Parkinson's disease, extranigral vascular or neuronal degenerative brain changes which have previously been considered mainly as etiological criteria are now attaining new clinical relevance in practice as course-modifying factors in terms of Parkinson plus.

The term Parkinson plus used here has developed from progressive observations; it does not relate to heterogeneous systemic diseases in the course of which parkinsonian symptoms may also occur [76].

As a rule, in advanced cases of the disease and largely in immobile terminal stages of PD, symptoms of extranigral cerebral changes become increasingly dominant. Psychopathological, but above all, demential changes and disturbances of the autonomic nervous system are of particular importance. Complex clinical pictures in which the symptoms of parkinsonism only account for the blurred core then develop.

Parkinson's disease is treated in relation to its symptoms and stage in any individual plan of therapy. In the individual case, there is a complex situation in which one must take into consideration the preceding features of the disease course, the present concomitant cerebral and internal diseases, and also the multifarious factors of the sociopsychological life situation, as well as the nature and severity of the symptoms. When choosing a method for treating the individual case, various factors are considered which are not always comparable to the severity of the parkinsonian symptoms. The therapy of parkinsonism can therefore be considered in schematic terms only to a certain extent. In incipient, mild PD, there is the greatest range of choice, since an adequate improvement can be attained in various ways and with all the anti-parkinsonian agents mentioned.

L-dopa therapy is the most effective method of treatment and is the yardstick and point of reference for all the parkinsonian agents. The problems during long-term L-dopa therapy have led to a tendency to abandon monotherapy and to give preference to primary combinations of L-dopa with other anti-parkinsonian agents. In this connection, it is still controversial as to which combination of medication should be used to commence treatment of PD. A combination of L-dopa plus peripherally active decarboxylase inhibitors with a dopamine agonist or a monoamine oxidase B inhibitor or the combination of all three therapeutic principles is preferred at present for the first treatment of parkinsonian patients. In the long-term course, it is frequently necessary to

P

increase the dose of the anti-parkinsonian agents administered. The terminal stages of the disease and Parkinson plus cases are often characterized by a decrease in tolerance to the anti-parkinsonian medication, so that their dose has to be reduced. At the same time, treatments of concomitant mental symptoms and multifarious disorders of the autonomic nervous system and complex interactions between the medication used are becoming of increasing significance.

References

[1] Kleist K. Beiträge zur Kenntnis der psychomotorischen Bewegungsstörungen. Zit nach K Kleist 1908; 1918.
[2] Kleist K. Zur Auffassung der subkortikalen Bewegungsstörungen (Chorea, Athetose, Bewegungsausfall, Starre, Zittern). Arch Psychiatr 1918; 59: 790–803.
[3] Naville F. Les complications et les sequelles mentales de L'encéphalite épidémique. Encéphale 1922; 17: 396–375, 423–436.
[4] Albert ML, Feldmann RG, Willis AL. The subcortical dementia of progressive supranuclear palsy. J Neurol Neurosurg Psychiatry 1974; 37: 121–130.
[5] Parkinson J. An Essay on the Shaking Palsy. Sherwood, Neely and Jones, London 1817.
[6] Fischer P-A, editor. Spätsyndrome der Parkinson-Krankheit. Editiones Roche, Basel 1986.
[7] Mayeux R. Mental State. In: Handbook of Parkinson's Disease. Koller WC, editor. Dekker New York-Basel 1987: 127–144.
[8] Russ M, Fischer P-A. Vergleichende testpsychologische Untersuchungen zur intellektuellen Leistungsfähigkeit von Parkinson-Patienten. Nervenarzt 1990; 61: 88–93.
[9] Fischer P-A, editor. Vegetativstörungen beim Parkinson-Syndrom. Editiones Roche, Basel 1984.
[10] Tanner CM, Goetz CG, Klawans HL. Autonomic nervous system disorders. In: Handbook of Parkinson's Disease. Koller WC, editor. M. Dekker, New York 1987: 145–170.
[11] Bateson MC, Gibber FB, Wilson RSE. Salivary Symptoms in Parkinson's Disease. Arch Neurol 1973; 29: 274–275.
[12] Cros P, Parret J, Peyrin J, Freidel M, Dumas P. Sialorrhées, apport des examens isotopiques. Revue Stomat Chir maxillofac 1979; 80/6: 319–324.
[13] Hoehn MM, Yahr MD. Parkinsonism: Onset, Progression and Mortality. Neurology (Minneap.) 1967; 17: 427–442.
[14] Fischer P-A, Schneider E, Jacobi P. Verlaufsformen und Verlaufsfaktoren beim Parkinson-Syndrom. In: Parkinson-Syndrom. Kombinations- und Begleittherapien. Fischer P-A, editor. Schattauer Stuttgart-New York 1980: 97–115.
[15] Jakob H. Neuropathologie des Parkinson-Syndroms und die Seneszenz des Gehirns. In: Langzeitbehandlung des Parkinson-Syndroms. Fischer P-A, editor. Schattauer Stuttgart-New York 1978: 5–25.
[16] Birkmayer W, Riederer P. Die Parkinson-Krankheit. 2. Aufl. Springer Wien-New York 1985.
[17] Fischer P-A, Schneider E, Jacobi P. Klinische Bilder des Parkinson-Syndroms und ihre Verläufe. In: Pathophysiologie, Klinik und Therapie des Parkinsonismus. Gänshirt H, editor. Editiones Roche, Basel 1983: 51–65.
[18] Birkmayer W, Knoll J, Riederer P, Youdim MBH, Hars V, Marton J. Increased life expectancy resulting from addition of L-deprenyl to madopar treatment in Parkinson's disease: a longterm study. J Neural Transm 1985; 64: 113–127.
[19] Parkinson Study Group. DATATOP: a multicenter controlled clinical trial in early Parkinson's disease. Arch Neurol 1989a; 46: 1052–1060.
[20] Parkinson Study Group. Effect of deprenyl on the progression of disability in early Parkinson's disease. New Engl J Med 1989b; 321: 1364–1371.
[21] Tetrud JW, Langston JW. The effect of deprenyl (selegiline) on the natural history of Parkinson's disease. Science 1989; 245: 519–522.

[22] Birkmayer W, Hornykiewicz O. Der L-3,4-Dioxyphenyl-alanin (L-dopa) Effekt bei der Parkinson-Akinese. Wien Klin Wschr 1961; 73: 787–788.

[23] Barbeau A, Murphy GS, Sourkes TL. Excretion of dopamine in diseases of basal ganglia. Science 1961; 133: 1706–1708.

[24] Fischer P-A, Schneider E, Jacobi P, Maxion H. Langzeitstudie zur Effektivität der L-Dopa-Therapie bei Parkinson-Kranken. Nervenarzt 1973; 44: 128–135.

[25] Guillard A, Chanstang C. Maladie de Parkinson. Les facteurs de prognostic à long term. Rev Neurol 1978; 134: 341–354.

[26] Marsden CD, Parkes JD. Success and problems of long-term Levodopa therapy in Parkinson's disease. Lancet 1977; 1: 345–349.

[27] Yahr MD. Evaluation of Long-term-Therapy in Parkinson's Disease: Mortality and Therapeutic Efficacy. In: Advances in Parkinsonism. Birkmayer W, Hornykiewicz O, editors. Roche, Basel 1976: 435–443.

[28] Birkmayer W. Experimentelle Ergebnisse über die Kombinationsbehandlung des Parkinson-Syndroms mit L-Dopa und einem Decarboxylase-Hemmer (Ro4-462). Wien Klin Wschr 1969; 81: 677–679.

[29] Fischer P-A, Schneider E, Jacobi P, Maxion H. Kombinationsbehandlung des Parkinson-Syndroms mit L-Dopa und Decarboxylase-Hemmer. Med Welt 1973; 24 (NF): 1742–1746.

[30] Marsden CD, Parkes JD, Ress JE. Long-term-Treatment of Parkinson's disease with an extracerebral dopa decarboxylase inhibitor (L-alpha-methyl-hydrazine. MK 486) and levodopa. Advances in Neurology 1973; 3: 79–93.

[31] Poewe W. Klinik und Klassifikation der L-Dopa-induzierten Dyskinesien beim Parkinson-Syndrom. Spätsyndrome der Parkinson-Krankheit. Fischer P-A, editor. Editiones Roche, Basel 1986: 257–265.

[32] Poewe W, Lees AJ. The Pharmacology of Foot Dystonia in Parkinsonism. Clin Neuropharmacol 1987; 10: 47–56.

[33] Erni W, Held K. The hydrodynamically balanced system: a novel principle of controlled drug release. Eur Neurol 1987; 27 (suppl. 1): 21–27.

[34] Yeh KC, August TE, Bush DF et al. Pharmacokinetics and bioavailability of Sinemet CR: A summary of human studies. Neurology 1989; 39: 25–38.

[35] Hornykiewicz O. The mechanism of action of L-dopa in Parkinson's Disease. Life Sci 1974; 15: 1249–1259.

[36] Hornykiewicz O. Bedeutung von cerebralen Neurotransmitter-Wechselwirkungen für das Parkinson-Syndrom. In: Parkinson-Syndrom: Kombinations- und Begleit-Therapien. Fischer P-A, editor. Schattauer Verlag Stuttgart-New York 1980: 5–25.

[37] Nutt JG, Woodward WR, Carter JH, Trotmann TL. Influence of fluctuations of plasma large neutral amino acids with normal diets on the clinical response to levodopa. J Neurol Neurosurg Psychiatry 1989; 52: 481–487.

[38] Yahr MD. Aspekte zur Pathogenese und Behandlung des Parkinsonismus. In: L-Dopa-Substitution der Parkinson-Krankheit. Riederer P, Umek H, editors. Springer Wien-New York 1985: 97–104.

[39] Schneider E, Fischer P-A, Jacobi P, Grotz A. Exogene Psychosen beim Parkinson-Syndrom. Häufigkeit und Entstehungs-bedingungen. Fortschr Neurol Psychiat 1984; 52: 207–214.

[40] Calne DB, Teychenne PF, Claveria LE, Eastman R, Greenacre JK, Petrie A. Bromocriptine in parkinsonism. Br Med J 1974; 4: 442–444.

[41] Fischer P-A, Frieling B, editors. Morbus Parkinson – Neue Möglichkeiten mit Lisurid. W de Gruyter, Berlin, 1989.

[42] Jankovic J. Long-term-study of pergolide in Parkinson's disease. Neurology 1985; 35: 296–299.

[43] Lees AJ, Stern GM. Sustained bromocriptine therapy in previously untreated patients with Parkinson's Disease. J Neurol Neurosurg a Psychiatry 1981; 44: 1020–1023.

[44] Schneider E, Fischer P-A. Bromocriptin in der Behandlung der fortgeschrittenen Stadien des Parkinson-Syndroms. Dtsch med Wschr 1982; 107: 175–179.

[45] Fischer P-A, Przuntek H, Majer M, Welzel D. Kombinations-behandlung früher Stadien des Parkinson-Syndroms mit Bromocriptin und Levodopa. Ergebnisse einer multizentrischen Studie. Dtsch Med Wschr 1984; 109: 1279–1283.

[46] Rinne UK. The importance of an early combination of a dopamine agonist levodopa in the treatment of Parkinson's disease. In: Lisuride: A New Dopamine Agonist and

Parkinson's Disease. van Hanen J, Rinne UK, editors. Excerpta Medica, Amsterdam 1986: 64–71.

[47] Rinne UK. Combined bromocriptine-levodopa therapy early in Parkinson's disease – a 5 years follow up. Neurol 1987; 37: 826–828.

[48] Rinne UK. Lisuride, a dopamine agonist in the treatment of early Parkinson's disease. Neurol 1989; 39: 336–339.

[49] Schwab RS, England AC, Poskanzer DC, Young RR. Amantadine in the treatment of Parkinson's Disease. JAMA 1969; 1168–1170.

[50] Wesemann W. Aspekte zum Wirkungsmechanismus von Amantadinen. In: Amantadin Workshop. Danielczyk W, Wesemann W, editors. Edition Materia Medica Gräfelfing 1984: 15–23.

[51] Kornhuber J, Bormann J, Retz W, Hübers M, Riederer P. Memantine displaces MK-801 at therapeutic concentrations in postmortem human frontal cortex. European Journal of Pharmacology 1989; 166: 589–590.

[52] Ordenstein L. Sur la paralysis agitante et la Sclérose en plaques généralisée. Doctoral Thesis, Martinet, Paris 1987.

[53] Duvoisin RC. Cholinergic-anticholinergic antagonism in parkinsonism. Archives of Neurology 1967; 17: 124–136.

[54] Lloyd KG. Neurochemical compensation in Parkinson's Disease. In: Parkinson's Disease, concepts and prospects. Lakke JPF, Korf J, Wesseling H, editors. Excerpta Medica Amsterdam-Oxford 1977: 61–72.

[55] Syndulko K, Gilden ER, Hansch EC, Potvin AA, Tourtellotte WW, Potvon JH. Decreased verbal memory associates with anti-cholinergic treatment in Parkinson's disease. Internat J Neurosci 1981; 14: 61–66.

[56] Johnston JP. Some observations upon a new inhibitor of monoamine oxidase in brain tissue. Biochem Pharmacol 1968; 17: 1285–1297.

[57] Riederer P, Konradi C, Schay K, Wenziel W, Birkmayer G, Danielczyk W, Sofic E, Youdim MBH. Localization of MAO-A- and MAO-B in Human Brain: A Step in Understanding the Therapeutic Action of L-Deprenyl. In: Parkinson's Disease. Yahr MD, Bergmann KJ, editors. Raven Press, New York 1987: 111–118.

[58] Birkmayer W, Riederer P, Youdim MBH. The potentiation of the antiakinetic effect of L-dopa treatment by an inhibitor of MAO-B, deprenyl. J Neural Transm 1975; 36: 303–326.

[59] Spiegel EA, Wycis HT, Marks M, Lee AJ. Stereotaxie apparatus for operations on the human brain. Science 1947; 106: 349–350.

[60] Mundinger F. 30 Jahre stereotaktische Hirnoperationen beim Parkinsonismus. In: Pathophysiologie, Klinik und Therapie des Parkinsonismus. Gänshirt H, editor. Editiones Roche, Basel 1983: 331–357.

[61] Lindvall O, Brundin P, Widner H, Rehncrona S, Gustavii B, Frakkoviak R, Leenders K, Sawle G, Rothell JC, Marsden CD, Björklund A. Grafts of fetal dopamine neurons survive and improve motor function in Parkinson's disease. Science 1990; 247: 574–577.

[62] Lindvall O, Rehncrona S, Brundin P, Gustavii B, Astedt B, Widner H, Lindholm T, Björklund A, Leenders K, Rothwell JC, Frackowiak F, Marsden CD, Johnels B, Steg G, Freedman R, Barry JH, Seiger A, Bygdeman M, Strömberg I, Olson L. Human fetal dopamine neurons grafted into the striatum of two patients with severe Parkinson's disease. A detailed account of methodology and a 6-months follow up. Arch Neurol 1989; 46: 615–631.

[63] Lindvall O. Transplantation into the human brain: present status and future possibilities. J Neurol Neurosurg Psychiatry 1989; (spec. supp.): 39–54.

[64] Oertel W, Kupsch A. Transplantation von Dopamin-synthetisierenden Zellen und trophische Faktoren – zukünftige Behandlungsverfahren des idiopathischen Parkinson-Syndroms? In: Parkinson-Syndrom und Nigra-Prozesse. Fischer P-A, editor. Editiones Roche, Basel 1991: 207–241.

[65] Fahn St, Bressmann SB. Should Levodopa therapy for Parkinsonism be started early or late? Evidence against early treatment. Can J Neurol Sci 1984; 11: 200–206.

[66] Fischer P-A. Aktuelle Parkinson-Therapie: Heutiges Konzept für die Anwendung von L-Dopa. Akt Neurol 1988; 15: 38–41.

[67] Markham CH, Diamond SG. Evidence of support early Levodopa therapy in Parkinson's disease. Neurology 1981; 31: 125–131.

[68] Muenter MD. Should Levodopa therapy be started early or late? Can J Neurol Sci 1984; 11: 195–199.
[69] Rinne UK. Combination of a dopamine agonist, MAO-B inhibitor and Levodopa – a new strategy in the treatment of early Parkinson's disease. Acta Neurol Scand 1989; 126: 165–169.
[70] Birkmayer W, Riederer P, Youdim MBH. Distinction between benign and malignant type of Parkinson's disease. Clin Neurol Neusurg 1979; 158: 81–83.
[71] Fischer P-A, Jacobi P, Schneider E, Maxion H. Correlation between Clinical and CT-Findings in Parkinson's Syndrome. In: Computerized Tomography. Lanksch N, Kazner E, editors. Springer Berlin-Heidelberg-New York-Tokyo 1976: 244–248.
[72] Schneider E, Becker H, Fischer P-A, Grau H, Jacobi P. The course of brain atrophy in Parkinson's disease. Arch Psychiat Nervenkr 1979; 227: 89–95.
[73] Schneider E, Fischer P-A, Jacobi P, Becker H, Beyer M. Cerebral atrophy and long-term response to Levodopa in Parkinson's disease. J Neurol 1979; 222: 37–43.
[74] Fischer P-A, editor. Parkinson plus. Zerebrale Polypathie beim Parkinson-Syndrom. Springer-Heidelberg-New York-Tokyo 1984: 159.
[75] Fischer P-A. Long-term course in Parkinson's syndrome and cerebral polypathy (Parkinson plus). Raven Press, New York, Adv Neurol 1987; 45: 235–238.
[76] Fahn St. Secondary Parkinsonism. In: Scientific approaches to Clinical Neurology. Goldensohn ES, Appel SH, editors. Lea and Febinger, Philadelphia 1977: 1159–1189.

Chemistry and Pharmacology of Monoamine Oxidase B Inhibitors

Inhibitors of Monoamine Oxidase B
Pharmacology and Clinical Use in Neurodegenerative Disorders
ed. by I. Szelenyi
© 1993 Birkhäuser Verlag Basel/Switzerland

CHAPTER 4
Medicinal Chemistry of Present and Future MAO-B Inhibitors

J. Gaál and I. Hermecz

Dedicated to the Memory of Tamás Keleti and Zoltán Mészáros, our Mentors in Research

1   Introduction
2   Theoretical Basis of Selective Inhibition
2.1   Enzyme
2.2   Substrate
2.3   Types of Enzyme Inhibition
2.3.1 Reversible Inhibition
2.3.2 Irreversible Inhibition
3   Measurement of the Enzyme Activity and the Inhibition
3.1   *In Vitro* Determination
3.1.1 Application of Purified Enzyme System
3.1.2 Application of Selective Substrates
3.2   *In Vivo* Determination of Selective Inhibition
4   Reversible Inhibitors
5   Irreversible Inhibitors
5.1   Acetylenic Compounds
5.2   Allylamine Derivatives
5.3   Cyclopropylamine Derivatives
5.4   Pyridopyrimidine Derivatives
5.5   Silyl Compounds
5.6   Allenic Amines
6   Partly Irreversible Inhibitors
6.1   MPTP and Its Analogs
6.2   Oxazolidone Derivatives
7   Stereoselectivity
8   Outlook
       Summary
       References

1. Introduction

The first monoamine oxidase (MAO) inhibitor was described 26 years before the discovery of the enzyme itself. As late as the mid-1900s millions of patients still suffered from tuberculosis. Then, several groups of chemists synthesized molecules with different chemical structures in attempts to create an efficient treatment for this illness. One of these compounds, isonicotinyl hydrazide (isoniazid) was originally synthe-

sized as a necessary intermediary but was later described as an antitu-
berculotic agent. This substance was, in essence, the first MAO inhibitor, and it had been described as early as 1912, without regard to its
biological activity. Among its monoalkyl derivatives the 2-isopropyl-1-
isonicotinyl hydrazide (iproniazid) was the most effective in clinical
practice. Its unwanted "lightening" side-effect had been the starting
point for pharmacological therapy of depression [1].

Zeller and coworkers discovered the connection between the antidepressant action of iproniazid and its MAO inhibitor potential [2, 3].
MAO catalyzes the oxidative deamination of biogenic amines and, in
this way, has a role in their biological inactivation *in vivo*. The inhibition of MAO results in increased brain levels of the biogenic amines
including noradrenaline and serotonin which pathologically decreased
in depression. The 1950s and early 1960s saw the first classic use of
MAO inhibitors. However, the discovery of their side-effects, particularly their ability to potentiate the sympathomimetic action of indirectly
acting amines, thus causing hypertensive crises after patients consumed
tyramine-containing food (especially cheese, hence the so-called cheese
effect) temporarily curtailed the use of MAO inhibitors in clinical
practice [4, 5].

A new era began when deprenyl was synthesized in 1962, and was
found to be a selective irreversible inhibitor of MAO [6]. Later, in 1968,
Johnston differentiated multiple forms of MAO into subtypes A and B
using clorgyline as a selective MAO-A inhibitor [7]. After clarification of
the substrate specificity of the two enzyme forms, it became clear that the
dangerous blood-pressure increasing effect of the MAO inhibitors can be
avoided when only the B form is inhibited, because in the intestine
tyramine is metabolized by the A form. Deprenyl was found to fulfill
these requirements as the first selective MAO-B inhibitor [8]. The
selective inhibition of the B form preferentially decreases the deamination
of dopamine. This makes it a useful drug in the treatment of Parkinson's
disease (PD), because the dopamine level of the parkinsonian human
brain basal ganglia is dramatically decreased. In the last 20 years efforts
have focused on finding more potent and selective MAO inhibitors.

2. Theoretical Basis of Selective Inhibition

2.1. Enzyme

Monoamine oxidase {(amine: oxygen oxidoreductase); (deaminating),
(flavin-containing); (EC 1.4.3.4)} catalyzes the following overall oxidative deamination reaction:

$$RCH_2NH_2 + H_2O + O_2 \rightarrow RCHO + NH_3 + H_2O_2 \qquad (1)$$

The enzyme covalently binds the cofactor, flavin adenine nucleotide (FAD). Because the FAD actively participates in the enzyme reaction the process contains three identical steps:

$$RCH_2NH_2 + E\text{-}FAD \rightarrow RCH{=}NH + E\text{-}FADH_2 \quad \text{(FAD reduction)}$$
$$(2)$$

$$RCH{=}NH + H_2O \rightarrow RCHO + NH_3 \quad \text{(deamination)} \qquad (3)$$

$$E\text{-}FADH_2 + O_2 \rightarrow E\text{-}FAD + H_2O_2 \quad \text{(FAD oxidation)} \qquad (4)$$

The precise mechanism of these processes has been described by Silverman [9]. The deamination of phenylethylamine (PEA) involves a two-fold electron-abstraction by the electrophilic prosthetic group FAD-*ox*, which is intercalated by a proton abstraction through a nucleophilic group of apoenzyme, leading to an iminium ion. Subsequently, the latter is hydrolyzed and yields benzylic aldehyde and ammonia. The reduced FAD*red* is enzymatically reoxidized by molecular oxygen. The regeneration sequence of FAD*ox* results in the formation of H_2O_2.

From the medical point of view, it is important that the enzymatic reaction requires molecular oxygen and produces aldehyde and hydrogen peroxide. The consequences of these are that, under hypoxic conditions, the activity of the enzyme will decrease or, conversely, the increased enzyme activity may cause higher oxygen consumption or local hypoxia. The aldehyde product will be rapidly reduced either to alcohol or oxidized to carboxylic acid by aldehyde reductase or dehydrogenase, respectively. It has been hypothesized that, in different pathological stages under particular circumstances, the dopamine turnover of basal ganglia of the brain will be increased and an excessive formation of hydrogen peroxide is caused. This might lead to the production of a cytotoxic hydroxyl radical ($^{\cdot}$OH) and could impose oxidative stress on neurons, causing local cell death in most enzyme-containing brain regions.

In tissues, MAO is an integral protein of the outer mitochondrial membrane (except of the erythrocyte). It exists in two forms which can be distinguished by differences in substrate preference, inhibitor specificity, tissue distribution, immunological properties, and amino acid sequences [7, 10–16]. The existence of two different forms of enzyme has been proven by cloning and sequencing cDNA coding for human liver and showing that these two proteins are derived from separate genes [17]. By definition, the selective substrate of the A form is the serotonin (5-HT) and can be selectively inhibited by clorgyline; that of the B form is β-phenylethylamine (PEA) and can be inhibited by *l*-deprenyl. The molecular weight of the enzyme is 100 000–115 000 and contains one mol FAD/subunit FAD [18, 19]. A direct comparison of subunits of highly purified MAO-A and -B reveals that the molecular mass of the A form is 59 700 and that of the B form is about 58 800 [15, 20]. Because the

Table 1. Distribution of MAO-A and MAO-B in tissues of different species

Species and tissues	% of total MAO activity	
	A	B
Brain		
Human	20	80
Cat	25	75
Pig	40	50
Guinea pig	20	80
Rat	55	45
Liver		
Human	55	45
Cat	35	65
Pig	20	80
Cow	5	95
Rat	50	50
Platelet		
Human	5	95
Pig	5	95
Placenta		
Human	>90	10
Intestine		
Human	75	25
Rat	70	30
Adrenal medulla		
Human	35	65
Cow	30	70
Rat	40	60
Cromaffin cell		
Human	<5	>95

based on Youdim and Finberg [4]

overall structural homology of the two enzymes is 70%, their physical separation has been elucidated only recently [17]. The measured MAO activity in different animal and human tissues consists mainly of the activity of both two forms. Furthermore, the composition of the two forms changes in different species, and is tissue-specific (Table 1), e.g., placenta expresses MAO-A, whereas platelets contains only MAO-B.

The active site of MAO consists of the FAD residue that is covalently bound to an identical cysteinyl-peptide fragment [Ser-Gly-Gly-(Cys-FAD)-Tyr] in both forms of the enzyme [20–24]. Because a monoclonal antibody can discriminate between MAO-A and MAO-B in human liver [11], there must be structural differences separate from the catalytic site of the enzyme where the aromatic ring of a substrate binds (Figure 1) [25]. It seems that specificity of the binding is determined by a specific relationship among the ring moiety, side-chain nitrogen, and its substitution [25].

In recent years the two main proposed theories were that differences between A and B enzymes arise from different phospholipid environments of active centers [26, 27]. Different procedures were used to

Type A MAO (Active site)

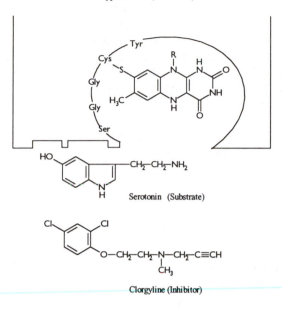

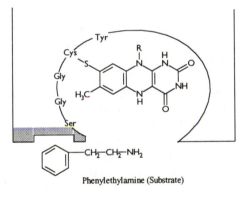

Serotonin (Substrate)

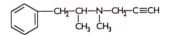

Clorgyline (Inhibitor)

Type B MAO (Active site)

Phenylethylamine (Substrate)

Deprenyl (Inhibitor)

Figure 1. Schematic representation comparing and contrasting the active site and accessory binding sites of monoamine oxidase (MAO) types A and B which account for the selectivity of substrates and inhibitors. The active site of both forms is identical and consists of a flavin residue that is attached covalently to a pentapeptide. The remaining sequence of the active site has not yet been determined. The accessory sites which bind the ring groups of the substrates or inhibitors are hypothesized to be different: compare the stippled area of type B with the unshaded area of type A. (Adapted from Kalir et al. [25].)

reduce the phospholipid content of the enzyme: using gentle, not denaturating processes only slight activity losses were found [28] Husain et al. [29] essentially delipidated beef kidney MAO-B without activity losses. Naoi and Yagi [26] used unfolding agents (dithiothreitol, sodium dodecyl sulfate) for delipidation, which denaturated the protein structure, but they obtained contradictory results. Huang and Foulkner [30] found a reduction of activity during delipidation, but when the phospholipid was replaced a complete reconstruction was seen.

As in the case of several other membrane-bound enzymes, the activity of MAO-B may well be influenced by lipid environment, but no direct evidence exists that the phospholipid would be an integral component of enzyme.

2.2. Substrate

MAO deaminates a wide variety of monoamines such as aliphatic amines with structure $CH_3(CH_2)_n NH_2$ if $n > 1$ [31–34], isoamylamine, isobutylamine [35], and amines containing an aralkyl group [31]. Furthermore, MAO can also catalyze the oxidative deamination of secondary and tertiary amines. Among these, a tertiary amine, 1-methyl-4 phenyl-1,2,3,6 tetrahydropyridine (MPTP) is interesting, because this compound is metabolized mostly by MAO-B and thus it becomes a potent neurotoxin that causes a Parkinson-like syndrome in humans and nonhuman primates. The most important substrates of MAO are neurotransmitters such as adrenaline, noradrenaline, dopamine, 5-HT, PEA, and tyramine. In the brain serotonin is the predominant substrate of MAO-A, while PEA and dopamine are those of MAO-B. Tyramine, adrenaline, noradrenaline, octopamine, and tryptamine are metabolized by both forms of the enzymes. Some other substrates and their specificity are listed in Table 2. The substrates do not show absolutely specific binding to a single enzyme form, but interact with both forms. The observed activity is the overall result of the K_m and V_{max} values of an enzyme form toward the given substrate. The specificity of the substrate also depends on its concentration and was found to vary considerably from tissue to tissue [36–43].

The kinetic equation of the MAO reaction is

$$v = \frac{V_{max}}{1 + \dfrac{K_a}{[amine]} + \dfrac{K_o}{[oxygen]}}, \qquad (4)$$

where V_{max} is the maximum velocity, K_a and K_o are the concentration of amine and oxygen, respectively, which give half-maximum velocity

Table 2. Substrates of MAO-A and MAO-B

A	B	A + B
Serotonin	Benzylamine	Tyramine
Octopamine	Phenylethylamine	Adrenaline
	Methyl-histamine	Noradrenaline
	N-Acetylputrescine	Dopamine
	MPTP	Tryptamine
	n-Phenylamine	Kynuramine
	Decylamine	3-Methoxy-tyramine
	Octylamine	
	Milacemide	

based on Youdim and Finberg [4]

at saturating concentration of the other substrate, and the square brackets indicate the equilibrium concentration. At low concentration of the amine substrate and with oxygen concentration close to the K_m value (which under the normal experimental conditions is fulfilled [44]) Eq. (4) can be reduced to:

$$v = V_{max}[amine]/K_a \tag{5}$$

$$= k_{cat}[enzyme][amine]/K_a. \tag{6}$$

The constant k_{cat}/K_a thus represents the apparent second-order rate constant of the enzyme amine combination. The flux in the case of two competing substrates is given in one-enzyme form as follows:

$$\frac{v_{S_1}}{v_{S_2}} = \frac{(k_{cat}/K_m)_{S_1}[S_1]}{(k_{cat}/K_m)_{S_2}[S_2]}, \tag{7}$$

where S_1 and S_2 are the indexes of first and second substrates and $[S_1]$ and $[S_2]$ are their equilibrium concentrations.

In the case of two enzymes competing for the same substrate, the relative flux will be given by:

$$\frac{v_A}{v_B} = \frac{V_{max\ A}(K_B + [S])}{V_{max\ B}(K_A + [S])}, \tag{8}$$

where the subscripts A and B refer to the two enzyme species. At high substrate concentration the relative flux will depend only on the ratio of $V_{max\ A}$ and $V_{max\ B}$, whereas at very low substrate concentration the flux ratio will be given by:

$$\frac{v_A}{v_B} = \frac{(k_{cat}[enzyme]/K_m)_A}{(k_{cat}[enzyme]/K_m)_B}. \tag{9}$$

As is shown above, the competition will depend on the relative concentration of two enzymes.

2.3. *Types of Enzyme Inhibition*

In any case of MAO inhibition by chemical substances, the first question to clarify is the reversible or irreversible nature of inhibition. The most successful way to do this is by equilibrium dialysis. If the enzyme activity is restored during the dialysis, then the inhibition is reversible, if not, then an irreversible inhibitor is present. Technically and theoretically, the two cases require different treatments.

But between these two end-points several intermittent forms of inhibition were discovered and described.

The difference between *in vitro* and *in vivo* actions of inhibitors is noteworthy from another respect. Some of them are active *in vitro* and *in vivo*, and others are activated only metabolically [45–49]. In the following the different categories and the main representatives will be discussed. The chemical structures of inhibitors are summarized in Table 4.

2.3.1. *Reversible inhibition:* In the case of reversible selective inhibition the inhibitor has a selective binding capacity to the active site of the enzyme, thus preventing the binding of a real substrate. This action can be realized by "wrong" substrate analogs which are degraded very slowly, but are bound strongly.

The reversible inhibition can be described by the following equation:

$$[E] + [I] \underset{k_{-1}}{\overset{k_{+1}}{\rightleftharpoons}} [EI], \tag{10}$$

where E is the enzyme, I is the inhibitor, EI is the reversible enzyme inhibitor complex, and $K_i = k_{-1}/k_{+1}$ is the dissociation constant.

The calculation of the numerical value of inhibitor constants (IC_{50} or K_i) is possible from the concentration dependency of the inhibition. In a series of experiments the inhibitor potency of test material has to be measured in a broad concentration range (usually $10^{-4}–10^{-8}$ M). From a plot of percent of inhibition against the logarithmic concentration of the inhibitor, the concentration that causes 50% inhibition (IC_{50}) can be determined. In the case of MAO enzymes the majority of reversible inhibitors is competitive and, in this case, we can use Eq. (11) to calculate the real dissociation constant of the enzyme inhibitor complex:

$$K_i = \frac{IC_{50}}{1 + \dfrac{K_m}{[S]}}. \tag{11}$$

We remind that this gives a truly correct result only in those cases when the inhibition is competitive. If the inhibition is noncompetitive, $K_i = IC_{50}$. The type of inhibition can be determined by measuring the function of substrate concentration to the inhibition.

2.3.2. Irreversible inhibition: The irreversible inhibitors bind covalently to the active site of the enzymes, mostly to the FAD moiety. The selectivity of the irreversible inhibition is composed of two factors: 1) from the selective binding of the inhibitor to the adequate form of the enzyme, and 2) from the velocity difference of the irreversible inactivation of the two enzyme forms. Thus, the irreversible inhibitors of MAO-B inhibit the enzyme time-dependently. In the abscence of a preincubation they seem to be reversible inhibitors. The reaction can be generally described as:

$$[E] + [I] \underset{k_{-1}}{\overset{k_{+1}}{\rightleftharpoons}} [EI] \overset{k_2}{\to} EI^*, \tag{12}$$

where E is the enzyme, I is the inhibitor, EI is the reversible enzyme-inhibitor complex, and EI^* is the irreversible, covalent enzyme-inhibitor complex. The observed selectivity of an inhibitor consists of either differences in the affinities of the two forms for reversible interaction with an inhibitor, or differences in the rates of reaction within the noncovalent complexes to form the irreversibly-inhibited adduct, or a combination of these factors. Therefore, the relationship between the K_i and k_2 values for the A and B forms of enzyme is a characteristic factor of selectivity, but it is hard to make predictions about how the chemical structure can influence it. It results from this theoretical consideration that the irreversible inhibitors are also not absolutely selective. An inhibitor, depending on the experimental conditions and the applied concentration, might seem to be highly selective or could lose its selectivity absolutely. The irreversible phase of inhibition shown in Eq. (12) has been analyzed by Kitz and Wilson [50]. They showed that if the rate of the formation of EI^* is slower than the dissociation of EI reversible complex, such that the concentration of EI remains in thermodynamic equilibrium with the free enzyme and the inhibitor and the inhibitor concentration is not significantly depleted during the reaction, then the rate of irreversible inhibition can be described by:

$$\frac{d[EI^*]}{dt} = k_2[EI] = \frac{k_2([E_t] - [EI^*])}{\frac{K_i}{[I]} + 1}, \tag{13}$$

where ($[I]$, $[EI]$, $[EI^*]$, and k_2 are defined in Eq. (12)) $[E_t]$ is the total enzyme concentration, and K_i is the dissociation constant of the EI complex (k_{-1}/k_{+1}). Under adequate experimental conditions Eq. (13) can be integrated to give:

$$-k't = \ln \frac{[E_t] - [EI^*]}{[E_t]} = 2.303\{\log_{10}(\% \text{ activity remaining}) - 2\},$$
$$\tag{14}$$

where the apparent first-order rate constant for activity loss k′ is given by:

$$k' = \frac{k_2}{\dfrac{K_i}{[I]} + 1}.$$ (15)

The k′ can be obtained from a graph delineated logarithm of the percent remaining activity versus the preincubation time.

The half-life of enzyme activity at a saturating inhibitor concentration may be calculated according to [51]:

$$t_{1/2} = (\ln 2)/k_2 = 0.693/k_2.$$ (16)

3. Measurement of the Enzyme Activity and the Inhibition

Based on Eqs. (2–4), there are different theoretical possibilities to measure the enzyme activity: the disappearance of the substrate, utilization of the oxygen, the appearance of metabolites such as ammonia and hydrogen peroxide, and the isolation or further derivation of the aldehyde product (see Table 3) [52]. Because of the large variety of enzyme sources and of the wide range of substrates there is no generally useful method; each method has its own advantages and disadvantages and it is impossible to discuss all of them. We describe some of the most applicable methods, but, depending on the aim of the determination and the nature of the enzyme used and of the substrate, modifications may be required.

3.1. In Vitro Determination

In an *in vitro* experiment it is possible to determine the binding capacity of a reversible inhibitor to the selected form of the enzyme using a given substrate. In this experiment a purified enzyme subtype or selective substrates have to be used. A first possibility is the use of placenta MAO-A [53] or human platelet MAO-B [54] and highly purified bovine liver MAO-B [53, 55]. Other sources of the enzyme are mostly problematic and the physical separation of the two forms was only elucidated recently [11].

3.1.1. Application of purified enzyme system: Chromogenic substrates can be used in this case and the concentration of the end product can be determined photometrically or fluorometrically. The most frequently used chromogenic substrates are the kynuramine-HBr and benzylamine-HCl in 1 mM and 3 mM final concentration, respectively. The reaction mixtures are placed in a quartz cuvette thermostated at 30°C and enzyme is added to start the reaction. Rates are measured at 314 nm

Table 3. Assay of monoamine oxidase (from [52])

Principle	Method
Consumption of oxygen	Manometry
	Oxygen electrode
Disappearance of amine substrates	Direct UV measurement (Kynuramine)
	Ninhydrin reagent (spectrophotometry)
	2,4,6-Trinitrobenzene-1-sulphonic acid (TNBS) reagent (spectrophotometry)
	HPLC (electrochemical)
Formation of ammonium	Nessler's color reaction (spectrophotometry)
	Indolephenol color reaction (spectrophotometry)
	Coupled with glutamate dehydrogenase system (spectrophotometry)
	Fluorometry
	Ammonium sensitive
Formation of aldehydes	Direct UV measurement with various amine derivatives as substrates
	p-Dimethylaminobenzalamine as substrate (colorimetry)
	2,4-Dinitrophenylhydrazine reagent (colorimetry)
	Formation of 4-hydroxyquinoline from kynuramine (fluorometry)
	Formation of 4,5-dihydroxyquinoline from 5-hydroxykynuramine (fluorometry)
	Coupled with aldehyde dehydrogenase system (spectrophotometry)
	Fluorometry
	Bioluminesence
	HPLC (Spectrophotometry)
	HPLC (Fluorophotometry)
	HPLC (Electrochemical detection)
Formation of H_2O_2	Amperometry
	Homovanillic acid as fluorescent acceptor (fluorometry)
	Seueo-2′,7′-dichlorofluorescein as fluorescent acceptor (fluorometry)
	Seopolin as fluorescent acceptor (fluorometry)
Formation of acid or alcohol metabolites	Direct fluorometry of indoleacetic acid or 5-hydroxyindoleacetic acid
	Radioenzymatic (solvent extraction)
	Radioenzymatic (ion exchange chromatography)
	Radioenzymatic (liquid chromatography)
	Gas chromatography
	HPLC

with kynuramine and MAO-A [56, 57] and at 250 nm with benzylamine and MAO-B [58]. The unit of activity is expressed as the formation of 1 μmol of product/minute.

The *bioluminescence* method [59] is a coupled process in which the product of the MAO reaction is a substrate for the second enzyme system, the bacterial luciferase. The light-emitting reaction needs a long-chain aliphatic aldehyde which is produced by the MAO reaction. The bioluminescence is very sensitive, thus, even the formation of 5 pmol of aldehydes per min can be detected with a continuous registration. In this system n-octyl-, nonyl-, or decanyl amine are used as substrates.

3.1.2. Application of selective substrates: For a non-purified enzyme system, selective substrates (preferably 5-HT for MAO-A and PEA for MAO-B) have to be used. The final concentrations in the reaction mixtures are 1 mM and 10 μM, respectively. The disadvantage of this method is that the concentration of the reaction product can only be measured radioactively, as described by Wurtman and Axelrod [60] and others [61, 62], and, in this case, continuous detection of the activity change is not possible.

3.2. In Vivo Determination of Selective Inhibition

In the *brain*, one of the interesting possibilities to determine the selective inhibition of MAO-B in animal experiments is the use of ^{14}C methylphenylethanolamine (MPEOA) as substrate. The MPEOA rapidly enters the mouse brain after its intravenous injection and it is metabolized specifically by MAO-B. The measurement of radioactivity shows that metabolite produced in the brain is proportional to the MAO-B activity. Thus, the rate of production of labeled metabolite is highly sensitive to *l*-deprenyl treatment, but insensitive to clorgyline. The above result indicates that ^{14}C-MPEOA can be used for measurement of selective *in vivo* inhibition of the brain MAO-B activity [63]. The same process can be performed with use of N-[methyl-^{14}C]N,N-dimethylphenylethylamine (DMPEA) [64].

[^{13}N]-β-phenylethylamine ([^{13}N]PEA) was found to be a radiotracer for measuring mouse *heart* MAO-B activity *in vivo*. After intravenous administration, [^{13}N]PEA is deaminated by MAO-B. The resulting ^{13}NH$_3$ is taken up by amino acids and trapped in the heart. The relation between the radioactivity trapped in the heart and activity of MAO-B is proportional. The radioactivity in the heart can be reduced in a dose-dependent manner by pretreatment with deprenyl, but not with clorgyline. [^{13}N]PEA as substrate is a useful radiotracer for the noninvasive measurement of heart MAO-B activity and its inhibition [65].

4. Reversible Inhibitors

In contrast to MAO-A, the reversible inhibitors of MAO-B (see Table 4) are rather scarce, and have only a moderate degree of selectivity for this enzyme form. This deviation might be due to differences in the active centers of MAO-A and MAO-B. Structure-activity relationship studies suggested that MAO-A has both an electrophilic and a hydrophobic site, whereas only the hydrophobic site is present in the active center of MAO-A [66, 67]. According to these suggestions, a selective MAO-A inhibitor is able to bind to MAO-A, but is sterically hindered from binding to the active center of MAO-B. On the other hand, an inhibitor of MAO-B having high affinity for the hydrophobic site is not sterically prevented from binding to that of MAO-A.

Benzylamine is a good substrate of MAO-B (see Table 2), thus, it is not surprising that some analogs (such as benzylalcohol, benzylcyanide, and 4-cyanophenol) have been found to be reversible selective inhibitors of MAO-B *in vitro* [68, 69].

The *tricyclic antidepressant* uptake inhibitors such as imipramine and amitriptyline have been shown to be selective inhibitors of MAO-B. Their K_i values for inhibition were 4×10^{-5} and 5×10^{-6}, respectively [70, 71]. The N-demethyl and N-didemethyl derivatives of imipramine and chlorpromazine were as effective as the parent compound. But they are, overall, poor inhibitors of MAO and have no place in the therapy of parkinsonism.

The racemic *salsolinol* is an endogenous compound which might be formed by condensation of dopamine with acetaldehyde or pyruvic acid. Salsolinol is a competitive inhibitor of MAO-A ($K_i = 110\ \mu M$) and noncompetitively inhibits MAO-B ($K_i = 53$ mM) [72]. Other simple isoquinoline alkaloids which are analogs of salsolinol were found not to be substrates for either enzyme, but many of these could stereoselectively inhibit either of the two forms of MAO [73].

Vincristine (VCR) and *vinblastine* (VBL) are widely used antitumor agents. There is a common structural feature between the vindoline portion of the vinca alkaloid dimers and the tertiary allyl amine moiety within the piperidine ring of MPTP. The presence of the tertiary allyl amine moiety in vinca alcaloids prompted studies on their inhibitory potential in the MAO system [74]. Measurements on intact rat brain mitochondrial preparation using 0.1 mM benzylamine as a MAO-B selective substrate have shown that the relative inhibitory effects at 0.2 mM inhibitor concentrations were $VBL = VCR > MPTP = MPP^+ > $ vindoline $> MPDP^+ > $ 16-α-carbometoxy-cleavamine. For the oxidation of 0.1 mM kynuramine as a non-selective substrate at the same inhibitor concentration the order of inhibition was changed to the following: $MPP^+ > MPDP^+ > VCR > MPTP > $ vindoline $>$ 16-α-carbometoxy-cleavamine. In a purified beef liver mitochondrial enzyme system the VBL was found to be a competitive, reversible, time-independent inhibitor with an estimated K_i of 77 μM. No detectable metabolite was produced during the incubation time, and there was no oxygen consumption. Thus, while MPTP, VBL, and VCR are comparable in their ability to inhibit the initial velocity of benzylamine oxidation catalyzed by MAO-B, VBL and VCR differ from MPTP in that the two vinca alkaloids are not substrates of the enzyme. In the only report published to date, elevated serum levels of MAO activity in some forms of lung cancer were decreased after treatment with VCR [75].

Many reversible selective MAO-A inhibitors are simple α-methylated analogs of the substrates [76, 77, 126]. On the other hand, there have been very few useful reversible MAO-B-selective inhibitors. *In vitro* 5-fluoro-α-methyltryptamine (5-FMT) reversibly and competitively inhibits the MAO-A in mouse brain; in contrast, the *p*-chloro-β-methylphenethylamine (*p*CMPEA) selectively inhibits MAO-B activity. Kinetic data obtained in rat brain *in vitro* showed that 5-FMT exhibited about a 18 000-fold higher sensitivity to MAO-A than to MAO-B, while *p*CMPEA had a 620-fold higher selectivity to MAO-B. Using 5-FMT and *p*CMPEA as inhibitors *in vivo* the inhibition of MAO-A and MAO-B were dose-dependent and reversible, with a complete recovery time of 24 h and 45 min, respectively, after the treatment [78].

N-(2-Aminoethyl)(het)arylcarboxamides are moclobemide analogs. *Ro-19-6327* [*N*-(2-aminoethyl)-5-chloro-2-pyridinecarboxamide] (lazabemide) and *Ro-41-1049* [*N*-(2-aminoethyl)-5-*m*-fluorophenyl)-4-thiazole-carboxamide] are close structural analogs and are the prototypes of a new series of time-dependent, mechanism-based, reversible MAO-B and MAO-A inhibitors, respectively. Both molecules behave as selective substrates of MAO and produce intermediates with high affinity to the enzymes. The MAO inhibition induced by Ro-41-1049 and MAO Ro-19-6327 *in vitro* is rapidly reversed by dialysis. Despite their structural similarity, they are able to exclusively bind to the active site of the appropriate enzymes. The IC_{50} values of Ro-41-1049 were 2×10^{-8} M and 1.2×10^{-5} M and, in the case of Ro-19-6327, they were $> 10^{-3}$ M and 6×10^{-8} M for MAO-A and MAO-B, respectively, using 5-HT and PEA as substrates [79, 80]. The high selectivity appears to depend on the aromatic moiety, whereas the 2-aminomethyl-carboxamide residue seems to play the key role in stabilization of the reversible enzyme-inhibitor adduct. *In vivo*, after a very low p.o. dose of Ro-19-6327 (236 μg/kg = 1 μmol/kg), almost complete MAO-B inhibition was obtained in rat brain and liver. In contrast, even at very high doses (1 mmol/kg) Ro-19-6327 was virtually ineffective in inhibiting rat brain and liver MAO-A. At 3 mg/kg, Ro-19-6327 induced complete MAO-B inhibition in rabbit striatum, cortex, liver, and platelets which lasted about 12 h. In healthy volunteers, complete but short-lasting inhibition of platelet MAO-B was obtained already with 5 mg doses. After 40- and 200-mg doses of Ro-19-6327 the duration of complete MAO-B inhibition in platelets lasted 12 and 24 h, respectively. Positron emission tomography (PET) studies using ^{11}C-*l*-deprenyl showed that, 12 h after a single dose of 50 mg Ro-19-6327, more than 90% MAO-B inhibition had developed in the brain and in platelets. Therefore, the compounds are possibly useful in treating depression and PD [81].

5. Irreversible Inhibitors

5.1. Acetylenic Compounds

The acetylenic compounds such as k_{cat} "suicide inhibitors" follow the reaction described in Eq. (12). In the first step of the reaction (as with a substrate) the inhibitor interacts reversibly with the enzyme. The product of this reaction is a highly reactive diazene intermediate which, in a subsequent reaction, reacts covalently with the N5 position of FAD-ox and, possibly, also with the apoenzyme [82]. The velocity of this reaction is represented by k_2 in Eq. (12). Because the enzyme actively participates in the production of the irreversible inhibitor, this type of inhibition is termed "suicide inhibition" [83].

l-Deprenyl (($-$)E-250, selegiline; for chemical name, see Table 4). Selegiline was the first, selective, irreversible MAO-B inhibitor [8]. In the first, reversible step of the reaction, using PEA as substrate, deprenyl seems to be a competitive inhibitor, thus indicating its substrate nature. The K_i values for the A and B forms of MAO are 38 and 0.97 μM, respectively [84]. Thus, the K_i value of l-deprenyl for the B form of MAO is only about 40-fold lower than that of the A-form, and other factors must also play a role in its selectivity.

In determining kinetic parameters of irreversible inhibition of l-deprenyl the k_2 values (min^{-1}) were found to be 0.14 ± 0.05 and >0.99; the $t_{1/2}$ values were 7 min ± 3 and <0.7 for MAO-A and MAO-B, respectively, at 200 nM. The combination of selective binding and the different rates of irreversible inactivation is responsible for the selectivity of l-deprenyl.

It was reported by several authors that l-deprenyl loses its selectivity at higher doses during long-term treatment [85, 86]. In animal experiments the selective dose is 0.25 mg/kg (s.c.) and in human therapy it is between 5 and 10 mg/day (p.o.) [84]. In humans, after administration of this dose range the blood level of l-deprenyl is 1–5 nM/ml. Under these conditions the inactivation rate of MAO-B is "fast" enough to produce a significant level of inhibition, but the inactivation of the A-form is very "slow"; it is practically in equilibrium with the de novo synthesis of the enzyme. In such a treatment regimen selegiline does not lose its selectivity for MAO-B. In animals or humans treated with a higher dose of selegiline than necessary, the inactivation rate of both enzyme forms will be increased. This offers no advantage in the case of MAO-B, because it is otherwise completely inhibited, but the inhibition of MAO-

A becomes "faster" than its *de novo* synthesis and the selectivity of treatment will disappear.

Because of selective MAO-B inhibition and adjuvant tyramine uptake inhibitor potential of selegiline, it is free from the "cheese effect" (see Chapters 6, 7). In clinical practice selegiline is used in monotherapy [87] and in combined therapy with L-dopa to treat PD [88] (see Chapter 13). It can also be used to treat depression and Alzheimer's disease [89, 90] (see Chapter 16). It seems that factors other than MAO inhibitory potential also play a significant role [91, 92, 125] in the effectiveness of selegiline.

A newer, effective derivative of selegiline, *fludepryl* has been synthesized, which contains a *p*-fluorine atom in the phenyl ring and has the same selectivity against MAO enzymes but a different profile of uptake inhibition. The pharmacodynamic properties and the main metabolites of fludepryl differ from selegiline, which also suggests a different clinical profile [91].

Starting from the structure of *l*-deprenyl other selegiline analogs, i.e., aromatic-N-propargyl (acetylenic) compounds were synthesized and tested for their inhibitory action on MAO. Among these, one of the most potent compounds was AGN 1133 (*N*-methyl-*N*-propargyl-1-amino indane) which was described under different names (J-508 and Su-11-739) by three research groups [93–95]. This compound is a highly effective inhibitor of MAO-B, both *in vitro* and *in vivo* [25, 96, 127]. A greater selectivity for MAO-B with reduction in potency was shown by *N*-desmethyl analog AGN 1135 as compared with AGN 1133 [25, 97].

5.2. Allylamine Derivatives

The β-halomethylene analogs of the substrates which are deaminated through imine and aldehyde formation act as suicide substrates, leading to irreversible inactivation [98]. The mechanism seems to be identical to that of β,γ-acetylenic amines. This series of compounds contains both selective MAO-A and -B inhibitors. The metatyramine derivative MDL 72392 and dopamine analog MDL 72394 show modest selectivity (up to 10-fold) for the A-form of the enzyme.

MDL 72638 [(*Z*)-2-(2,4-dichlorophenoxy)methyl-3-fluoroallylamine], surprisingly, is a potent and very selective MAO-B inhibitor in spite of its close structural relationship to clorgyline. The K_i values of MDL 72638 for MAO-A and -B are 30 times higher and 660 times lower, respectively, than those of clorgyline. The minimum half-life ($t_{1/2}$) at saturating conditions and the apparent dissociation constant (K_i) were for MAO-A 8.9 min and 1.75 μM, and for MAO-B 2.9 min and 0.088 μM [99].

MDL 72145 [2-(3,4,-dimethoxyphenyl)-3-fluoroallylamine] is also a selective enzyme-activated suicide inhibitor of MAO-B both *in vitro* and *in vivo*. The minimum half-life ($t_{1/2}$) at saturating concentration and the apparent dissociation constant (K_i) of MDL 72145 determined at 10°C are 14.5 min and 130 μM, and 1.7 min and 40 μM for the A- and B-forms of MAO, respectively [100]. It does not influence the cardiovascular actions of intravenously-administered tyramine. In contrast to selegiline, it does not inhibit the amine uptake and release [101].

MDL 72.974A [(*E*)-4-fluoro-β-fluoromethylene benzenebutanamine] is an enzyme-activated inhibitor of the B-type enzyme. Comparison with the *in vitro* IC_{50} values for inhibition of rat brain mitochondrial MAO-A and MAO-B indicates a selectivity ratio of 190 in favor of MAO-B [102]. The inhibition of platelet MAO activity was dose-dependent over a range from 0.1 to 0.5 mg. The profile of inhibition following administration of doses of 1 mg and above includes a maximal inhibition of enzyme occurring within 1 h of dosing, and gradual recovery to normal levels during 14 days [102].

5.3. Cyclopropylamine Derivatives

Of particular interest are the cyclopropylamines which can inhibit the MAO enzymes in different ways, depending on their structure. Tranylcypromine reacts through a radical intermediate with the cysteine-containing peptide of the apoenzyme. However, *N*-(1-methylcyclopropyl)-benzylamine has been shown to form a stable bond at position 5 of FAD. 1-Phenylcyclopropylamine inhibits the enzyme in both ways. It reacts reversibly with cysteine and irreversibly at N5 of FAD [22, 103, 104].

5.4. Pyridopyrimidine Derivatives

Pyridopyrimidines containing the 3-amino-2-*oxazolidone moiety* displayed pronounced, irreversible MAO-inhibitory activity *in vivo*, but they were practically inactive *in vitro* [45–49, 105]. Without the above moiety they did not possess any inhibitory potential. The 6-methyl derivatives proved to be more effective than the 6-desmethyl derivatives [47–49]. The inhibitory activity was higher for liver than for brain enzyme. The onset of action of these derivatives was fast and the duration of the effect was very long. The recovery period of MAO-B was complete at 7 days.

5.5. Silyl Compounds

Some of the aromatic silicon amines are potent, new types of enzyme-activated inhibitors of MAO-B. Benzyl-dimethyl-silyl-methanamine and its p-fluoro and p-chloro derivatives are time-dependent inhibitors. The most potent member of this series is 4-fluorobenzyl-dimethyl-silyl-methanamine: the dissociation constant (K_i) of its reversible phase is 11 μM, and the $t_{1/2}$ value of its reversible inactivation is 2.3 min. It therefore has a 1000-fold selectivity for the B form of MAO [106].

5.6. Allenic Amines

Allenic amines are another type of MAO inhibitor [107–110]. The MAO-B selective R-enantiomer of N-2,3-pentadienyl-N-methylbenzyl amine was found to be 2–7 times as active as the nonselective S-form in vivo, and 25 times as active in vitro. While the R-enantiomer was found to be a time-dependent, irreversible inhibitor, the S-enantiomer acted as a reversible, competitive inhibitor.

6. Partly Irreversible Inhibitors

6.1. MPTP and Its Analogs

The first report about the neurotoxic action of 1-methyl-4-phenyl-1,2,3,6-tetrahydropyridine (MPTP) [111] and the possible prevention of its action by l-deprenyl [112] opened a new perspective on MAO inhibitors. The report [113] that brain mitochondria oxidize MPTP was followed shortly by the demonstration that MPTP is an excellent substrate of MAO-B and is reasonably well oxidized by MAO-A [114–116]. Furthermore, the MPTP in vitro was found to be a strong $(K_i = 9 \ \mu M)$, competitive, reversible inhibitor of MAO-A and a less potent $(K_i = 106 \ \mu M)$, noncompetitive, not fully reversible inhibitor of MAO-B [117]. The irreversible part of inhibition is like those k_{cat} ("suicide") inhibitors which are acted upon by an enzyme to produce a reactive product that can covalently attach to the enzyme [116]. In order for the MPTP to be neurotoxic to dopaminergic cells, it must be oxidized by one form of MAO. This is a two-step reaction:

$$\text{MPTP} \xrightarrow{\text{MAO}} \text{MPDP}^+ \xrightarrow[\text{chem. ox.}]{\text{disproportionation, (MAO?)}} \text{MPP}^+ \qquad (17)$$

The first oxidation step is faster and is catalyzed by MAO [118], and the second step can be the result of a spontaneous disproportionation or chemical oxidation [119]. The mechanism-based inactivation of MAO forms by MPDP$^+$ is a time-dependent reaction and is due to the processing MPDP$^+$ by these enzymes. The end product of the reaction is MPP$^+$, a competitive reversible inhibitor of MAO-A and MAO-B with $K_i = 3.0 \, \mu M$ and $230 \, \mu M$, respectively [120]. All neurotoxic MPTP analogs examined are good substrates of MAO-A and MAO-B or both. Among these compounds 2-methyl-MPTP is especially interesting because, in contrast with MPTP, it is metabolized mostly by MAO-A. An excellent summary of the action of these types of tertiary amines is given by Singer and Remsey [120] along with a kinetic description of actions. The structure-activity relationship was discussed by Dostert et al. [121].

6.2. Oxazolidone Derivatives

MD 780236 [3-(4-((3-chlorophenyl)methoxy)phenyl-5-((methylamino)-methyl-2-oxazolidone) methansulphonate] inhibits MAO-B selectively and irreversibly *in vitro*, whereas inhibition *ex vivo* consists of a reversible and irreversible component. Further studies have indicated that MDL 780236 is, in fact, a substrate for MAO-A ($K_m = 1.1 \, \mu M$), and a substrate and irreversible "suicide inhibitor" for MAO-B. The reaction mechanism can be summarized as follows:

$$[E] + [I] \underset{}{\overset{K_i}{\rightleftharpoons}} [EI] \xrightarrow{k_2} [EI'] \xrightarrow{k_4} EI^*$$
$$\downarrow k_3 \qquad\qquad (18)$$
$$E + P,$$

where E is the concentration of enzyme, I is the concentration of MDL 780236, EI is the reversible enzyme inhibitor complex, EI' is the reactive intermediate leading to the irreversible complex EI*, and free enzyme and the product (P). The ratio of k_4/k_3 is about 1/530, but it can be strongly influenced by MAO-A inhibitors [122]. Further experiments have suggested that this ratio is stereoselective [123], and the two enantiomers of the compound show different degrees of reversibility. More detailed explanation of the stereoselectivity is given in a recent, excellent review [121].

7. Steroselectivity

A review of stereochemical aspects of various MAO substrates and inhibitors was published by Tenne and Youdim [124], Strolin Benedetti, Dostert [138] and in Chapter 5 of this book.

Table 4. Some selective inhibitors of the MAO-B enzyme

Chemical name used in chemical abstracts	Synonyms	Structure	Reference
N-Methyl-N-2-propynyl-benzenemethanamine	Pargyline		128
N-2-Propynylbenzenemethanamine	NPB		129
(−)(R)-N,α-Dimethyl-N-2-propynyl-benzeneethanamine	Selegeline l-Deprenyl		93
(−)(R)-α-Methyl-N-2-propynyl-benzeneethanamine			130
(−)(R)-4-Fluoro-N-,α-dimethyl-N-2-propynylbenzeneethanamine	CHINOIN-175 Fludepryl		131

Table 4 (continued)

Chemical name used in chemical abstracts	Synonyms	Structure	Reference
(−)(R)-4-Fluoro-,α-methyl-N-2-propynylbenzeneethanamine			132
N-Methyl-N-2-propynyl-benzeneethanamine	TZ-650		93
(±)2,3-Dihydro-N-methyl-N-2-propynyl-1H-inden-1-amine	AGN-1133 J-508 Su-11,739		93–95
(±)2,3-Dihydro-N-propynyl-1H-inden-1-amine	AGN-1135		94, 126

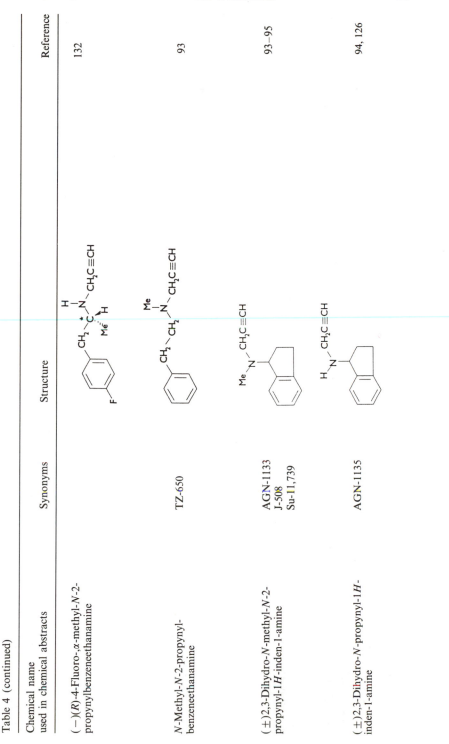

Table 4 (continued)

Chemical name used in chemical abstracts	Synonyms	Structure	Reference
(±)-N,α-Dimethyl-N-2-propynyl-2-furanethamine	U-1424		93
(Z)-2-[(2,4-Dichlorophenoxy)-methyl]-3-fluoro-2-propen-1-amine	MDL 72 638		99
(E)-β-(Fluoromethylene)-3,4-dimethoxybenzeneethanamine	MDL 72 145		100

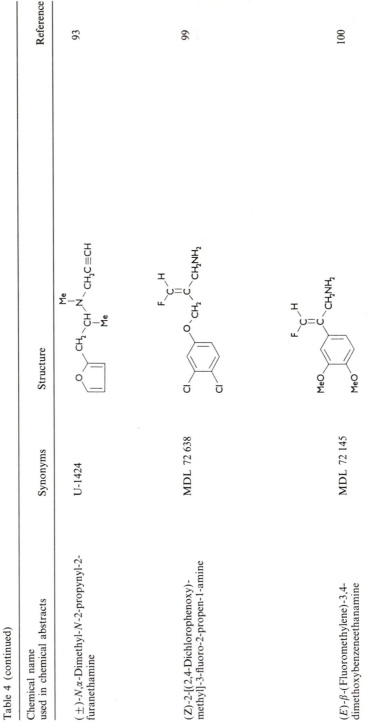

Table 4 (continued)

Chemical name used in chemical abstracts	Synonyms	Structure	Reference
(E)-2-(2-(4-Fluorophenethyl)-3-fluoro-2-propen-1-amine	MDL 72 974		102
(R)-3-[4-[(3-Chlorophenyl)-methoxy]-phenyl]-5-[(methylamino)methyl]-2-oxazolidinone	MD 240928		123
(±)-3-[4-[(3-Chlorophenyl)-methoxy]-phenyl]-5-[(methylamino)methyl]-2-oxazolidinone	MD 780236		122

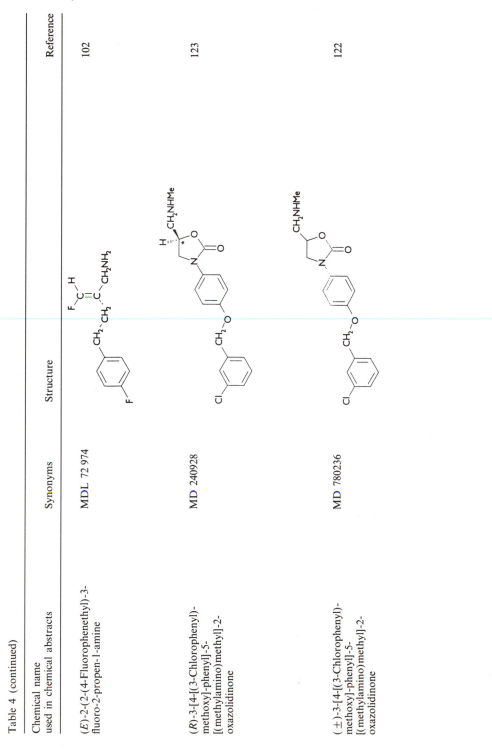

Table 4 (continued)

Chemical name used in chemical abstracts	Synonyms	Structure	Reference
N'-(2-Aminoethyl)-4-chlorobenzamide	Ro 16-6491		133
N'-(2-Aminoethyl)-5-chloropyridine-carboxamide	Ro 19-6327		79
2-(Cyclopropylamino)-1-phenyletanone	L 54761 LY 54761 Lilly 54761		134
(±)4-Chloro-β-methylbenzeneethanamine	p-CMPEA		77

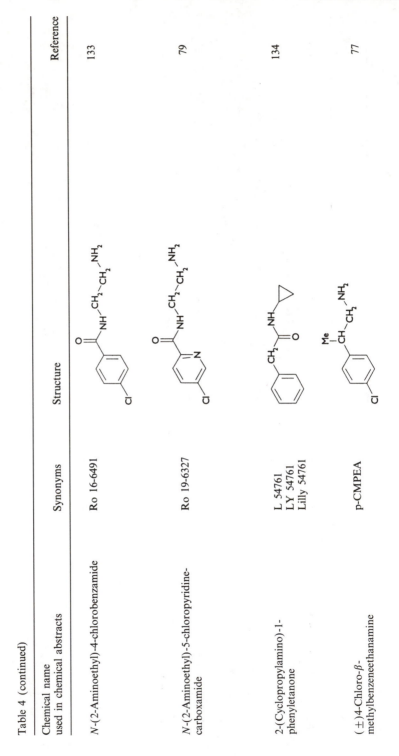

Table 4 (continued)

Chemical name used in chemical abstracts	Synonyms	Structure	Reference
(±)-(1-Methyl-2-phenylethyl)hydrazine	Pheniprazine		135
(R)-N-Methyl-N-2,3-pentadienylbenzenemethanamine			110
[(4-Fluorophenyl)methyl]-dimethylsilylmethanamine			106
2-(Pentylamino)acetamide	Milacemide		136

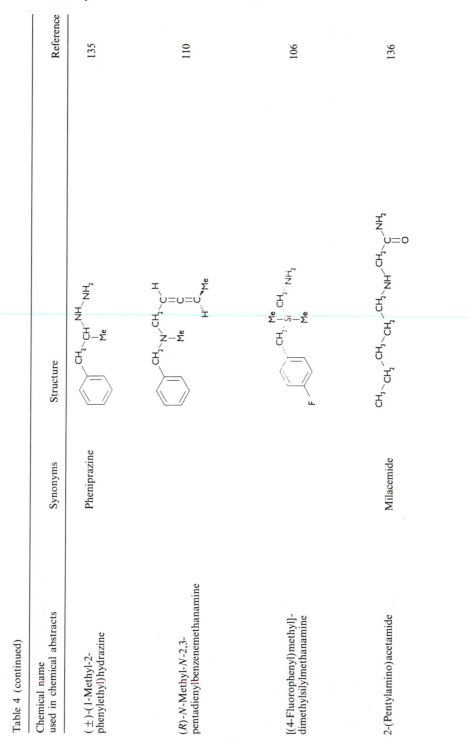

Table 4 (continued)

Chemical name used in chemical abstracts	Synonyms	Structure	Reference
Liposomes of phosphatidylserine L-Serine, esters; 2,3-bis[(1-oxooctadecyl)oxy]propyl hydrogen phosphate	PS		137
10,11-Dihydro-*N*,*N*-dimethyl-5*H*-dibenzo(*b*,*f*)azepine-5-propanamine	Imipramine		70, 71
3-(10,11-Dihydro-5*H*-dibenzo(*a*,*d*)cyclohepten-5-ylidene)-*N*,*N*-dimethyl-1-propanamine	Amitryptyline		70, 71

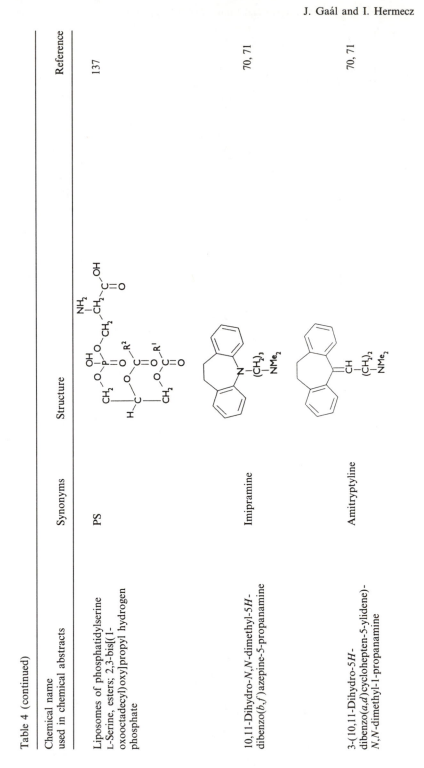

Table 4 (continued)

Chemical name used in chemical abstracts	Synonyms	Structure	Reference
2-Chloro-*N*-,*N*-dimethyl-10-*H*-phenothiazine-10-propanamine	Chloropromazine		70, 71
Vinblastine (R = Me)	VBL		74
Vincristine (R = CHO)	VCR		74

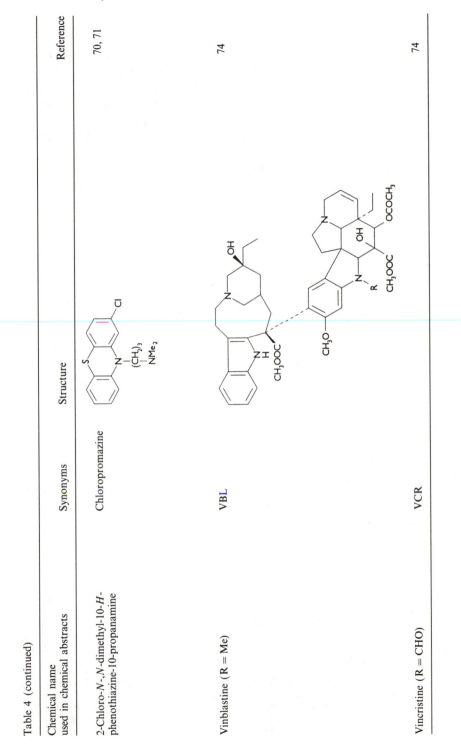

8. Outlook

The therapeutic use of different selective MAO inhibitors has changed over the course of time, as our knowledge has progressed. Initially, their anti-depression action was noted. After discovery of the "cheese effect", their application was virtually halted. Discovery of selective inhibitors opened a new therapeutic venue, including the treatment of Parkinson's disease. Since the creation of *l*-deprenyl many different MAO inhibitors have been discovered, but their therapeutic value has not attained that of *l*-deprenyl. Therefore, we consider it possible that MAO inhibitory potential is a very important component of the pharmacological action of *l*-deprenyl, but that its action is complex and might involve other components not directly related to the MAO inhibitory potential.

Summary

The theoretical and methodological basis of selective monoamine oxidase type-B (MAO-B) inhibition has been discussed in this chapter. The widespread use of MAO inhibitors in clinical practice requires a deeper theoretical base in order to understand the activity and side-effects of different drugs. The major types of inhibitors, such as reversible, mechanism-based, irreversible, and partly irreversible inhibitors, and their chemical structure and relationship to selective inhibition have been discussed.

Acknowledgements

The authors are grateful to Mr. A. C. Bonis for his valued assistance in preparing the manuscript and to Katalin Botos for her outstanding assistance in creating the final version.

References

[1] Crane GE. Psychiatric side effects of iproniazid. Am J Psychiatry 1956; 112: 494–497.
[2] Zeller AA, Barsky J. *In vivo* inhibition of liver and brain monoamine oxidase by 1-isonicotinyl-2-isopropyl hydrazine. Proc Soc Exp Biol Med 1952; 81: 459–461.
[3] Zeller EA, Barsky J, Fouts JR, Kirchheimer WF, van Orden LS. Influence of isonicotinic acid hydrazide and 1-isonicotinyl-2-isopropylhydrazide on bacterial and mammalian enzymes. Experientia 1952; 8: 349–350.
[4] Youdim MBH, Finberg JMP. Monoamine oxidase inhibitors. In: Grahame-Smith DG, Cowen PE, editors. Psychopharmacology. Part 1, Preclinical Psychopharmacology. Amsterdam: Excerpta Medica, 1983: 37–51.
[5] Murphy DL, Garrick NA, Aulakh CS, Cohen RM. New contributions from basic science to understanding the effects of monoamine oxidase inhibiting antidepressants. J Clin Psychiatry 1984; 45: 37–43.

[6] Knoll J, Ecsery JG, Nievel J, Knoll B. Phenylisopropylmethylpropinylamine HCl (E-250), egy új hatásspektrumú psychoenergetikum. MTA V Oszt Közl 1964; 15: 231–239.

[7] Johnston JP. Some observations upon a new inhibitor of monoamine oxidase in brain tissue. Biochem Pharmacol 1968; 17: 1285–1297.

[8] Knoll, J, Magyar K. Some puzzling pharmacological effects of monoamine oxidase inhibitors. Adv Biochem Psychopharm 1972; 5: 393–408.

[9] Silverman RB, Hoffman SJ, Catus WB. III. A mechanism for mitochondrial monoamine oxidase catalyzed amine oxidation. J Amer Chem Soc 1980; 102: 7126–7128.

[10] White HL, Tansik RL. Characterization of multiple substrate binding sites of MAO. In: Singer TP, Von Korff RW, Murphy DL, editors. Monoamine oxidase: structure, function and altered functions. London: Academic Press, 1979: 129–144.

[11] Denney RM, Fritz RR, Patel NT, Abell CW. Human liver MAO-A and MAO-B separated by immunoaffinity chromatography with MAO-B-specific monoclonal antibody. Science 1982; 215: 1400–1403.

[12] Kochersperger LM, Waguespack A, Patterson JC, Hsieh CC, Weyler W, Salach JI, et al. Immunological uniqueness of human monoamine oxidase A and B; new evidence from studies with monoclonal antibodies to human monoamine oxidase A. J Neurosci 1985; 5: 2874–2881.

[13] Kinemuchi H, Arai Y, Toyoshima Y, Tadano T, Kisara K. Studies on 5-fluoro-alpha-methyltryptamine and p-chloro-beta-methylphenethylamine: Determination of the MAO-A or MAO-B selective inhibition *in vitro*. Jap J Pharmac 1988; 46: 197–199.

[14] Westlund KN, Denney RM, Kochersperger LM, Rose RM, Abell CW. Distinct monoamine oxidase A and B populations in primate brain. Science 1985; 230: 181–183.

[15] Cawthon RM, Pintar JE, Haseltine FP, Breakefield XO. Differences in the structure of A and B forms of human monoamine oxidase. J Neurochem 1981; 37: 363–372.

[16] Smith D, Filipowicz C, McCauley R. Monoamine oxidase A and monoamine oxidase B activities are catalyzed by different proteins. Biochim Biophys Acta 1985; 831: 1–7.

[17] Bach AWJ, Lan NC, Johnson DL, Abbel CW, Bembenek ME, Kwan S-W, et al. cDNA cloning of human liver monoamine oxidase A and B: Molecular basis of differences in enzymatic properties. Proc Natl Acad Sci 1988; 85: 4934–4938.

[18] Chuang HYK, Patek DR, Hellerman L. Mitochondrial monoamine oxidase. J Biol Chem 1974; 249: 2381–2384.

[19] Powell JF, Hsu Y-PP, Weyler W, Chen S, Salach J, Andrikopoulos K, Mallet J and Breakefield XO. The primary structure of bovine monoamine oxidase type A. Comparison with peptide sequences of bovine monoamine oxidase type B and other flavoenzymes. Biochem J 1989; 259: 407–413.

[20] Weyler W, Salach JI. Purification and properties of mitochondrial monoamine oxidase type A from human placenta. J Biol Chem 1985; 260: 13199–13207.

[21] Von Korff RW. Monoamine oxidase: unanswered questions. In: Singer TP, Von Korff RW, Murphy DL, editors. Monoamine oxidase: structure, function and altered functions. New York: Academic Press, 1979: 1–6.

[22] Kyburz E. New development in the field of MAO inhibitors. ND&P 1990; 3: 592–599.

[23] Yu PH. Studies on the pargyline-binding site of different types of monoamine oxidase. Can J Biochem 1981; 59: 30–37.

[24] Kearney EB, Salach JI, Walker WH, Seng RL, Kenney W, Zeszotek E, et al. The covalently-bound flavin of hepatic monoamine oxidase. I. Isolation and sequence of a flavin peptide and evidence for binding at the 8 position. Eur J Biochem 1971; 24: 321–327.

[25] Kalir A, Sabbagh A, Youdim MBH. Selective acetylenic "suicide" and reversible inhibitors of monoamine oxidase types A and B. Br J Pharm 1981; 73: 55–64.

[26] Naoi M, Yagi K. Effects of phospholipids on beef heart mitochondrial monoamine oxidase. Arch Biochem Biophys 1980; 205: 18–26.

[27] Singer TP. Perspectives in MAO: past, present and future. J Neurol Transm 1987 [suppl.]; 23: 1–23.

[28] Erwin VG, Hellerman L. Mitochondrial monoamine oxidase. I. Purification and characterization of the bovine kidney enzyme. J Biol Chem 1967; 242: 4230–4238.

[29] Husain M, Edmondson DE, Singer TP. Catalytic mechanism of MAO from liver. In: Usdin E, Weiner N, Youdim MBH, editors. Function and regulation of monoamine enzymes. London: Macmillan, 1981; 477–487.

[30] Huang RH, Faulkner R. The role of phospholipids in the multiple forms of brain monoamine oxidase. J Biol Chem 1981; 256: 9211–9215.
[31] Blaschko H, Richter D, Schlossmann H. The oxidation of adrenaline and other amines. Biochem J 1937; 31: 2187–2196.
[32] Pugh CEM, Quastel JH. Oxidation of aliphatic amines by brain and other tissues. Biochem J 1937; 31: 286–291.
[33] Kohn HI. Tyramine oxidase. Biochem J 1937; 31: 1693–1704.
[34] Alles GA, Heegaard EV. Substrate specificity of amine oxidase. J Biol Chem 1943; 147: 487–503.
[35] Bhagvat K, Blaschko H, Richter D. Amine oxidase. Biochem J 1939; 33: 1338–1341.
[36] Fowler CJ, Callingham BA, Mantle TJ, Tipton KF. Monoamine oxidase A and B: a useful concept? Biochem Pharmacol 1978; 27: 97–101.
[37] Neff NH, Yang H-YT, Goridis C, Bialek D. The metabolism of indolealkylamines by type A and B monoamine oxidase of brain. Adv Biochem Psychopharmacol 1974; 11: 51–58.
[38] Fowler CJ, Tipton KF. Concentration dependence of the oxidation of tyramine by the two forms of rat liver mitochondrial monoamine oxidase. Biochem Pharmacol 1981; 30: 3329–3332.
[39] Strolin Benedetti M, Boucher Th, Carlsson A, Fowler CJ. Intestinal metabolism of tyramine by both forms of monoamine oxidase in the rat. Biochem Pharmacol 1983; 32: 47–52.
[40] Schoepp DD, Azzaro AJ. Specificity of endogeneous substrates for types A and B monoamine oxidase in rat striatum. J Neurochem 1981; 36: 2025–2031.
[41] Kinemuchi H, Wakui Y, Kamijo K. Substrate selectivity of type A and B monoamine oxidase in rat brain. J Neurochem 1980; 35: 109–115.
[42] Parkinson D, Lyles GA, Browne BJ, Callingham BA. Some factors influencing the metabolism of benzylamine by type A and B monoamine oxidase in rat heart and liver. J Pharm Pharmacol 1980; 32: 844–850.
[43] Guffroy C, Fowler CJ, Strolin Benedetti M. The deamination of n-pentylamine by monoamine oxidase and a semicarbazide-sensitive amine oxidase of rat heart. J Pharm Pharmacol 1983; 35: 416–420.
[44] Tipton KF. Some properties of monoamine oxidase. Adv Biochem Psychopharmacol 1972; 5: 11–24.
[45] George T, Kaul CL, Grewal RS, Tahilramani R. Antihypertensive and monoamine oxidase inhibitory activity of some derivates of 3-formyl-4-oxo-4H-pyrido[1,2-a]-pyrimidine. J Med Chem 1971; 14: 913–915.
[46] Kaul CL, Grewal RS. Antihypertensive and monoamine oxidase inhibitory activity of 3-amino-2-oxazolidinone (3AO) and its condensation product with 2-substituted-3-formyl-4-oxo-4H pyrido [1,2-a]pyrimidines. Biochem Pharmacol 1972; 21: 303–316.
[47] Magyar K, Sátory E, Mészáros Z, Knoll J. Uj homopirimidazol származékok monoaminooxidáz-benitó hatása. Orvostudomány 1974; 25: 143.
[48] Magyar K, Sátory E, Mészáros Z, Knoll J. The monoamine oxidase inhibitory effect of new homopyrimidazole derivates. Med Biol 1974; 52: 384–389.
[49] Sátory E, Mészáros Z, Magyar K, Knoll J. The monoamine oxidase inhibitory effect of new homopyrimidazole derivatives. Congr Hung Pharmacol Soc 1974 (Proc.); 1976; 2: 43.
[50] Kitz R, Wilson IB. Esters of methanesulfonic acid as irreversible inhibitors of acetylcholinesterase. J Biol Chem 1962; 237: 3245–3249.
[51] Tipton KF. Kinetics and enzyme inhibition studies. In: Sandler M, editor. Enzyme Inhibitors as Drugs. London: Macmillan, 1980: 1–23.
[52] Yu PH. Monoamine oxidase. In: Boulton AA, Baker GB, Yu PH, editors. Nuromethods Vol. 5. Neurotransmitter enzymes. New Jersey: Humana Press, 1986; 235–272.
[53] Salach IJ, Weyler W. Preparation of flavin containing aromatic amine oxidases of human placenta and beef liver. In: Colowick SP, Kaplan NO, editors. Methods in Enzymology. London: Academic Press, 1987; 142: 627–637.
[54] Ansari GAS, Patel NT, Fritz RR, Abell CW. Purification of human platelet monoamine oxidase B by high performance liquid chromatography. J Liq Chromatogr 1983; 6: 1407–1419.
[55] Youdim MBH, Tenne M. Assay and purification of liver monoamine oxidase. In: Colowick SP, Kaplan NO, editors. Methods in Enzymology. London: Academic Press, 1987; 142: 617–637.

[56] Weissbach H, Smith TE, Daly JW, Witkop B, Udenfriend S. A rapid spectrophoto-metric assay of monoamine oxidase based on the rate of disappearance of kynuramine. J Biol Chem 1960; 235: 1160–1163.

[57] Kraml M. Rapid microfluorometric determination of monoamine oxidase. Biochem Pharmacol 1965; 14: 1683–1685.

[58] Tabor CW, Tabor H, Rosenthal SM. Purification of amine oxidase from beef plasma. J Biol Chem 1954; 208: 645–661.

[59] Tenne M, Finberg JP, Youdim MBH, Ulitzur S. A new rapid and sensitive biolu-minescence assay for monoamine oxidase activity. J Neurochem 1985; 44: 1378–1384.

[60] Wurtman RJ, Axelrod J. A sensitive and specific assay for the estimation of monoamine oxidase. Biochem Pharmacol 1963; 12: 1439–1440.

[61] Tipton KF, Youdim MBH. Assay of monoamine oxidase. Ciba Found Symp (New Ser.) 1976; 39: 393–403.

[62] Otsuka S, Kobayashi Y. Radioisotopic assay for monoamine oxidase determinations in human plasma. Biochem Pharmacol 1964; 13: 995–1006.

[63] Inoue O, Tominaga T, Yamasaki T, Kinemuchi H. A new method for in vivo measurement of brain monoamine oxidase activity. Prog Neuropsychopharmacol Biol Psychiatry 1984; 8: 385–395.

[64] Inoue O, Tominaga T, Yamasaki T, Kinemuchi H. Radioactive N,N-dimethyl-phenylethylamine: selective radiotracer for in vivo measurement of monoamine oxi-dase-B activity in the brain. J of Neurochem 1985; 44: 210–216.

[65] Tominaga T, Inoue O, Suzuki K, Yamasaki T, Hirobe M. [^{13}N]-β-phenethylamine ([^{13}N]PEA): A prototype tracer for measurement of MAO-B activity in heart. Biochem Pharmacol 1987; 36: 3671–3675.

[66] Severina IS. On the substrate-binding sites of the active centre of mitochondrial monoamine oxidase. Eur J Biochem 1973; 38: 239–246.

[67] Severina IS. Multiplicity of mitochondrial monoamine oxidases and ways of selective blocking of the enzyme activity. Biokhimiia 1976; 41: 955–967.

[68] Fowler CJ, Callingham BA, Mantle TJ, Tipton KF. The effect of lipophilic com-pounds upon the activity of rat liver mitochondrial monoamine oxidase-A and -B. Biochem Pharmacol 1980; 29: 1177–1183.

[69] Houslay MD, Tipton KF. A kinetic evaluation of monoamine oxidase activity in rat liver mitochondrial outer membranes. Biochem J 1974; 139: 645–652.

[70] Roth JA. Inhibition of human brain type B monoamine oxidase by tricyclic psycho-active drugs. Mol Pharmacol 1978; 14: 164–171.

[71] Edwards DJ, Burns MO. Effects of tricyclic antidepressants upon human platelet monoamine oxidase. Life Sci 1974; 15: 2045–2058.

[72] Meyerson LR, McMurtrey KD, Davis VE. Neuroamine-derived alkaloids: substrate-preferred inhibitors of rat brain monoamine oxidase in vitro. Biochem Pharmacol 1976; 25: 1013–1020.

[73] Bembenek ME, Abell CW, Chrisey LA, Rozwadowska MD, Gessner W, Brossi A. Inhibition of monoamine oxidase A and B by simple isoquinoline alkaloids: racemic and optically active 1,2,3,4-tetrahydro-, 3,4-dihydro-, and fully aromatic isoquinolines. J Med Chem 1990; 33: 147–152.

[74] Freidinger RM, Williams PD, Tung RD, Bock MG, Pettibone DJ, Clineschmidt BV, et al. Vinblastine and vincristine are inhibitors of monoamine oxidase B. J Med Chem 1990; 33: 1845–1848.

[75] Kaminski KA, Bodziony J, Kozielski J. Monitoring treatment of pulmonary car-cinomas by serial determination of monoamine oxidase and diamine oxidase in blood serum. Arch Geschwulstforsch 1984; 54: 377–385.

[76] Mantle TJ, Tipton KF, Garrett NJ. Inhibition of monoamine oxidase by am-phetamine and related compounds. Biochem Pharmac 1976; 25: 2073–2077.

[77] Kinemuchi H, Arai Y. Selective inhibition of monoamine oxidase A and B by two substrate-analogues. 5-fluoro-alpha-methyltryptamine and p-chloro-beta-methyl-phenethylamine. Res Commun Chem Pathol Pharmacol 1986; 54: 125–128.

[78] Kim SK, Toyoshima Y, Arai Y, Kinemuchi H, Tadano T, Oyama K, et al. Inhibition of monoamine oxidase by two substrate-analogues with different preferences for 5-hy-droxytryptamine neurons. Neuropharmacology 1991; 30: 329–335.

[79] Da Prada M, Kettler R, Keller HH, Cesura AM, Richards JG, Saura Marti J, et al. From moclobemide to Ro 19-6327 and Ro 41-1049: the development of a new class

of reversible, selective MAO-A and MAO-B inhibitors. J Neural Trans 1990; 29: 279–292.

[80] Dostert P, Strolin-Benedetti M. Structure-modulated recognition of substrates and inhibitors by monoamine oxidase A and B. Biochemical Society Transactions, Amine Oxidases 1990; 19: 207–211.

[81] Bench CJ, Price GW, Lammertsma AA, Cremmer JC, Luthra SK, Turon D, et al. Measurement of human cerebral monoamine oxidase type B (MAO-B) activity with positron emission tomography (PET): a dose ranging study with the reversible inhibitor Ro 19-6327. Eur J Clin Pharmacol 1991; 40: 169–173.

[82] Kenny WC, Nagy J, Salach JI, Singer TP. Structure of the covalent phenylhydrazine adduct of monoamine oxidase. In: Singer TP, editor. Monoamine oxidase: structure, function and altered function. New York: Academic Press, 1979: 25–37.

[83] Abeles RH, Maycock AL. Suicide enzyme inactivators. Acc Chem Res 1976; 9: 313–319.

[84] Fowler JC, Mantle TJ, Tipton KF. The nature of inhibition of rat liver monoamine oxidase types A and B by the acetylenic inhibitors clorgyline, l-deprenyl and pargyline. Biochem Pharmacol 1982; 31: 3555–3561.

[85] Waldmeier PC, Felner AE. Deprenyl: loss of selectivity for inhibition of B-type MAO after repeated treatment. Biochem Pharmacol 1978; 27: 801–802.

[86] Ekstedt B, Magyar K, Knoll J. Does the B form selective monoamine oxidase inhibitor lose selectivity by long term treatment? Biochem Pharmacol 1979; 28: 919–923.

[87] Csanda E, Tárczy M. Selegiline in the early and late phases of Parkinson's disease. J Neural Trans 1987; 25(suppl.): 105–113.

[88] Birkmayer W, Marton J, Hárs V, Reiederer P, Knoll J, Youdim MBH. l-Deprenyl increases the life expectancy of patients with Parkinson's disease. In: Markey, Sanford P, editors. MPTP: neurotoxin producing a parkinsonian syndrome. Orlando, Fla: Academic Press, 1986; 599–606.

[89] Tariot PN, Cohen RM, Sunderland T, Newhouse PA, Yount D, Mellow AM, et al. l-Deprenyl in Alzheimer's disease: preliminary evidence for behavioral change with MAO-B inhibition. Arch Gen Psychiatry 1987; 44: 427–433.

[90] Tariot PN, Sunderland T, Weingartner H, Murphy DL, Welkowitz JA, Thomson K, et al. Cognitive effects of l-deprenyl in Alzheimer's disease. Psychopharmacology 1987; 91: 489–495.

[91] Fejér E, Gaál J. Does deprenyl inhibit dopamine uptake? 18th FEBS Meeting: 1987 Jun 28–Jul 3; Ljubljana-Yugoslavia. Abstract: p. 273.

[92] Cserhalmi M, Fejér E, Réffy A, Gaál J. Deprenyl binding site in human brain? In: Tucek S, Stipek S, Stastny F, Krivanek J, editors. Molecular basis of neural function. Abstracts of the sixth ESN general meeting in Prague 1986; N5: 320.

[93] Knoll J, Ecsery Z, Magyar K, Sátory E. Novel (−)deprenyl-derived selective inhibitors of B-type monoamine oxidase. The relation of structure to their action. Biochem Pharmacol 1978; 27: 1739–1747.

[94] Huebner CF, Donoghue EM, Plummer AJ, Furness PA. N-methyl-N-2-propynl-1-indanamine. A potent monoamine oxidase inhibitor. J Med Chem 1966; 9: 830–832.

[95] Maitre L. Monoamine oxidase inhibiting properties of SU-11,739 in the rat. Comparison with pargyline, tranylcypromine and iproniazid. J Pharm Exp Ther 1967; 157: 81–88.

[96] Riederer P, Reynolds GP, Youdim MBH. Selectivity of MAO inhibitors in human brain and their clinical consequences. In: Youdin MBH, Paykel ES, editors. Monoamine oxidase inhibitors – The state of the art. Chichester: Wiley, 1981: 63–76.

[97] Youdim MBH, Finberg JPM. MAO type B inhibitors as adjunct to L-dopa therapy. Adv in Neurol 1986; 45: 127–136.

[98] Palfreyman MG, McDonald IA, Bey P, Danzin C, Zreika M, Lyles GA, et al. The rational design of suicide substrates of amine oxidases. Biochem Soc Trans 1986; 14: 410–413.

[99] McDonald I, Palfreyman MG, Zreika M, Bey P. (Z)-2-(2,4-dichlorophenoxy)methyl-3-fluoroallylamine: a clorgyline analogue with surprising selectivity for monoamine oxidase type B. Biochem Pharmacol 1986; 35: 349–351.

[100] Bey P, Fozard J, Lacoste JM, McDonald J, Zreika M, Palfreyman MG. (E)-[2-(3,4-dimethoxyphenyl)-3-fluoroallylamine]: A selective enzyme-activated inhibitor of type B monoamine oxidase. J Med Chem 1984; 27: 9–10.

[101] Fozard JR, Palfreyman GM, Robin M, Zreika M. Selective inhibition of monoamine oxidase type B by MDL 72145 increases the central effects of L-dopa without modifying its cardiovascular effects. Br J Pharmacol 1986; 87: 257–264.

[102] Zreika M, Fozard JR, Dudley MW, Bey P, McDonald IA, Palfreyman MG. MDL 72.974A: a potent and selective enzyme activated irreversible inhibitor of monoamine oxidase type B with potential for use in Parkinson's disease. J Neurol Trans 1989; 1: 243–254.

[103] Silverman RB. Mechanism of inactivation of monoamine oxidase by trans-2-phenyl-cyclopropylamine and the structure of the enzyme-inactivator adduct. J Biol Chem 1983; 258: 14766–14769.

[104] Silverman RB, Hiebert CK. Inactivation of monoamine oxidase A by the monoamine oxidase B inactivators 1-phenylcyclopropylamine, 1-benzylcyclopropylamine, and N-cyclopropyl-alpha-methylbenzyl amine. Biochemistry 1988; 27: 8448–8453.

[105] Hermecz I, Mészáros Z. Pyridol[1,2-a]pyrimidines; new chemical entities in medicinal chemistry. Med Res Rev 1988; 8: 203–230.

[106] Danxin C, Collard P, Schirlin D. Selective inactivation on MAO-B by benzyl-dimethyl-silyl-methanamine in vitro. Biochem Biophys Res Com 1989; 160: 540–544.

[107] Hallyday RP, Davis CS, Heotis JP, Pals DT, Watson EJ, Bickerton RK. Allenic amines: a new class of nonhydrazine MAO inhibitors. J Pharm Sci 1968; 53: 430–433.

[108] White RL, Smith RA, Krantz A. Differential inactivation of mitochondrial monoamine oxidase by stereoisomers of allenic amines. Biochem Pharm 1983; 32: 3661–3664.

[109] Sahlberg C, Ross SB, Fagervall I, Ask A-L, Claesson A. Synthesis of monoamine oxidase inhibitory activities of alpha allenic amines in vivo and in vitro. Different activities of two enantiomeric allenes. J Med Chem 1983; 26: 1036–1042.

[110] Smith RA, White RL, Krantz A. Stereoisomers of allenic amines as inactivators of monoamine oxidase type B. Stereochemical probes of the active site. J Med Chem 1988; 31: 1558–1566.

[111] Davis GC, Williams AC, Markey SP, Ebert MH, Caine ED, Reichert CM, et al. Chronic Parkinsonism secondary to intravenous injection of meperidine analogues. Psychiatry Res 1979; 1: 249–254.

[112] Heikkila RE, Manzino L, Cabbat FS, Duvoisin RC. Protection against the dopaminergic neurotoxicity of 1-methyl-4-phenyl-1,2,3,6-tetrahydropyridine monoamine oxidase inhibitors. Nature 1984; 311: 467–469.

[113] Chiba K, Trevor A, Castagnoli N, Jr. Metabolism of the neurotoxic tertiary amine, MPTP, by brain monoamine oxidase. Biochem Biophys Res Commun 1984; 120: 574–578.

[114] Salach JI, Singer TP, Castagnoli N, Jr, Trevor A. Oxidation of the neurotoxic amine 1-methyl-4-phenyl-1,2,3,6-tetrahydropyridine (MPTP) by monoamine oxidases A and B and suicide inactivation of the enzymes by MPTP. Biochem Biophys Res Commun 1984; 125: 831–835.

[115] Singer TP, Salach JI, Castagnoli N, Jr, Trevor A. Interactions of the neurotoxic amine 1-methyl-4-phenyl-1,2,3,6-tetrahydropyridine with monoamine oxidases. Biochem J 1986; 235: 785–789.

[116] Tipton KF, McCrodden JM, Youdim MBH. Oxidation and enzyme-activated irreversible inhibition of rat liver monoamine oxidase-B by 1-methyl-4-phenyl-1,2,3,6-tetrahydropyridine (MPTP). Biochem J 1986; 240: 379–383.

[117] Fuller RW, Hemrick-Luecke SK. Inhibition of types A and B monoamine oxidase by 1-methyl-4-phenyl-1,2,3,6-tetrahydropyridine. J Pharm Exp Ther 1985; 232: 696–701.

[118] Peterson LA, Caldera PS, Trevor A, Chiba K, Castagnoli N, Jr. Studies on the 1-methyl-4-phenyl-2,3-dihydropyridinium species 2,3-MPDP+, the monoamine oxidase catalyzed oxidation product of the nigrostriatal toxin 1-methyl-4-phenyl-1,2,3,6-tetrahydropyridine (MPTP). J Med Chem 1985; 28: 1432–1436.

[119] Singer TP, Salach JI, Castagnoli N, Jr, Trevor A. Interactions of the neurotoxic amine 1-methyl-4-phenyl-1,2,3,6-tetrahydropyridine with monoamine oxidases. Biochem J 1986; 235: 785–789.

[120] Singer TP, Ramsay R. The interaction of monoamine oxidases with tertiary amines. Biochemical Society Transactions, Amine Oxidases 1990; 19: 211–215.

[121] Dostert PL, Strolin-Benedetti S, Tipton KF. Interaction of monoamine oxidase with substrate and inhibitors. Med Res Rev 1989; 9: 45–89.

[122] Tipton KF, Fowler CJ, McRodden JM, Strolin-Benedetti M. The enzyme-activated irreversible inhibition of type-B monoamine oxidase by 3-{4-[(3-chlorophenyl)methoxy]phenyl}-5- [(methyl-amino)-methyl]-2-oxazolidinone methansulphonate (compound MD 780236) and the enzyme-catalyzed oxidation of this compound as competing reactions. Biochem J 1983; 209: 235–242.

[123] Dostert P, Strolin-Benedetti M, Guffroy C. Different stereoselective inhibition of monoamine oxidase-B by the R- and S-enantiomers of MD 780236. J Pharm Pharmacol 1983; 35: 161–165.

[124] Tenne M, Youdim BH. MAO-inhibiting drugs: stereochemical aspects. In: Smith D, editor. CRC Handbook of Stereoisomers: Drugs in Psychopharmacology; Boca Raton, FL: CRC, 1984; 285–296.

[125] Finnegan KT, Skratt JJ, Irwin I, DeLanney LE, Langston JW. Protection against DSP-4 induced neurotoxicity by deprenyl is not related to its inhibition of MAO-B. Eur J Pharmacol 1990; 184: 119–126.

[126] Tipton KF, McCrodden JM, Kalir AS, Youdim MBH. Inhibition of rat liver monoamine oxidase by alpha-methyl- and N-propargyl-amine derivatives. Biochem Pharmacol 1982; 31: 1251–1255.

[127] Heikkila RE, Davoison JP, Finberg M, Youdim MBH. Prevention of MPTP-induced neurotoxicity by AGN-1133 and AGN-1135, selective inhibitors of monoamine oxidase-B. Eur J Pharmacol 1985; 116: 313–317.

[128] Swett LR, Martin WB, Taylor JD, Everett GM, Wykers AA, Gladish YC. Structure-activity relations in the pargyline series. Ann NY Acad Sci 1963; 107: 891–898.

[129] Karoum F. N-Propargylbenzylamine, a major metabolite of pargyline, is a potent inhibitor of monoamine oxidase type-B in rats in vivo: a comparison with deprenyl. Br J Pharmacol 1987; 90: 335–345.

[130] Martin YC, Martin WB, Taylor JD. Regression analysis of the relationship between physical properties and the in vitro inhibition of monoamine oxidase by propynyl-amines. J Med Chem 1975; 18: 883–888.

[131] Ecsery Z, Knoll J, Somfai É, Török Z, Szinnyei É, Mozsolits K. Phenylizopropylamine derivative. PCT Int Appl WO 85 05,617 (1986; CA 105: 78632).

[132] Plenevaux A, Dewey SL, Fowler JS, Guillaume M, Wolf AP. Synthesis of (R)-$(-)$ and (S)-$(+)$-4-fluorodeprenyl and (R)-$(-)$ and (S)-$(+)$-[N-^{11}C-methyl]-4-fluorodeprenyl and positron emission tomography studies in baboon brain. J Med Chem 1990; 33: 2015–2019.

[133] Kettler R, Keller HH, Bonetti EP, Wyss PC, DaPrada M. Ro 16-6491: a new highly selective and reversible MAO-B inhibitor. J Neurochem 1985; 44: (Suppl.) S94.

[134] Fuller RW, Henrick SK, Mills J. Inhibition of monoamine oxidase by N-phenacil-cyclo-propylamine. Biochem Pharmacol 1978; 27: 2255–2261 C.

[135] Colpaert FC, Niemegeers, Carlos JE, Janssen PAJ. Evidence that a preferred substrate for type-B monoamine oxidase mediates stimulus properties of MAO inhibitors: a possible role for beta-phenylethyl-amine in the cocaine cue. Pharm Biochem Behav 1980; 13: 513–517.

[136] Roba J. Milacimide: a novel anti-convulsant. In: Meldum BS, Porter RR, editors. New anticonvulsant drugs. London: Libbey J and Co., 1966; 179–190.

[137] Buckman TD, Eiduson S, Boscia R. Investigation of the mechanism of selective inhibition of type-B mitochondrial monoamine oxidase by phoshatidylserine. Biochem Pharmacol 1983; 32: 3639–3647.

[138] Strolin Benedetti M, Dostert P. Stereochemical aspects of MAO interaction: reversible and selective inhibitors of monoamine oxidase. Trends in Pharm Sci 1985; 6: 246–251.

Inhibitors of Monoamine Oxidase B
Pharmacology and Clinical Use in Neurodegenerative Disorders
ed. by I. Szelenyi
© 1993 Birkhäuser Verlag Basel/Switzerland

CHAPTER 5
l-Deprenyl: A Unique MAO-B Inhibitor

E. E. Polymeropoulos

1 Introduction
2 Deprenyl and Its Metabolites
3 Comparison of *l*-Deprenyl to Other MAO-B Inhibitors
4 Formation of Inhibitor-FAD Complexes
5 Discussion
  Summary
  References

1. Introduction

Monoamine oxidase (MAO) is a flavin-adenosine-dinucleotide (FAD)-containing enzyme located on the outer mitochondrial membrane [1–3]. Its function is to catalyze the oxidative deamination of biogenic amines to the corresponding aldehyde [4]. It is generally accepted that it exists in two functional isoenzyme forms, MAO-A and MAO-B, each of which shows preferential affinity for substrates and specificity towards inhibitors [3, 5]. Available evidence suggests that two different proteins are responsible for the activity of the isoenzymes [6–8]. Although the role of the FAD cofactor in the oxidative process seems to be quite clear, the position of FAD relative to the substrate recognition and binding site has not yet been resolved. However, the structure of the flavin peptide has been determined, and it has been shown that for the liver and brain enzymes FAD is covalently linked at the 8α-carbon atom of the isoalloxazine ring to a cystein via a thioether bridge [9]. The sequence of the peptide together with the bound flavin is shown in Figure 1.

Severina [10] has attempted an identification of the binding sites which participate in the binding of substrates in the active center of MAO. She proposes three main interaction centers, namely, a hydrophobic pocket, a nucleophilic region, and an electrophilic group. Her conclusions are mainly based on the possible interactions that MAO can have with its various substrates. The importance of these binding sites differs for MAO-A and MAO-B. Thus, it is suggested that MAO-A inhibitors preferentially block a hydrophobic and an electrophilic site, whereas MAO-B inhibitors block a different hydrophobic site. The

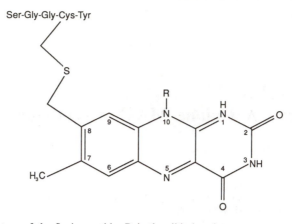

Figure 1. Structure of the flavin peptide. R is the ribityl moiety.

significance of these lipophilic binding sites is further emphasized by the assumption that, due to the lack of steric hindrance, MAO-B may bind to the lipophilic binding sites of both type A and B oxidases, while MAO-A inhibitors are sterically hindered from binding to the type B oxidase [11, 12].

The generally accepted mechanism for amine oxidation is shown in Figure 2 [13]. According to this scheme the flavin in FAD is fully reduced in a two-step electron transfer process by the bound amine with the simultaneous formation of an amine radical cation during the first electron transfer, and of an iminium cation during the second electron transfer. Subsequently, the flavin is reoxidized and the cyclic process is restored to its initial phase. To interrupt this cyclic process inhibitors have been designed that can bind to the active site and react with the flavin in FAD. The reaction is brought about by a nucleophilic attack upon a suitable center of the inhibitor. Such a center is the acetylenic group of *l*-deprenyl (selegiline) (MAO-B) or clorgyline (MAO-A). After formation of the iminium cation the N5 nitrogen (see Figure 1 for

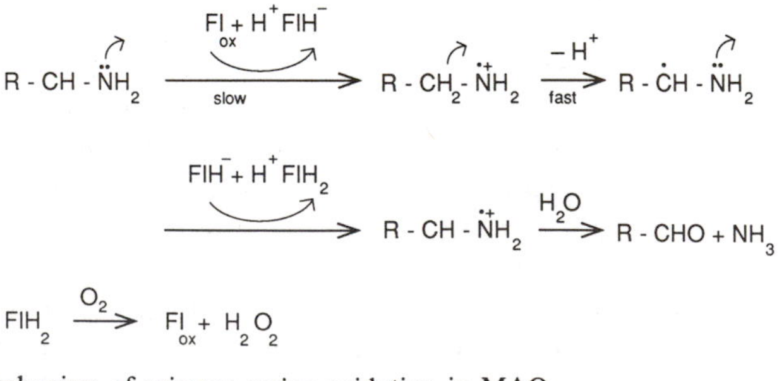

Figure 2. Mechanism of primary amine oxidation in MAO.

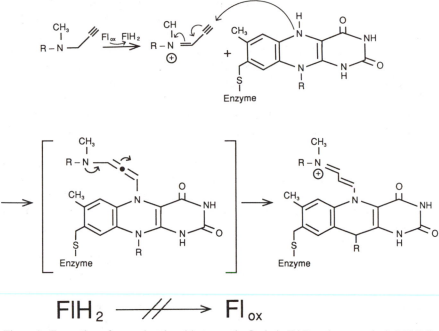

Figure 3. Formation of a covalent bond between the flavin in FAD and an acetylenic MAO-B inhibitor.

numbering) of the flavin in FAD attacks the acetylenic group and an allene intermediate is built which leads to the formation of an irreversible covalent bond between the inhibitor and the flavin (Figure 3) [14]. Thus, FAD is rendered inactive and amine oxidation can no longer take place.

Since most acetylenic inhibitors react irreversibly and stoichiometrically with FAD, it can be concluded that the selectivity of such compounds is not directly associated with FAD itself, but rather with the different substrate or inhibitor recognition sites situated near the active center. However, the proper positioning of the inhibitor relative to FAD is of great importance if inhibition is to take place. Therefore, in order to explain the action of MAO inhibitors, one has to take two factors in account. Firstly, the topology of the binding site, and secondly, the possibility that an irreversible or reversible reaction with FAD can take place.

2. Deprenyl and Its Metabolites

It is well known that many drugs display enantioselectivity in their therapeutic activity. Deprenyl is an excellent example of such a drug.

l-deprenyl (or *R*-deprenyl; selegiline) is a more potent inhibitor of MAO-B than is *d*-deprenyl (or *S*-deprenyl) [15, 16]. *l*-Deprenyl is metabolized to *l*-amphetamine (*R*-), and to *l*-metamphetamine (*R*-) [17]. Both metabolites show no inhibition of MAO-B, but have weak stimulatory effects on the CNS, whereas *d*-deprenyl is metabolized to *d*-amphetamine (*S*-) and *d*-metamphetamine (*S*-) which also show no inhibition of MAO-B, but are strong stimulants of the CNS [18]. Since *l*-deprenyl is a strong MAO-B inhibitor it is quite certain that it fits into the binding site of the active center and also binds covalently to FAD. The inactivity of *d*-deprenyl can be explained either by a steric hindrance in the enzyme binding site – which cannot recognize the inhibitor – or mechanistically by assuming that *d*-deprenyl cannot form an irreversible covalent bond with the flavin. The latter argument may also involve a steric hindrance that prevents a favorable relative position of the flavin and *d*-deprenyl, with the consequence that no covalent bond can be formed.

The crystal structure of deprenyl has been determined by Simon et al. [19]. If we perform conformational analysis on the two enantiomers of deprenyl we can show that the conformations in the crystal are indeed energetically low lying ones and, therefore, can be considered as possible candidates for the biologically active conformations. The structural comparison of the *l*- and *d*-enantiomers (Figure 4a,b) clearly shows that, as expected, there is no way in which the two configurations can be completely superimposed.

These observations may be rather obvious, but they may help in understanding why *d*-deprenyl is inactive towards MAO-B. The position of the methyl substituent on the chiral carbon atom hinders *d*-deprenyl from fitting into the binding site and, as a consequence, the acetylenic group cannot come near the N5 of the flavin for an eventual nucleophilic attack, as depicted in Figure 3.

If we now compare the structure of *l*-deprenyl to the structure of its metabolite *l*-amphetamine (similar considerations can be made for *l*-metamphetamine), we see that there is no conformational difference between the two molecules up to the amine nitrogen (Figure 5a). So why is *l*-amphetamine not a MAO-B inhibitor? We suggest that the difference in activity cannot be explained by structure alone. Let us assume that, according to the mechanism presented in Figure 2, *l*-amphetamine is oxidized by MAO-B and an iminium cation is formed. Furthermore, if *l*-amphetamine were able to build a covalent bond with the flavin, then the nucleophilic attack by the flavin N5 nitrogen atom would have to take place at the α-amine carbon atom.

Taking this into account, we compare the structures of the *l*-deprenyl and *l*-amphetamine iminium cations (Figure 5b). We observe that the two available centers for nucleophilic attack are approximately 4.8 Å away from each other. This means that the α-amine carbon atom of

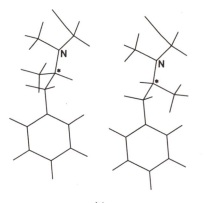

(a)

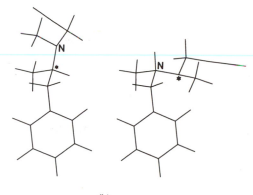

(b)

Figure 4. Structural comparison of *l*-and *d*-deprenyl. The structures have first been superimposed and then one enantiomer has been translated horizontally. If we superimpose the phenyl rings, the amine nitrogens, and the acetylenic moieties, then the methyl substitutes on the chiral carbon atom (marked with an asterisk) have different orientations in space (Figure 4a). On the other hand, if we superimpose the phenyl and the methyl substitute on the chiral carbon, then the acetylenic moieties have completely different orientations in space (Figure 4b).

l-amphetamine is too far away from the flavin for any nucleophilic attack to take place. In addition, due to the presence of the methyl substitute this carbon atom must have a higher electron density than the corresponding acetylenic carbon in *l*-deprenyl and, thus, it should be less suitable for nucleophilic attack. In section 4 we will further discuss the question of inactivity of *l*-amphetamine in conjunction with the formation of complexes between the reduced flavin and the iminium cations of inhibitors that lead to the creation of covalent bonds between the two partner molecules.

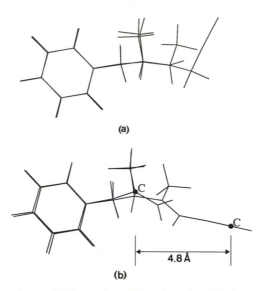

(a)

(b)

4.8 Å

Figure 5. a) Comparison of *l*-deprenyl and *l*-amphetamine. b) Comparison between the respective iminium cations of the molecules in a). No obvious structural difference can be observed, either between the two neutral molecules or their iminium cations. The distance between the center for nucleophilic attack in *l*-deprenyl and the corresponding center in *l*-amphetamine is 4.8 Å.

3. Comparison of *l*-Deprenyl to other MAO-B inhibitors

Among the MAO-B inhibitors (see also Appendix I) we have chosen MDL-72145 [20], Ro-166491 [21], U-1424 [22], AGN-1135 [23] and J-508 [24] as representative samples for comparison with *l*-deprenyl (Figure 6). The latter three also show optical isomerism, have an acetylenic group, and are irreversible inhibitors. Neither J-508 nor its *N*-demethyl derivative AGN-1135 are, however, metabolized to amphetamine. U-1424, a furan derivative, is an irreversible inhibitor that also exhibits optical isomerism. MDL-72145, a fluoroallylamine-substituted phenyl derivative, is also an irreversible inhibitor, but with a different center for nucleophilic attack than *l*-deprenyl. In this molecule an electron-withdrawing flourine atom is attached to an allylic carbon atom, thus, reducing its electron density and making it more nucleophilic. Finally, Ro-166491, an aminoethyl chlorbenzamide derivative with no apparent center for nucleophilic attack is a reversible inhibitor.

Since these compounds are selective MAO-B inhibitors, we can assume that they all bind to the same binding site of the active center. In addition, they probably all react with the flavin in FAD to produce a reversible or irreversible bond. This means that they must share some common structural and electronic characteristics which give them a common mode of action. It is quite obvious that all compounds have

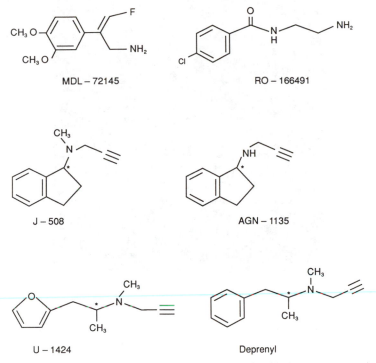

Figure 6. Structures of some selected MAO-B inhibitors. The chiral centers are marked with an asterisk.

a lipophilic ring system which is essential for MAO-B binding [10–12]. Furthermore, they all possess an amine nitrogen. If we consider the distance of this nitrogen from the lipophilic ring, we notice that *l*-deprenyl (5.09 Å), MDL-72145 (4.71 Å), and U-1424 (4.72 Å) differ from AGN-1135 (3.76 Å), J-508 (3.75 Å) and Ro-166491 (7.29 Å). For Ro-166491 the amine nitrogen is further away from the phenyl ring, whereas for AGN-1135 and J-508 the amine nitrogen is closer to the phenyl ring than in the case of *l*-deprenyl, MDL-72145 or U-1424. However, this difference does not seem to play a major role, and there should be a large tolerance in the binding site. Moreover, *l*-deprenyl, AGN-1135, U-1424, and J-508 possess acetylenic groups, while MDL-72145 has a fluorine-substituted allylic group which can act as a center for a nucleophilic attack. Finally, Ro-166491 has no such obvious center. For U-1424, AGN-1135, and J-508 stereoselectivity is also of importance. If we take *l*-deprenyl as the active configuration that fits into the MAO-B binding site then only *R*-U-1424, *R*-AGN-1135, and *R*-J-508 would fit this configuration. All of these considerations are taken into account in the structural comparison of the optimized structures of these compounds shown in Figure 7 (structure optimiza-

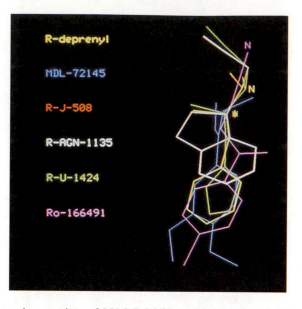

Figure 7. Structural comparison of MAO-B inhibitors. Name and optical isomer are color coded. Hydrogen atoms have been ommitted for clarity. The chiral carbon atom is marked with an asterisk. The yellow nitrogen (N) indicates the position of the superimposed amine nitrogen atoms of all inhibitors except Ro-166491 whose amine nitrogen is violet. The amine chains of all molecules except Ro-166491 (violet) are well superimposed. For this compound, however, the amine nitrogen falls in the vicinity of the other amine nitrogens. The lipophilic ring systems share a common region in space, although two orientations can be distinguished: one is assumed by deprenyl (yellow), MDL-72145 (blue), Ro-166491 (violet), and U-1424 (green), and the other by J-508 (red) and AGN-1135 (white). Due to their structural similarity the latter two structures cannot be distinguished from each other. The importance of enantioselectivity is emphasized by the fact that the saturated methylene carbon atom of the indane (AGN-1135, J-508) ring systems points in the direction of the methyl substitute on the chiral carbon atom of *l*-deprenyl.

tions were performed with the AM1 method [25], and computer graphics were carried out with the program MOLCAD [26] on a Silicon Graphics 4D80/GT workstation). Since we have chosen the crystal structure of *l*-deprenyl as a model for "optimal" binding to the active site, we have investigated the possibility that all other MAO-B inhibitors can assume similar low energy conformations.

Here, we have attemted to superimpose the lipophilic ring systems, the amine chains and the amine nitrogens while taking into account the optical isomerism of the molecules. It is evident that the spatial orientation of these characteristics is roughly the same for all molecules. Most important is the orientation of the indane (AGN-1135, J-508) ring systems which point in the direction of the methyl substitute of the chiral carbon in *l*-deprenyl. This indicates the significance of stereoselectivity in MAO-B inhibition. If these rings had the opposite orientation they would have fitted the *d*- and not the *l*-configuration of deprenyl.

Table 1. Calculated values for water/octanol partition coefficient log P^a.

Inhibitor	log P	Inhibitor	log P
l-Deprenyl	2.87	U-1424	2.72
J-508	2.65	MDL-72145	0.96
AGN-1135	2.30	Ro-166491	0.85

a) See [27, 28].

Although the fit of the ring systems of AGN-1135 and J-508 to the rest of the molecules appears to be only moderate, it can be shown by means of conformational analysis that a better fit of energetically acceptable conformations is possible. This means that there exists a common lipophilic binding site for all inhibitors. The amine nitrogens for all but Ro-166491 fall in the same region of space, despite the differences in distance from the benzene ring mentioned above. For Ro-166491 the amine nitrogen is in the vicinity of the acetylenic group. The consequence of this will be discussed later on in conjunction with the reaction of these inhibitors with the flavin in FAD.

The lipophilic character of the chosen inhibitors was also investigated by calculating the water/octanol partition coefficient by means of the method of Crippen et al. [27, 28]. We have used this method instead of the more widely applied method of Hansch [29] because, with the latter, it was not possible to calculate log P values for all the inhibitors. Although the obtained results (Table 1) cannot be taken absolutely, they are indicative of the existing differences in lipophilicity. Thus, we can assert that *l*-deprenyl is more lipophilic than MDL-72145 or Ro-166491, and slightly more lipophilic then AGN-1135 and U-1424. In addition, *l*-deprenyl and J-508 are the most lipophilic compounds. This may contribute favorably to their binding properties to the active center of MAO-B and, consequently, to their superior inihibtory potency, in view of the fact that a lipophilic binding site seems to be one of the primary binding sites of the enzyme [11].

Since inhibition takes place in most cases via a reaction with FAD, we suggest as a further criterion (that is at least as important as the structural considerations discussed above) the relative position of the flavin moiety to the iminium cation formed during oxidation of the amine, and particularly to the available site for nucleophilic attack of the inhibitors. This aspect will be disscussed in the next section.

4. Formation of Inhibitor-FAD Complexes

According to the reaction scheme shown in Figures 2 and 3 acetylenic inhibitors react irreversibly with the flavin portion of the enzyme.

Initially, the inhibitor is oxidized to form an iminium cation which subsequently reacts with the N5 nitrogen of the flavin isoalloxine ring to form a covalent bond. This last step involves a nucleophilic attack of the reduced flavin upon the acetyl moiety of the iminium cation. We regard this process, which leads to the formation of the covalent bond, as decisive for MAO inhibition. Should it take place, then the two reaction partners must be positioned in such a relative way to each other as to facilitate nucleophilic attack.

We have tried to explore the differences in mechanism for the various MAO-B inhibitors by building supermolecular complexes of the reduced flavin cofactor and the iminium cation intermediate. To build up these complexes we first optimized the structures of the reduced flavin and the iminium cations. In contrast to the neutral molecules the geometry of the iminium cation moiety is planar due to the $C=NR_2^+$ double bond. To start the calculation we positioned the flavin at a distance of approximately 3.0 Å above and near the middle of the chain that extends from the lipophilic ring system to the amine nitrogen. Subsequently, we allowed the complexes to become geometrically optimized; this optimization takes into account both geometric and electronic factors. Our aim was to show that electron transfer and covalent bonding would take place at the predicted positions, thus forming different compounds for the acetylenic irreversible inhibitors l-deprenyl, U-1424, AGN-1135, and J-508 on the one hand, and MDL-72145 on the other hand, however, by means of the same mechanism. This mechanism was further exploited in order to understand why Ro-166491 is a reversible MAO-B inhibitor.

Before we proceed with the results for the flavin-inhibitor complexes we would like to consider once again the question of why l-amphetamine is not a MAO-B inhibitor. To study this effect we have built the supermolecular complex of l-amphetamine with flavin and have optimized its geometry. The resulting structure is shown in Figure 8. It is obvious that nucleophilic attack on the α-carbon adjacent to the amine nitrogen is not favored. Instead, regardless of what starting geometry we choose, the interaction takes place between the N5 nitrogen of the flavin and the NH_2^+ moiety of amphetamine. These calculation indicate that, even if l-amphetamine were able to bind to the MAO-B active center, it would not form a bond to the flavin and, consequently, would not inhibit the enzyme activity.

For interpreting the results obtained for the flavin-inhibitor complexes we have made the assumption that FAD must be situated somewhere on the surface of the enzyme. As mentioned above, the structure of the flavin peptide has been established, and the flavin is bound to the peptide through a thioether bridge (Figure 1). Since the volume occupied by FAD is quite large, we assume that it resides on the outer part of the binding site of the enzyme. Recent experimental

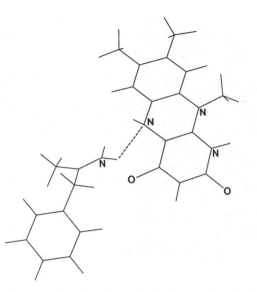

Figure 8. Optimized structure of the *l*-amphetamine-flavin complex. The interaction between the two molecules takes place preferentially between the N5 nitrogen of the flavin and the NH_2^+ group of *l*-amphetamine. The formation of a covalent bond is not possible.

evidence suggests that the binding site is well exposed, thus strengthening the argument that FAD itself could also be well exposed to the outside [30]. This would give FAD a greater rotational degree of freedom around the thioether bridge.

Figure 9 shows the optimized structures of the complexes for *l*-deprenyl, *R*-U-1424, *R*-AGN-1135, *R*-J-508, Ro-166491, and MDL-72145. We have superimposed only the flavin part of the complexes in order to see whether the inhibitory parts also coincide. The results show that all molecules actually share the same part of space relative to the flavin, and that either the acetylenic carbon atom or the allylic carbon atom (for MDL-72145) are the preferred centers of nucleophilic attack for irreversible inhibitors. Ro-166491 is known to be a reversible inhibitor of MAO-B. The exact mechanism has not yet been elucidated, but it has been suggested that the iminium cation (Figure 10a) first reacts with a nucleophilic group in the enzyme, and after reduction becomes a stable derivative [20]. If the nucleophilic group is a nitrogen – such as the N5 of flavin – then after formation of the iminium cation the most possible center for nucleophilic attack is the α-amine carbon atom. If this is the case, then an aminal can be formed (Figure 10b). Such reactions, however, are known to be reversible, and this could explain the fact that Ro-166491 is a reversible MAO-B inhibitor. In Figure 9 it can be seen that the flavin is indeed positioned near the end of the amine chain of Ro-166491 with the free election pair of the N5 nitrogen pointing in the direction of the α-amine carbon atom which

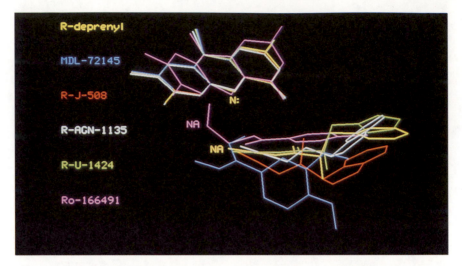

Figure 9. Structural comparison of optimized inhibitor-flavin complexes. Name and optical isomer are color coded. Hydrogen atoms have been ommitted for clarity. The ribityl moeity has been replaced by a methyl group. Only the flavin part has been superimposed. The yellow N: is the N5 nitrogen atom of the flavin. NA (yellow) is the center for nucleophilic attack of all inhibitors except Ro-166491 whose center is violet. With the exception of MDL-72154 (blue), the spatial coincidence of the inhibitor structures is rather good. Even in the case of MDL-72145, if we take the rotational flexibility of the flavin into account, we can assert that this inhibitor shares the same part of "space" as do the other inhibitors. For the compounds having an acetylenic group the N5 nitrogen atom of the reduced flavin resides over the acetylenic group, with the free electron pair pointing towards the electron-density-deficient carbon atom which is the center of nucleophilic attack, whereas for MDL-72145 the preference for the allylic carbon atom is quite obvious. The irreversible covalent bonds are formed at these positions. For Ro-166491 (violet) nucleophilic attack takes place at the α-amine carbon atom which results in the formation of a reversible aminal bond.

is the available center for nucleophilic attack, thus favoring the formation of an aminal. This hypothesis is also supported by the proximity of this carbon atom to the acetylenic carbon atoms of the other inhibitors, which, in turn, indicates that a common volume in space can be defined in which the centers for nucleophilic attack should be positioned.

5. Discussion

Deprenyl is a stereoselective MAO-B inhibitor. Neither enantiomer of its metabolites amphetamine and metamphetamine shows MAO-B inhibition. This can be attributed to the fact that the metabolites are not able to form a reversible or irreversible covalent bond to the FAD coenzyme factor. The mode of action of the active enantiomer *l*-deprenyl is characterized by a good fit into the binding site of the enzyme active center, and by the formation of an irreversible covalent

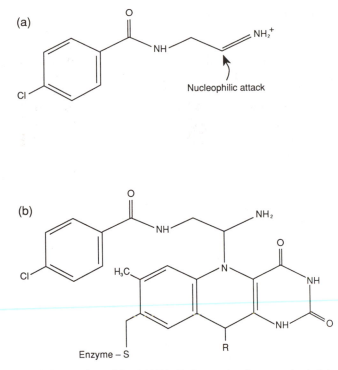

Figure 10. a) Iminium cation of Ro-166491. b) Interaction between the iminium cation of Ro-166491 and flavin leads to the formation of an aminal.

bond with FAD. Other inhibitors possessing an acetylenic group as the center for nucleophilic attack may also bind covalently to the flavin, but their potency may be affected by the degree of affinity towards the MAO-B binding site. U-1424 differs from *l*-deprenyl only in the lipophilic ring. Perhaps the slight decrease in lipophilicity influences its binding to the lipophilic receptor binding site in such a way that causes a slight decrease in its *in vitro* potency in comparison to *l*-deprenyl [31]. J-508 and its *N*-demethyl derivative AGN-1135 have a rather rigid geometry caused by the presence of the indane ring system. *In vitro* J-508 is a more potent inhibitor of MAO-B than *l*-deprenyl [31]. AGN-1135 is *in vitro* less potent than J-508 [32]. Both compounds are stereoselective and the geometry of the *R*-enantiomer is comparable to that of *l*-deprenyl. The fact that J-508 is more lipophilic than AGN-1135 may contribute to its greater potency as a result of better binding to the lipophilic pocket of MAO-B. Since *l*-deprenyl is a potent MAO-B inhibitor, we can assume that the flavin-*l*-deprenyl complex, which leads to the formation of a covalent bond, has an "optimal" geometry. Then, the presence of the *N*-methyl group in *R*-J-508 gives the geometry of the flavin complex of this compound a greater similarity to the "optimal" flavin-*l*-deprenyl complex than to the corresponding complex of R-AGN-1135. This can be expressed quantitatively by first superimposing the complexes and then calculating the root-mean-square (rms) deviation in the positions of the superimposed atoms. The rms values are 0.54 Å and 0.75 Å for the J-508 and AGN-1135 complexes, respectively, in accordance with the *in vitro* potency of these compounds. MDL-72145 is a structurally novel reversible MAO-B inhibitor that binds covalently to the flavin, and shows selectivity both *in vitro* and *in vivo* towards MAO-B [33]. Finally, Ro-166491 is a reversible MAO-B inhibitor whose mode of action is not yet well understood. A possible explanation for the reversibility may be the formation of an aminal with the flavin. Since such reactions are known to be reversible, the flavin could be released and become reoxidized in a later step, thus once again triggering the amine oxidation cycle.

Summary

The differences in potency towards monoamine oxidase type-B inhibitors (MAO-B) of the optical isomers of deprenyl and its metabolites have been discussed from structural and mechanistic points of view. In addition, the structures of a series of selective reversible and irreversible MAO-B inhibitors (MDL-72145, AGN-1135, J-508, U-1424, Ro-166491) were compared with the structure of *l*-deprenyl. The ability of these compounds to form a complex with the flavin in the flavin-adenosine-dinucleotide (FAD) enzyme cofactor, resulting in the formation of a covalent bond, and as a consequence in MAO-B inhibition, has been investigated by means of semiempirical quantum mechanical methods.

References

[1] Schnaitman C, Erwin VG, Greenawalt JW. The submitochondrial localisation of MAO. An enzymatic marker for the outer membrane of rat liver mitochondria. J Cell Biol 1967; 32: 719–35.
[2] Igaue I, Gomes B, Yasunobu KT. Beef mitochondrial monoamine oxidase, a flavin dinucleotide enzyme. Biochem Biophys Res Commun 1967; 29: 562–70.
[3] Edwards DJ, Molecular properties of the monoamine oxidases. Schizophr Bull 1980; 6: 275–81
[4] Singer TP, Von Korff RW, Murphy DL, editors. Monoamine Oxidase: Structure, Function and Altered Functions. New York: Academic Press, 1979.
[5] Johnston JP. Some observations upon a new inhibitor of monoamine oxidase in brain tissue. Biochem Pharmacol 1968; 17: 1285–97.
[6] Cawthan RM, Breakfield XO. Differences in A and B forms of monoamine oxidase revealed by limited proteolysis and peptide mapping. Nature 1979; 281: 692–94.
[7] Denney RM, Fritz RR, Patel NT, Abell CW. Human liver MAO-A and MAO-B separated by immunoaffinity chromatography with MAO-B specific antibody. Science 1982; 215: 1400–03.

[8] Smith D, Filipowicz C, McCauley R. Monoamine oxidase A and monoamine oxidase B activities are catalyzed by different proteins. Biochim Biophys Acta 1985; 831: 1–7.

[9] Walker WH, Kearney EB, Seng R, Singer TP. Sequence and structure of a cysteinyl flavin peptide from monoamine oxidase. Biochem Biophys Res Commun 1971; 44: 287–92.

[10] Severina IS. Multiplicity of mitochondrial monoamine oxidases and methods of selective blocking of enzyme activity. Biochemisty (Biokhimiya) 1976; 41: 785–94.

[11] Severina IS. Possible mechanism of selective inhibition of rat liver mitochondrial monoamine oxidase by chlorgyline and deprenyl. Biochemistry (Biokhimiya) 1979; 44: 151–60.

[12] Severina IS. Mechanism of inhibition of chlorgyline and deprenyl of oxidative deamination of tyramine by rat liver mitochondrial monoamine oxidase. Biochemistry (Biokhimiya) 1980; 45: 1443–52.

[13] Silverman RB, Hoffman SJ, Catus III WB. A mechanism for mitochondrial monoamine oxidase catalyzed amine oxidation. J Am Chem Soc 1980; 102: 7126–28.

[14] Maycock AL, Abeles RH, Salach JI, Singer TP. The action of acetylenic inhibitors on mitochondrial monoamine oxidase: structure of the flavin site in the inhibited enzyme. In: Wolstenholme GEW, Knight J, editors. Monoamine Oxidase and its Inhibition. Amsterdam: Elsevier, 1976: 33–47.

[15] Magyar K, Vizi ES, Ecseri Z, Knoll J. Comparative pharmacological analysis of the optical isomers of phenyl-isopropyl-methyl-propylamine (E-250). Acta Physiol Hung 1967; 32: 377–87.

[16] Tenne M, Youdim MBH. MAO-Inhibiting drugs: Stereochemical aspects. In: Smith DF, editor. CRC Handbook of stereoisomers: Drugs in psychopharmacology. Boca Raton: CRC, 1984: 285–96.

[17] Karoum F, Chuang LW, Eisler MST, Calne DB, Liebowitz MR, Quitkin FM et al. Metabolism of (−)deprenyl to amphetamine and metamphetamine may be responsible for deprenyl's therapeutic benefit: A biochemical assessment. Neurology 1982; 32: 503–9.

[18] Berry CN, Griffiths RJ, Hoult JRS, Moore PK, Taylor GW. Identification of 6-oxo-prostaglandin El as a naturally occurring prostanoid generated by rat lung. Br J Pharmacol 1986; 87: 327–35.

[19] Simon K, Podanyi B, Ecsery Z. Absolute configuration and conformational analysis of R-deprenyl and its homologs. J Chem Soc, Perkin Trans 2, 1986; 111–15.

[20] Bey P, Fozard J, Lacoste JM, McDonald IA, Zreika M, Palfreyman MG. (E)-2-(3,4-dimethoxyphenyl)-3-fluroallylamine: a selective enzyme-activated inhibitor of type B monoamine oxidase. J Med Chem 1984; 27: 9–10.

[21] Cesura AM, Imhof R, Takacs B, Galva MD, Picotti GB, Da Prada M. [^{3}H]Ro-166491, a selective probe for affinity labelling of monoamine oxidase type B in human brain and platelet membranes. J Neurochem 1988; 50: 1037–43.

[22] Knoll J, Ecsery Z, Magyar K, Satory E. Novel (−)deprenyl-derived selective inhibitors of B-type monoamine oxidase. The relation of structure to their action. Biochem Pharmacol 1978; 27: 1739–47.

[23] Finberg JP, Tenne M, Youdim MB. Tyramine antagonistic properties of AGN-1135, an irreversible inhibitor of monoamine oxidase type B. Br J Pharmacol 1981; 73: 65–74.

[24] Magyar K, Foldi P, Ecseri Z, Held G, Zsilla G, Knoll J. Selective inhibition of B type MAO by the optical isomers of N-methyl-N-propargyl-(1-indanyl)-ammonium·HCl (J-508). 4th Meeting of the European Society for Neurochemistry, Catania, Abst. 490, 1982.

[25] MOPAC v. 5.0, QCPE No. 455.

[26] Brickman J, Waldherr-Teschner M. Interaktive Computergraphik und Molekuelmodellierung. Informationstechnik 1991; 33: 83–90.

[27] Ghose AK, Pritchett A, Crippen GM. Atomic physicochemical parameters for three dimensional structure directed quantitative structure-activity relationships III: Modeling hydrophobic interactions. J Comput Chem 1988; 9: 80–90.

[28] Viswanadhan VN, Ghose AK, Revankar GR, Robins RK. Atomic physicochemical parameters for three dimensional directed quantitative structure-activity relationships. 4. Additional parameters for hydrophobic and dispersive interactions and their application for an automated superposition of certain naturally occurring nucleoside antibiotics. J Chem Inf Comput Sci 1989; 29: 163–72.

[29] Hansch C, Leo A. Substituent constants for correlation analysis in chemistry and biology. New York: Wiley-Interscience, 1979.

[30] Nicholson BH. Symmetric constraints and the active site of MAO-B. Biochem Soc Trans 1991; 19: 24S.

[31] Magyar K, Ecseri Z, Bernath G, Satory E, Knoll J. Structure-activity relationship of selective inhibitors of MAO-B. In: Magyar K, editor. Monoamine oxidases and their selective inhibition. Budapest, Pergamon Press, 1980: 11–21.

[32] Youdim MB, Finberg JP. MAO type B inhibitors as adjunct to L-dopa therapy. Adv Neurol 1987; 45: 127–36.

Inhibitors of Monoamine Oxidase B
Pharmacology and Clinical Use in Neurodegenerative Disorders
ed. by I. Szelenyi
© 1993 Birkhäuser Verlag Basel/Switzerland

CHAPTER 6
Pharmacology of Monoamine Oxidase Type B Inhibitors

K. Magyar

1   Introduction
2   Multiplicity of MAO
3   Regional and Cellular Distribution of MAO
4   Pharmacology of MAO-B Inhibitors
4.1   Irreversible Inhibitors of MAO-B
4.2   Reversible Inhibitors of MAO-B
4.3   Pharmacokinetics and Metabolism of MAO-B Inhibitors
4.4   Pharmacological Activities of MAO-B Inhibitors
4.4.1   Dopamine Potentiating Effects of MAO-B Inhibitors
4.4.2   The Neuroprotective Effects of MAO-B Inhibitors
4.4.3   The Age-Dependent Increase of MAO-B Activity
5   MAO-B Inhibitors and the "Cheese Effect"
        Summary
        References

1. Introduction

Monoamine oxidase (MAO; EC 1.4.3.4.) plays an essential role in the oxidative deamination of biogenic and food-derived amines, both in the central nervous system and the peripheral tissues. The enzyme was first described by Hare as tyramine oxidase [1] and was called monoamine oxidase by Zeller [2] in 1938. MAO is prevalent in animals [3]. The early findings in the late 1950s that iproniazid, with its tuberculostatic activity, caused a mood-elevating effect and inhibited MAO [4] gave an impetus to the clinical application of MAO inhibitors (MAOIs) in the treatment of depression and also to the search for new inhibitors. Their effects were not only beneficial in the treatment of psychiatric disorders, but they substantiated the concept that certain psychiatric states derive from the same neurochemical imbalance. Although the inhibitors proved to be as effective as the tricyclic antidepressants in the treatment of major depression, they fell into disrepute in the early 1960s because of the severe, and sometimes unpredictable interactions between MAOIs and food-derived amines (tyramine), which lead to cardiovascular complications and even death in some cases, and came to be called the "cheese effect" [5, 6]. In recent decades many efforts have been made to avoid the cheese effect. New MAOIs were developed with no or less severe adverse cardiovascular reactions [7, 8]. The main effect of MAOIs is to increase the amine concentration at the vicinity of the postsynaptic receptors.

2. Multiplicity of MAO

MAO is tightly bound to the outer membrane of the mitochondrion [9]. It is a flavin-adenosine-dinucleotide (FAD)-containing enzyme [10], and differs from the Cu-containing benzylamine oxidase found in the plasma and blood vessels [11].

In 1968 Johnston discovered that MAO exist in two forms, types A and B, and that they possess different substrate specificities and inhibitor sensitivities [12]. MAO-A represents the form which is selectively and irreversibly inhibited by clorgyline, while MAO-B is relatively insensitive to this inhibitor. It was found later that MAO-B is selectively inhibited by selegiline [7]. The specific substrate for MAO-A is 5-hydroxytryptamine (serotonin, 5-HT), and MAO-B preferentially oxidizes 2-phenylethylamine (PEA). In addition, mixed types of substrates, like tyramine (TA), also exist; their oxidation shows a biphasic inhibition response curve to either clorgyline or selegiline.

Both the substrates and the inhibitors can be grouped according to substrate specificity and inhibitor sensitivity. Eventually, 5-HT, noradrenaline (NA), adrenaline, and octopamine became generally regarded as being the specific substrates for MAO-A; benzylamine and PEA are the substrates for MAO-B (for review see [13]). TA and dopamine (DA) are considered as mixed types of substrates; DA is preferentially oxidized by MAO-A in the rat brain, but by MAO-B in the human brain [14].

Recent work has indicated that the substrate specificity of the two forms of MAO is not absolute, but rather it overlaps. PEA is the specific substrate for MAO-B, but at higher concentrations it exhibited a biphasic inhibition response curve similar to the mixed type substrates [15]. 5-HT can also be oxidized by rat brain MAO-B, but with a much higher K_m value and a much lower maximum velocity (V_{max}) than substrates of the A-form. The kinetic parameters (K_m and V_{max} values) given in Table 1 well represent the relative specificities of substrates (5-HT, DA, PEA) in the rat liver [16].

The inhibitors of MAO probably outnumber most of the inhibitors of any enzymes, except cholinesterases. They can be grouped according to their sensitivity to the two forms of the enzyme. There are inhibitors which have no selective inhibitory potency towards MAO-A and MAO-B, and this group represents the first generation of MAOIs [17]. The selective inhibitors of MAO-A and MAO-B represent the second or new generation.

Table 1. K_m and V_{max} values of the rat liver MAO-A and MAO-B toward different substrates. (Data obtained from Fowler and Tipton 1982; ref. [16])

Substrates	MAO forms*	K_m (μmol)	V_{max}
5-HT	A + B	173	2.42
	A	161	1.96
	B	2032	0.22
DA	A + B	220	8.0
	A	140	3.6
	B	430	49.0
PEA	A + B	20	2.65
	A	280	0.35
	B	20	2.30

*When the parameters of MAO-A or MAO-B were determined, the other form of the enzyme was blocked by deprenyl or clorgyline, respectively.

Although MAO-A and MAO-B have long been recognized as being pharmacologically distinguishable, there is considerable debate about the structural and genetic bases for the functional differences. It is still not known whether it is encoded by different genes, or whether different conformations of a single protein depend on the lipid environment or post-translational modifications [18]. Some of the most recent pharmacological, physical, and immunological evidence support the view that MAO-A and MAO-B are structurally different enzymes (for review see [19]). It has been shown recently that the homology in the primary structures of MAO-A and MAO-B is about 70% [20].

3. Regional and Cellular Distribution of MAO

MAO-A and MAO-B are not equally distributed in the organs and cells [21]. The ratio of MAO-A and MAO-B in the human brain is 1:4; certain brain regions have higher enzyme concentration than the others [22]. The MAO-B concentration of the frontal cortex is twofold lower than that of the thalamus. The concentrations of both MAO-A and MAO-B are also high in the basal ganglia [23]. The liver has the highest specific activity of both forms [24], while the human placenta contains exclusively MAO-A, and the platelets exhibit only MAO-B activity. The intestinal mucosa is rich in MAO-A, as are the lungs and pancreas [25].

There are also well known species variations in the ratios of the two forms of the enzyme. In contrast to human brain, in the brain of the mice and the rats MAO-A is predominant [23, 26]. Enzyme radioautography revealed that in rat brain, MAO-A is concentrated in the locus coeruleus, paraventricular thalamus, solitary tract nucleus, inferior olives, interpeduncular nucleus, and claustrum. In contrast to MAO-A,

MAO-B is concentrated in the ependyma, all circumventricular organs, the paraventricular thalamus and the posterior pituitary gland in rats.

The distribution of MAO-A and MAO-B was studied with ^{3}H-Ro 41-1049 and ^{3}H-Ro 19-6327, respectively [27]. The brain of the guinea pig contains more MAO-B than the MAO-A [28], therefore, this species seems to be a suitable model for studying MAO activity and inhibition, as it well imitates the human brain situation [29]. (It is therefore unusual that the guinea pig is not frequently used for this purpose in preclinical studies.)

The regional distribution studies of MAO-A and MAO-B were substantiated by use of the specific substrate and the selective and irreversible MAO inhibitors [30]. The use of positron emission tomography (PET) in applying the selective positron-emitter-labeled "suicide inhibitors" resulted in a nondestructive method for studying the multiplicity of MAO in the intact and functioning human brain [22]. Due to the development of this technique, a fast progression can be predicted in this field in the near future.

For studying the subcellular distribution of MAO-A and B new approaches are available, including a special histochemical technique [31] and use of monoclonal antibodies [32]. Studies with monoclonal antibodies recently indicated that catecholamine-containing neurons are rich in MAO-A, while in 5-HT cell bodies MAO-B activity predominates. An analog situation exists in adrenal chromaffin cells in which MAO-B is completely localized in spite of the cells' high catecholamine content [33].

The question arises about the physiological role of MAO-B in 5-HT neurons or in platelets. Youdim suggested that an endogenous MAO-B substrate can be present and have a modulator function in the central nervous system. The MAO-B activity keeps its concentration low in order to avoid the presynaptic release of 5-HT [34]. It is accepted that MAO-A activity maintains the low intraneuronal cytoplasmic concentration of NA, 5-HT, and DA.

In the gut, MAO-A inactivates the indirectly acting sympathomimetic amines (TA, PEA or other amine releasers) produced by bacterial enzymic decarboxylation from amino acids [35]. The blood vessels and the lungs are also rich in MAO-B activity which can protect these organs from the toxic influence of circulating vasoactive monoamines [36].

4. Pharmacology of MAO-B Inhibitors

The physiological function of MAO-B activity in the peripheral and central tissues appears to be a protective role, i.e., the deamination of foreign amines in the blood or by preventing their entry into the circulation. The localization of MAO-B in the glia or in the brain ventricles constitutes a metabolic barrier to amines.

Serotonergic neurons contain almost exclusively the B form of the enzyme, which has a very low affinity for the endogenous transmitter. The major role of MAO-B in these neurons is the elimination of foreign amines in the cytoplasm and the protection of their access to the synaptic granules. Because of the low affinity of MAO-B to serotonin, its extravesicular concentration can be relatively high intraneuronally. The inhibited activity of the enzyme can become detrimental as a consequence of the disturbance of the protective function of MAO (for review see [19]).

4.1. Irreversible Inhibitors of MAO-B

The B-type, selective, irreversible MAOIs available today belong to the category of the mechanism-based "suicide inhibitors". At the initial stage of their effect they bind to the target enzyme where they are converted to an active compound at the second stage, which forms a covalent bond with the active center of the enzyme.

The selectivity of the MAO-B inhibitors is relative; maintenance of their selectivity *in vivo* during chronic administration depends on careful dosing. It was proved in rats undergoing long-term treatment that selegiline preserved its selectivity when it was administered subcutaneously in a dose of 0.05–0.25 mg/kg body weight, which is similar to the human dose of selegiline in clinical trials [37]. When 1.0 mg/kg of selegiline was repeatedly administered it also inhibited the A form of MAO. It is generally agreed that the B-type inhibitors are less selective for MAO-B than the A-type inhibitors are for MAO-A.

Pargyline was earlier considered to be a selective inhibitor of MAO-B. In an appropriate dose and after a single administration, pargyline shows some selectivity to MAO-B, but when it is given chronically it induces a non-selective inhibition of both enzyme types [38].

The best-known selective MAO-B inhibitor is selegiline ((−)-deprenyl), first decribed by Knoll and Magyar [7]. Selegiline, which is similar to pargyline, is a propargyl derivative and its irreversible inhibition is preceded by a reversible competitive phase, at which time the presence of its specific substrates can prevent the irreversible inactivation of the enzyme. The (−)-isomer of selegiline is a more potent inhibitor of MAO-B than is its (+)-enantiomer [39].

In addition to selegiline a number of other MAO inhibitors show stereoselectivity. In contrast to (−)-deprenyl, the (+)-isomer of tranylcypromine [40] and J-508 [41] have greater inhibitory potency to MAO. Both (+)-tranylcypromine and (+)-J-508 exhibit a certain preference to MAO-B activity.

A number of deprenyl analogs were synthesized during recent decades and structure-activity relationship studies were carried out with compounds chemically related to deprenyl [42, 43]. These studies revealed that:

1) The substitution of deprenyl in the side chain at the alpha-position with ethyl-isopropyl- or benzyl-group decreases the MAO inhibitory potency of the compounds.

2) Alterations on the ring (*m*- or *o*-halogenation, methoxy-substitution or saturation) generally diminished the inhibitory potency. The *p*-fluoro-substitution of deprenyl resulted in a type-B selective and potent inhibitor of MAO (*p*-fluoro-deprenyl). Mainly, its (−)-enantiomer has promising qualities [70].

3) Omitting the methyl group of deprenyl in the side chain at alpha-position   (N-methyl-N-propargyl-(2-phenyl)-ethyl-amine·HCl; TZ-650) does not significantly influence the inhibitory potency or the B-type selectivity of the new derivative.

4) Replacing the phenyl ring with furan (N-methyl-N-propargyl-(2-furyl-1-methyl)-ethyl-amine·HCl; U-1424) or indenyl group (± -2,3-dihydro-N-methyl-N-2-propinyl-1H-inden-1-amine·HCl; J-508) resulted in potent inhibitors to MAO-B. U-1424 proved to be slightly less potent, but J-508 exceeded by one order of magnitude the inhibitory potency of the parent compound [44].

J-508 – mainly its (+)-enantiomer – is one of the most effective inhibitors of MAO-B described thus far. Concerning its chemical structure, no amphetamine-like metabolites can be formed from the compound. AGN-1135, the N-desmethyl derivative of AGN-1133 (developed and thoroughly studied by Youdim and Finberg [45]) is slightly less potent in inhibiting MAO than is the parent compound, but it has even greater selectivity for MAO-B than AGN-1133, and is equivalent to J-508.

Recently, a new, potent, enzyme-activated, irreversible inhibitor of MAO-B, (E)-2-(3,4-dimethoxyphenyl)-3-fluoro-allylamine·HCl (MDL-72145) was developed, and it showed considerable selectivity both *in vitro* and *in vivo* [46]. MDL-72974, which is a 4-fluorophenethyl derivative of the (E)-3-fluoroallylamines, also belongs to this family of MAO-B blockers [47]. These inhibitors, unlike selegiline, have no amine-releasing and uptake inhibiting properties, and they cannot be metabolized to amphetamine [48]. In animal experiments these inhibitors do not potentiate the cardiovascular effect of tyramine and the central effects of L-dopa. MDL-72145 and MDL-72974 can be considered as a reliable tool to study the physiological consequence of pure MAO-B inhibition.

4.2. Reversible Inhibitors of MAO-B

The tricyclic antidepressants are able to produce a selective and reversible inhibition of MAO-B, but their potency is low and their therapeutic effect is questionable [49]. Structure-activity relationship studies described by Strolin-Benedetti and coworkers [50] revealed that an oxazolidine derivative, MD-780236, can be considered to be a selective inhibitor of MAO-B; it acted irreversibly *in vitro* (the inhibition was not reversed by dialysis), but *in vivo* its effect appeared to be reversible. Enzyme activity was shown to return to the control value after 24 h following injection [50].

The discovery of moclobemide, a short-acting MAO-A inhibitor (synthesized in 1972), led to the identification of a new chemical class of highly selective reversible MAO-B inhibitors. In recent years much literature about the pharmacology of these inhibitors has appeared (for review see [51]). Ro 16-6491 has been considered as a metabolite of moclobemide, while Ro 19-6327 is a structural analog of the former. Both compounds inhibit the enzyme, and they have an initial competitive phase followed by a time-dependent inhibition of MAO-B (i.e., they are mechanism-based inhibitors). The MAO inhibitory potency of Ro 19-6327 exceeds that of Ro 16-6491. The inhibition induced by Ro 19-6327 is short lasting (12–24 h) and it did not potentiate the TA-induced increase of the mean arterial blood pressure. Based on the binding interference of ^{11}C-selegiline and Ro 19-6327 on human cerebral MAO-B, elegant PET studies were carried out in order to determine the inhibitory concentration of Ro 19-6327 necessary to inhibit brain MAO-B almost completely [52].

4.3. Pharmacokinetics and Metabolism of MAO-B Inhibitors

Relatively little is known about the pharmacokinetics and metabolic conversions of MAO-B inhibitors. Selegiline is one of the most widely studied inhibitors in this respect in both animal and human experiments. It is highly soluble in lipids, and its distribution ratio between hexane and water is 82:18 [53]. Selegiline is well absorbed after oral or any kind of parenteral administration in rats, and it rapidly penetrates into the central nervous system. When ^{14}C-selegiline is given intravenously to mice its highest brain concentration is reached within 30 s (whole-body autoradiography studies), but most of the radioactivity rapidly (1–2 min) disappears from the brain [54]. It binds to serum protein and remains partially irreversibly bound to the proteins [55]. Selegiline is metabolized to methylamphetamine, amphetamine, and desmethyl-selegiline in rats, without producing any remarkable signs of psychostimulant activity when it is administered in doses sufficient to elicit selective MAO-B inhibition [54, 56].

Similar results were obtained in dogs by Salonen [57] with gaschromatography using a ^{63}Ni electron-capture detector. Pentafluorobenzyl derivates of amphetamine and related primary amines were determined with a good sensitivity. Reynolds and coworkers first published that biotransformation of selegiline produces amphetamine and methyl-amphetamine in man, both of which are excreted in urine and can be detected in brain tissue [58]. Heinonen confirmed a similar pattern of metabolic conversion of selegiline in man, but the concentration of the metabolites formed was very low during a continuous treatment that induced clinical effects [59]; for details see Chapter 10).

The lack of psychostimulant activity could partly be due to the distribution properties of selegiline, for example, a low detectable level of radioactivity in the mouse brain after 1–2 min following intravenous injection [54], and partly due to the fact that from selegiline are formed (−)-isomers of amphetamine derivatives which have less psychostimu-lant activity than the (+)-enantiomers [60]. (It was proved earlier in parkinsonian patients that racemase did not convert the (−)-am-phetamines to their (+)-forms [61].)

4.4. Pharmacological Activities of MAO-B Inhibitors

Before giving a detailed description of the pharmacological activities derived from MAO-B inhibition, it should be emphasized that some MAO-B inhibitors are probably simple enzyme inhibitors such as MDL-72145, while others have in addition to their enzyme inhibitory effect, further intrinsic pharmacological activities not related to the inhibition of MAO-B. These additional properties (like the uptake inhibitory potency) may be reversible and short-lasting.

4.4.1. Dopamine potentiating effect of MAO-B inhibitors: Although there is a considerable amount of confusion concerning the substrate specificity of MAO-A and MAO-B towards DA, it is generally agreed that DA is metabolized by both forms of the enzyme in the rat brain [62], but it is preferentially oxidized by MAO-B in the human brain [14]. Since DA is considered to be deaminated predominantly by MAO-B in the human brain, selegiline has been used as an adjunct to L-dopa therapy of Parkinson's disease [63–65]. The inhibition of MAO-B by selegiline impairs the degradation of DA and reduces the amount of L-dopa required to maintain the optimal DA level in the parkinsonian brain [66, 67]. The L-dopa sparing effect of selegiline seems to potentiate the antiakinetic effect of L-dopa and reduces the incidence of dyskine-sias and on-off phenomena (for review see [68]).

The inhibition of MAO-B primarily occurs in the glia, which leads to a considerable increase of DA in the synaptic gap. It is quite likely that DA from the glia overflows in a hormone-like process and that it recognizes its own synaptic receptor [69]. In addition to the selective inhibition of MAO-B, selegiline seems to interfere with DA regulation by several other mechanisms, e.g. inhibiting the uptake of NA and DA [7].

At higher doses than those needed for selective inhibition of MAO-B from selegiline, more amphetamine-like metabolites can be formed. Nevertheless, the releasing properties of the (−)-isomers of the amphetamines produced by the metabolism from selegiline are not equivalent to those of the (+)-enantiomers. This might partly be due to the fact that not directly the amphetamines, but rather their further metabolites ((+)-p-hydroxynorephedrine) are responsible for the release of NA from the depot granules [70]. Since only the (+)-p-hydroxyamphetamine is converted to (+)-p-hydroxy-norephedrine *in vivo* (the (−)-p-hydroxyamphetamine is not a substrate for beta-hydroxylase) this can explain the difference between the releasing potencies of the different enantiomers [71]. In respect of the release, the stereoisomers of the amphetamines are not equally potent; according to our latest findings both enantiomers are nearly equally effective in inhibiting the uptake process [72, 73].

According to Knoll, the main pharmacological influence of selegiline on the dopaminergic neurons is the increase of their sensitivity to physiological and pharmacological stimuli, which is the partial consequence of both the MAO-B inhibition and the inhibition of DA uptake [74]. After chronic treatment, selegiline reduces the number of beta-adrenoceptors and increases the turnover rate of DA [75, 76]. The MAO-B inhibition induced by selegiline could result in a) the potentiation of L-dopa effect, b) the reduction of the daily dose of L-dopa, and c) restoring the sensitivity to L-dopa when the response is diminished or lost [45].

A number of other MAO-B inhibitors are now available which cannot be metabolized to amphetamine. Animal experiments and clinical trials with these compounds ought to answer at least two important questions in the future: a) how much the antiparkinsonian action of selegiline is related to its metabolites; and b) whether the lack of the TA potentiation is a general property of MAO-B inhibitors or if it is a pharmacological quality unique to selegiline.

There is some evidence that the long-term treatment with selegiline in combination with L-dopa and peripheral decarboxylase inhibitor may prolong life and improve the life expectancy of parkinsonian patients in comparison to those treated with L-dopa or peripheral L-dopa decarboxylase inhibitor alone [77].

4.4.2. The neuroprotective effects of MAO-B inhibitors: Both forms of MAO play a general protective role by preventing the central and peripheral nervous systems from exogenous amines. The activation of 1-methyl-4-phenyl-1,2,3,6-tetrahydropyridine (MPTP) by MAO-B yields the 1-methyl-4-phenylpyridinium ion (MPP$^+$), the active neurotoxin, and can be considered to be the opposite mechanism of the normal function. MPTP is a preferential substrate for oxidation by MAO-B [78]. The mechanism of MPTP toxicity was reviewed by Glover et al. [79]. The oxidation of MPTP is highly sensitive to inhibition by selegiline, but not by clorgyline. A daily oral dose of 10 mg of selegiline is sufficient to inhibit MAO-B almost completely and also prevents MPTP oxidation and subsequent degeneration of dopaminergic neurons in the substantia nigra. Since the neurotoxicity of MPTP depends on the MAO-B activity which forms neurotoxin from the parent compound, all of the selective inhibitors of MAO-B can potentially prevent MPTP-caused neurodegeneration *in vivo*.

A line of evidence exists that potent inhibitors of DA uptake (mazin-dol) can also prevent MPP^+-caused neurodegeneration. In the rodent brain MAO-B is located in glial cells and 5-HT neurons, but not in the DA terminals. It was suggested that MPTP is taken up into the glial cells and oxidized to MPP^+ which is released and taken up by the dopaminergic neurons by an active reuptake mechanism, a process which can be inhibited by mazindol [80].

Selegiline and, mainly, its metabolites are considerably potent inhibitors of DA uptake. The inhibition of this process, in addition to the MAO-B inhibition, may play a preventive role in MPTP neurotoxicity [73, 81]. The uptake-inhibitory effect of selegiline might also be responsible for antagonizing the neurotoxic action of 6-hydroxydopamine in the substantia nigra [81].

It was published recently that, in mice, selegiline but not MDL 72974 protected against the neurodegenerative effects of the noradrenergic neurotoxin DSP-4 [82]. Since both selegiline and MDL 72974 produce a comparable degree of MAO-B inhibition, it seems doubtful that MAO-B activity plays any significant role in the neurotoxicity of DSP-4. Similar results were obtained in rats with selegiline and especially, with its *para*-fluoro-derivative (Chinoin Pharmaceutical and Chemical Works Ltd., Budapest, Hungary); mainly their metabolites were found to be potent in the prevention of DSP-4 toxicity [73]. The protective effect of the metabolites of selegiline and its *p*-fluoro-derivative against DSP-4 toxicity strengthens the role of the uptake inhibition in the neuroprotection. The positively charged aziridinium ion is responsible for the toxic effect of DSP-4 which can be formed spontaneously and actively taken up by noradrenergic neurons [83]. MDL 72974 lacks the reuptake blocking effects and fails to inhibit the DSP-4-induced neurotoxicity [82].

4.4.3. The age-dependent increase of MAO-B activity: The MAO-B-age relationship was widely studied and it appears that brain MAO-B activity increases with age in both humans and animals (for review see [84]). The increase of MAO-B activity with age may be associated with glial cell proliferation which is accompanied by neuronal loss, since microglia contains mostly the B form of MAO.

The enzyme MAO catalyzes the oxidative deamination of primary, secondary, and tertiary amines, including neuronal transmitters, when aldehydes, ammonia, and hydrogen peroxide are formed. All of them are considered to be cytotoxic when they are not neutralized. The low content of reduced glutathione and the increased amount of ferrous ion in the substantia nigra of parkinsonian patients, and the hydrogen peroxide formed by deamination of dopamine might lead to an increase of oxygen free radicals which can elicit lipid peroxidation, and cause membrane damage and cell degeneration (for review see [85]).

There are conflicting data, but MAO-B activity in the blood platelets of parkinsonian patients and those with Alzheimer-type dementia (both of which are considered to be neurodegenerative diseases) is significantly higher than that in controls [86]; for review see [69]).

MAO-B inhibitors, by reducing the formation of hydrogen peroxide from dopamine, might decrease the risk of neurodegeneration of the aging brain [87, 88]. In addition to the oxidative stress caused by the age-dependent increase of MAO-B activity, further reactions between endogenous amines and aldehydes produced by MAO-B can also play a role in neurodegeneration [79].

The formation of hydroxy radicals by hydrogen peroxide through the Fenton or the Haber-Weiss reaction may also contribute to the neuronal damage [84]. It was published recently by Knoll that selegiline specifically increases the activity of superoxide dismutase (SOD) in the striatum of the rats, a finding which was confirmed by Carrillo and his coworkers [89, 90], The increase in the radical scavenging activity of SOD after long-term treatment with selegiline additionally supports the existence of the neuroprotective activity of selegiline. Based on the above observations, it seems rational to use selective MAO-B blockers to prevent the age-dependent increase of MAO-B activity and, in this way, prevent the subsequent oxidative damage in the aging brain.

5. MAO Inhibitors and the "Cheese Effect"

The dominant opinion about the efficacy and safety of MAOIs has changed over recent decades. Their benefits have been frequently under-estimated, but their side-effects have been overemphasized [91]. It is generally agreed that the non-selective, irreversible (first generation) MAOIs and the MAO-A blockers are effective drugs in treating psychic depression [92], but their interactions with TA-containing foodstuffs lead to serious complications [93–95]. MAO-B inhibitors generally lack the cheese effect, but their effectiveness in treating depression is rather questionable [93, 96, 97].

The hypertensive crises which result from the potentiation of the indirectly acting sympathomimetic amines like TA have seriously hindered the clinical application of MAOIs. After the early popularity of these drugs, they fell into disrepute, and tricyclic antidepressants became the drugs of choice in treating depression [98]. Most of the early clinical trials were performed with the non-selective, irreversible MAOIs, e.g., iproniazid, phenelzine, isocarboxazid, tranylcypromine, and their antidepressive effects were associated with the pressor response to orally or intravenously administered TA [99]. Tranylcypromine is perhaps the most potent in provoking hypertensive crisis or autopotentiation [100].

More recently, reversible and selective MAO-A inhibitors have been developed for the effective treatment of the depressive illness, with the aim to lower the risk of the cheese effect. The most selective MAO-A inhibitors are moclobemide, brofaromine, and cimoxatone. The most distinctive characteristics of these drugs are the selectivity to MAO-A, competitive behavior, and reversibility (for review see [101, 102]). Due to their short-acting nature (24 h) they were found to be less likely to induce a large increase in the pressor response to TA, both in animals and man [103]. There is good reason to believe that the reversible inhibitors of MAO-A may not potentiate TA-induced side-effects, thereby diminishing the risk of hypertensive crisis and obviating the need for dietary restrictions [104]. Nevertheless, for final proof more clinical trials are required.

A particularly innovative approach to avoid the cheese effect is provided by a new MAO inhibitor, MDL 72394, which is a bioprecursor amino acid (E-beta-fluoromethylen-*m*-tyrosine) of a selective MAO-A inhibitor MDL 72392. The prodrug is decarboxylated by aromatic L-amino acid decarboxylase (AAAD) in order to liberate MDL 72392, the potent irreversible inhibitor of MAO-A. Combination of MDL 72394 with carbidopa, a peripherally selective inhibitor of AAAD, restricts MAO inhibition to the brain. Under these conditions the propensity to potentiate the cardiovascular effect of TA is greatly reduced and was proved in human volunteers [94].

Among the irreversible and selective MAO-B inhibitors, selegiline was the most widely used compound in clinical trials. Early reports demonstrated that selegiline, the potent and selective inhibitor of MAO-B, did not potentiate, but instead strongly antagonized the effects of TA on isolated rat vas deferens preparations [7, 105]. It was also shown that the pressor response of orally administered TA (up to 200 mg) in human volunteers was not potentiated by a dose of selegiline that was adequate for selective inhibition of MAO-B [25, 106]. Similar results were also obtained in clinical trials by Varga and Tringer, who were not able to provoke the hypertensive response with foods containing high concentration of TA [107]. Even a high dose of selegiline failed to increase the sensitivity to intravenous TA, whereas low doses of standard inhibitors increased the sensitivity to TA [108].

The lack of potentiation of sympathomimetic amines (TA, PEA) by selegiline could be attributed to several factors: a) selegiline does not inhibit the intestinal MAO in man; human intestine contains mainly MAO-A [28]; b) selegiline inhibits the neuronal amine reuptake in mouse cortical slices [7], in rat cortex [109] and heart tissue [110]; and c) selegiline, in contrast to pargyline and tranylcypromine, blocks the release of NA from the storage vesicles of the rat heart [7, 66].

The effects of various MAO-B inhibitors on rabbit arterial strip response to TA were studied recently [111]. In addition to selegiline, MDL-72145, Ro 16-6491, AGN-1135, J-508, U-1424, TZ-650 were included in these studies. All of the MAO-B selective inhibitors except selegiline potentiated the effect of TA on the pulmonary artery strip, and similar results were also obtained in anesthetized cats and rats *in vivo* regarding blood pressure response to TA [112]. Tranylcypromine, pargyline, and clorgyline were also shown to be strong potentiators of TA both *in vitro* and *in vivo*. Selegiline was the only exception, which indicates that the lack of TA potentiation is not a general characteristic of MAO-B inhibitors. The lack of "cheese effect" after selegiline treatment led many authors to the conclusion that inhibitors of MAO-B, do not potentiate the effects of TA. Considering the former results according to Abdorubo and Knoll [111] this conclusion might be misleading.

The exact pharmacological mechanism for the lack of "cheese effect" by selegiline is not fully known, however, its metabolic conversion to (−)-methamphetamine and (−)-amphetamine *in vivo* (the uptake inhibitory effect of the metabolites) should also be considered [54, 73].

TA is an indirectly acting sympathomimetic amine which should be taken up by the sympathetic neurons to release NA from stores. The NA release is a displacement into the neuronal cytoplasm, and when the intraneuronal MAO-A is blocked the transmitter is preserved from metabolism. The inhibition of intraneuronal MAO-A also reduces the metabolism of TA within the neuron, a process which leads to TA potentiation (for review see [40]).

In clinical cases all of the processes which create elevated blood concentration of TA can cause a blood-pressure response, in addition to neuronal mechanisms. Orally administered TA is metabolized by the gut before entering the circulation. Since the gastrointestinal tract contains mainly MAO-A [28], selegiline slightly influences its activity in the therapeutic dose regimen and leaves the metabolism of TA relatively unaffected. This could be partly the reason why clorgyline enhanced TA absorption in the cat while selegiline did not.

The human liver contains both forms of MAO in 1:1 proportion. Since TA as a mixed type of substrate is oxidized by both types of the enzyme, the separate inhibition of either form may not dramatically influence the systemic blood level of TA. The inhibition of liver MAO-B is seemingly insignificant at the systemic TA level, which is indicated by the lack of TA potentiation after selegiline treatment.

Most of the clinical experience concerning the blood-pressure response to TA is based on the administration of selegiline and to a much lesser degree the other MAO-B inhibitors. Since a fatal outcome in clinical cases caused by the "cheese effect" is rather infrequent, it is difficult without broad clinical experience, to form a reliable opinion about the inducibility of blood-pressure response by any type of inhibitor.

Summary

The multiplicity and distribution of monoamine oxidase (MAO) with the pharmacological mechanism of action of MAO type-B inhibitors have been reviewed above. The inhibitors increase the dopaminergic tone in the central nervous system by a complex mechanism. Like other drugs, in addition to their irreversible enzyme inhibitory effect, MAO-B inhibitors have an intrinsic pharmacological activity unrelated to the enzyme inhibition. MAO-B activity increases with age and the age-related changes lead to an overproduction of neurotoxic agents. The inhibition of the enzyme activity can play a preventive role against neurodegenerative brain disorders (Parkinson's disease, Alzheimer-type dementia). MAO-B blockers are effective in preventing the toxicity of MPTP and the presumably existing MPTP-like endogenous neurotoxins.

Selegiline is the most widely used MAO-B inhibitor in therapy, and it lacks the "cheese effect". The blood-pressure response to dietary tyramine is less frequent with the MAO-B inhibitors than with the type-A blockers. Nevertheless, the generalized former conclusion might be misleading, because the complex mechanism for the lack of "cheese effect" by selegiline is not fully known.

References

[1] Hare MLC. Tyramine oxydase: New enzyme in liver. Biochem J 1928; 22: 968–79.
[2] Zeller EA. Über den enzymatischen Abbau von Histamin und Diaminen. Helv Chim Acta 1938; 21: 880–90.
[3] Blaschko H. The natural history of the amine oxidases. Physiol Biochem Pharmac 1974; 70: 83–148.
[4] Zeller EA, Barsky J. In vivo inhibition of liver and brain monoamine oxidase by 1-isonicotinyl-2-isopropylhydrazine. Proc Soc Exp Biol Med 1952; 81: 459–61.
[5] Natoff IL. Cheese and monoamine oxidase inhibitors. Interaction in anaesthetized cats. Lancet 1964; i: 532–33.

[6] Blackwell B, Marley E, Price J. Hypertensive interactions between monoamine oxidase inhibitors and food stuffs. Br J Psychiatry 1967; 113: 349–65.

[7] Koll J, Magyar K. Some puzzling pharmacological effects of monoamine oxidase inhibitors. In: Costa E, Sandler M, editors. Monoamine Oxidises – New Vistas. Adv in Biochem Psychopharmacol. Raven Press, New York, 1972; 5: 393–408.

[8] Dollery CT, Brown MJ, Davies DS, Strolin-Benedetti M. Pressor amines and monoamine oxidase inhibitors. In: Tipton KF, Dostert P, Strolin-Benedetti M, editors. Monoamine oxidase and disease: Prospects for therapy with reversible inhibitors. New York: Academic Press, 1984; 430–41.

[9] Schnaitman C, Erwin VG, Greenawalt JW. The submitochondrial localisation of MAO. An enzymatic marker for the outer membrane of rat liver mitochondria. J Cell Biol 1967; 32: 719–35.

[10] Igaue I, Gomes B, Yasunobu KT. Beef mitochondrial monoamine oxidase, a flavin dinucleotide enzyme. Biochem Biophys Res Commun 1967; 29: 562–70.

[11] Lewinsohn R. Mammalian monoamine-oxidizing enzymes, with special reference to benzylamine oxidase in human tissues. Brazilian J Med Biol Res 1984; 17: 223–56.

[12] Johnston JP. Some observations upon a new inhibitor of monoamine oxidase in brain tissue. Biochem Pharmac 1968; 17: 1285–97.

[13] Dostert P, Strolin-Benedetti M, Tipton KF. Interaction of monoamine oxidase with substrates and inhibitors. Medicinal Research Reviews 1989; 9: 45–89.

[14] Glover V, Sandler M, Owen F, Riley GJ. Dopamine is a monoamine oxidase B substrate in man. Nature 1977; 265: 80–1.

[15] Kinemuchi H, Wakui W, Kamijo K. Substrate selectivity of type A and type B monoamine oxidase in rat brain. J Neurochem 1980; 35: 109–15.

[16] Fowler CJ, Tipton KF. Deamination of 5-hydroxytryptamine by both forms of monoamine oxidase in the rat brain. J Neurochem 1982; 38: 733–36.

[17] Quitkin F, Rifkin A, Klein DG. Monoamine oxidase inhibitors: A review of antidepressant effectiveness. Arch Gen Psychiatry 1979; 36: 749–60.

[18] Cesura AM, Imhof R, Glava MD, Kettler R, Da Prada M. Interaction of the novel inhibitors of MAO-B Ro 19-6327 and Ro 16-6491 with the active site of the enzyme. Pharmacol Res Commun Suppl IV, 1988; 20: 51–61.

[19] Denney RM, Denney CB. An update on the identity crisis of monoamine oxidase: new and old evidence for the independence of MAO A and B. Pharmacol Ther 1985; 30: 227–59.

[20] Bach AWJ, Lan NC, Johnson DL, Abell CW, Bembenek ME, Kwan SW, et al. cDNA cloning of human liver monoamine oxidase A and B: molecular basis of differences in enzymatic properties. Proc Natl Acad Sci USA 1988; 85: 4934–8.

[21] Lewinsohn R, Glover V, Sandler M. Development of benzylamine oxidase and monoamine oxidase A and B in man. Biochem Pharmacol 1980; 29: 1221–30.

[22] Fowler JS. Enzyme activity: monoamine oxidase. In: Frost JJ, Wagner HN, editors. Quantitative imaging: Neuroreceptors, neurotransmitters and enzymes. New York: Raven Press, 1990; 179–92.

[23] Oreland L, Arai Y, Strenström A, Fowler CJ. Monoamine oxidase activity and localization in the brain and the activity in relation to psychiatric disorders. In: Beckmann H, Riederer P, editors. Modern problems in pharmacopsychiatry monoamine oxidase and its selective inhibitors. Basel: Karger, 1983; 19: 246–54.

[24] Glover V, Sandler M. Clinical chemistry of monoamine oxidase. Cell Biochem Funct 1986; 4: 89–97.

[25] Elsworth JD, Glover V, Reynolds GP, Sandler M, Lees AJ, Phuapradit P, et al. Deprenyl administration in man: a selective monoamine oxidase B inhibitor without the "cheese effect". Psychopharmacology 1978; 57: 33–8.

[26] Garrick NA, Murphy DL. Species differences in the deamination of dopamine and other substrates for monoamine oxidase in brain. Psychopharmacology 1980; 72: 27–33.

[27] Marti JS, Kettler R, Da Prada M, Richards JG. Molecular neuroanatomy of MAO-A and MAO-B. J Neural Transm Suppl 1990; 32: 49–53.

[28] Squires RF. Multiple forms of monoamine oxidase in intact mitochondria as characterized by selective inhibitors and thermal stability: a comparison of eight mammalian species. In: Costa E, Sandler M, editors. Advances in biochemical psychopharmacology. Monoamine oxidases – new vistas. New York: Raven Press, 1972; 5: 355–70.

[29] Azzaro AJ, King J, Kotzuky J, Schoepp DD, Frost J, Schochet S. Guinea pig striatum as a model of human dopamine deamination: the role of monoamine oxidase isoenzyme ratio, localization, and affinity for substrate in synaptic dopamine metabolism. J Neurochem 1985; 45: 949–56.

[30] Ross SB. Distribution of the two forms of monoamine oxidase within monoaminergic neurons of the guinea pig brain. J Neurochem 1987; 48: 609–14.

[31] Uchida E, Koelle GB. Histochemical investigation of criteria for the distinction between monoamine oxidase A and B in various species. J Histochem Cytochem 1984; 32: 667–73.

[32] Levitt P, Pintar JE, Breakefield XO. Immunocytochemical demonstration of mono-amine oxidase B in brain astrocytes and serotonergic neurons. Neurobiology 1982; 79: 6385–9.

[33] Pollard HB, Ornberg R, Levine M, Kellner K, Morita K, Levine R, et al. Hormone secretion by exocytosis with emphasis on information from chromaffin cell system. Vitams Horm 1986; 42: 109–94.

[34] Youdim MBH. Platelet monoamine oxidase B: Use and misuse. Experientia 1988; 44: 137–41.

[35] Youdim MBH, Finberg JPM. Monoamine oxidase inhibitor antidepressants. In: Gra-hame-Smith DG, Hippius A, Winoker H, editors. Psychopharmacology. Amsterdam: Excerpta Medica, 1985; 37–71.

[36] Youdim MBH, Ben-Harari RR, Bakhle YS. Factors affecting monoamine inactivation in lung. In: Porter R, Knight J, editors. Metabolic aspects of the lung. Ciba Foundation Symposium, no.78, Amsterdam: Elsevier, 1980; 105–28.

[37] Ekstedt B, Magyar K, Knoll J. Does the B form selective monoamine oxidase inhibitor lose selectivity by long term treatment? Biochem Pharmacol 1978; 28: 919–23.

[38] Campbell IC, Robinson DS, Lovenberg W, Murphy DL. The effects of chronic regimens of clorgyline and pargyline on monoamine metabolism in the rat brain. J Neurochem 1979; 32: 49–55.

[39] Magyar K, Vizi ES, Ecseri Z, Knoll J. Comparative pharmacological analysis of the optical isomers of phenyl-isopropyl-methyl-propinylamine (E-250). Acta Physiol Hung 1967; 32: 377–87.

[40] Youdim MBH, Finberg JPM, Wajsbort J. Monoamine oxidase type B inhibitors in the treatment of Parkinson's disease. In: Ellis GP, West GB, editors. Progress in medicinal chemistry. Elsevier Science Publishers, B.V. 1984; 21: 137–67.

[41] Magyar K, Földi P, Ecseri Z, Held Gy, Zsilla G, Knoll J. Selective inhibition of B type MAO by the optical isomers of N-methyl-N-propargyl-(1-indanyl)-ammonium·HCl (J-508). 4th meeting of the European Society for Neurochemistry, Catania, Abst. 490, 1982.

[42] Magyar K, Knoll J. Selective inhibition of the "B form" of monoamine oxidase. Pol J Pharmacol Pharm 1977; 29: 233–46.

[43] Knoll J, Ecsery Z, Magyar K, Sátory É. Novel (−)deprenyl-derived selective inhibitors of B-type monoamine oxidase. The relation of structure to their action. Biochem Pharmac 1978; 27: 1739–47.

[44] Magyar K, Ecseri Z, Bernáth G, Sároty É, Knoll J. Structure-activity relationship of selective inhibitors of MAO-B. In: Magyar K, editor. Monoamine oxidases and their selective inhibition. Budapest: Pergamon Press, 1980; 11–21.

[45] Youdim MBH, Finberg JPM. MAO type B inhibitors as adjunct to L-dopa therapy. In: Yahr MD, Bergmann KJ, editors. Advances in Neurology 1986; 45: 127–36.

[46] Bey P, Fozard J, McDonald IA, Palfreyman MG, Zreika M. MDL 72145: a potent and selective inhibitor of MAO type B. Br J Pharmacol 1984; 81: p50

[47] Zreika M, Fozard JR, Dudley MW, Bey P, McDonald IA, Palfreyman MG. MDL 72 974: a potent and selective enzyme-activated irreversible inhibitor of monoamine oxidase type B with potential for use in Parkinson's disease. J Neural Transm Park Dis Dement Sect 1989; 1: 243–54.

[48] Bey P, Fozard J, Lacoste JM, McDonald IA, Zreika M, Palfreyman MG. (E)-2-(3,4-Dimethoxyphenyl)-3-fluoroallylamine: a selective, enzyme-activated inhibitor of type B monoamine oxidase. J Med Chem 1984; 27: 9–10.

[49] Roth JA. Inhibition of human brain type B monoamine oxidase by tricyclic psycho-active drugs. Mol Pharmacol 1978; 14: 164–71.

[50] Strolin-Benedetti M, Dostert P, Boucher T, Guffroy C. A new reversible selective type B monoamine oxidase inhibitor MD 780236. In: Kamijo K, Usdin E, Nagatsu T, editors. Monoamine oxidase, basic and clinical frontiers. Amsterdam: Excerpta Medica, 1982; p209.

[51] Da Prada M, Kettler R, Keller HH, Cesura AM, Richards JG, Marti JS, et al. From moclobemide to Ro 19-6327 and Ro 41-1049: the development of a new class of reversible, selective MAO-A and MAO-B inhibitors. J Neural Transm Suppl 1990; 29: 279–92.

[52] Bench CJ, Price GW, Lammertsma AA, Cremer JC, Luthra SK, Turton D, et al. Measurement of human cerebral monoamine oxidase type B (MAO-B) activity with positron emission tomography (PET): a dose ranging study with the reversible inhibitor Ro 19-6327. Eur J Clin Pharmacol 1991; 40: 169–73.

[53] Magyar K. Study of deprenyl metabolism. In: Kalász H, Ettre LS, editors. Chromatography: the state of the art 1984; 391–402.

[54] Magyar K, Szücs T. The fate of (−)-deprenyl in the body. Preclinical studies. In: Proceedings of the international symposium on (−)-deprenyl, Jumex. Szombathely, Hungary, 1982; 25–31.

[55] Szökő É, Kalász H, Kerecsen L, Magyar K. Binding of (−) deprenyl to serum proteins. Pol J Pharmacol Pharm 1984; 36: 413–21.

[56] Magyar K, Tóthfalusi L. Pharmacokinetic aspects of deprenyl effects. Pol J Pharmacol Pharm 1984; 36: 373–84.

[57] Salonen JS. Determination of the amine metabolites of selegiline in biological fluids by capillary gas chromatography. J Chromatography 1990; 527: 163–8.

[58] Reynolds GP, Elsworth JD, Blau K, Sandler M, Lees AJ, Stern GM. Deprenyl is metabolized to methamphetamine and amphetamine in man. Br J Clin Pharmacol 1978; 6: 542–4.

[59] Heinonen EH, Myllyla V, Sotaniemi K, Lammintausta R, Salonen JS, Anttila M, et al. Pharmacokinetics and metabolism of selegiline. Acta Neurol Scand 1989; 126: 93–9.

[60] Hoffman BB, Lefkowitz RJ. Catecholamines and sympathomimetic drugs. In: Gilman AG, Rall WT, Nies AS, Taylor P, editors. Goodman and Gilman's; the pharmacological basis of therapeutics. 8th ed. New York: Pergamon Press, 1990: 187–220.

[61] Schachter M, Marsden CD, Parkes JD, Jenner P, Testa B. Deprenyl in the management of response fluctuations in patients with Parkinson's disease on levodopa. J Neurol Neurosurg Psychiatr 1980; 43: 1016–21.

[62] Fowler CJ, Strolin-Benedetti M. The metabolism of dopamine by both forms of monoamine oxidase in the rat brain and its inhibition by cimaxatone. J Neurochem 1983; 40: 1534–41.

[63] Birkmayer W, Riederer P, Youdim MBH, Linauer W. The potentiation of the anti-akinetic effect of L-dopa treatment by an inhibitor of MAO-B, l-deprenyl. J Neural Transm 1975; 36: 303–36.

[64] Yahr M. Overview of present treatment of Parkinson's disease. J Neural Transm 1978; 43: 227–38.

[65] Rinne UK. A new approach to the treatment of Parkinson's disease. Acta Neurol Scand Suppl 95, 1983; 68: 5–144.

[66] Knoll J. The pharmacology of selective irreversible monoamine oxidase inhibitors. In: Seiler N, Jung MJ, Koch-Weser J, editors. Enzyme activated irreversible inhibitors. Amsterdam: Elsevier-North Holland, 1978; 253–69.

[67] Reynolds GP, Riederer P, Rausch WD. Dopamine metabolism in human brain: effects of monoamine oxidase inhibition in vitro by (−)deprenyl and (+) and (−)tranylcypromine. J Neural Transm Suppl 16, 1980; 173–8.

[68] Da Prada M, Keller HH, Pieri L, Kettler R, Haefely WE. The pharmacology of Parkinson's disease: basic aspects and recent advances. Experientia 1984; 40: 1165–72.

[69] Riederer P, Konradi C, Hebenstreit G, Youdim MBH. Neurochemical perspectives to the function of monoamine oxidase. Acta Neurol Scand 1989; 126: 41–5.

[70] Brodie BB, Cho AK, Gessa GL. Possible role of p-hydroxynorephedrine in the depletion of norepinephrine induced by d-amphetamine and in tolerance to this drug. In: Costa E, Garattini S, editors. Amphetamines and related compounds. New York: Raven Press, 1970; 217–30.

[71] Goldstein M, Anagnoste B. The conversion *in vivo* of d-amphetamine to (+)-p-hydroxy-norephedrine. Biochim Biophys Acta 1965; 107: 166–8.

[72] Magyar K, Knoll J. Effect of phenyl-isopropyl-methyl-propionylamine (deprenaline) on the subcellular distribution of ^{3}H-noradrenaline. Acta Physiol Hung 1970; 37: p414

[73] Magyar K. Neuroprotective effect of deprenyl and p-fluor-deprenyl. In: Paneuropean Society of Neurology, Second Congress, Vienna, 1991: 26.

[74] Knoll J. (−)Deprenyl (selegiline): the history of its development and pharmacological action. Acta Neurol Scand Suppl 95, 1983; 57–80.

[75] Zsilla G, Barbaccia ML, Gandolfi O, Knoll J, Costa E. (−) Deprenyl, a selective MAO-B inhibitor increased ^{3}H-imipramine binding and decreased beta-adrenergic receptor function. Eur J Pharmacol 1983; 11: 117.

[76] Zsilla G, Knoll J. The action of (−)deprenyl on monoamine turnover rate in rat brain. Adv Biochem Psychopharmacol 1982; 31: 211–7.

[77] Birkmayer W, Knoll J, Riederer P, Youdim MBH, Hars V, Martin J. Increased life expectancy resulting from addition of *l*-deprenyl to Madopar® treatment in Parkinson's disease: A long-term study. J Neural Transm 1985; 64: 113–28.

[78] Salach JI, Singer TP, Castagnoli N, Trevor A. Oxidation of the neurotoxic amine 1-methyl-4-phenyl-1,2,3,6-tetrahydropyridine (MPTP) by monoamine oxidases A and B and suicide inactivation of the enzymes by MPTP. Biochem Biophys Res Comm 1984; 125: 831–5.

[79] Glover V, Gibb C, Sandler M. The role of MAO in MPTP toxicity – A review. J Neural Transm Suppl XX 1986; 65–76.

[80] Javitch JA, d'Amato RJ, Strittmatter SM, Snyder SH. Parkinsonism-inducing neuro-toxin, N-methyl-4-phenyl-1,2,3,6-tetrahydropyridine: uptake of the metabolite N-methyl-4-phenylpyridine by dopamine neurons explains selective toxicity. Proc Natl Acad Sci USA 1985; 82: 2173–7.

[81] Hársing,LG, Magyar K, Tekes K, Vizi ES, Knoll J. Inhibition by deprenyl of dopamine uptake in rat striatum: a possible correlation between dopamine uptake and acetyl-choline release inhibition. Pol J Pharmacol Pharm 1979: 31: 297–307.

[82] Finnegan KT, Skratt JJ, Irwin I, DeLanney LE, Langston JW. Protection against DSP-4-induced neurotoxicity by deprenyl is not related to its inhibition of MAO B. Eur J Pharmacol 1990; 184: 119–26.

[83] Ross SB. Long-term effects of N-(2-chloroethyl)-N-ethyl-2-bromobenzylamine hy-drochloride on noradrenergic neurons in the rat brain and heart. Br J Pharmacol 1976; 58: 521–27.

[84] Strolin-Benedetti M, Dostert P. Monoamine oxidase, brain ageing and degenerative diseases. Biochem Pharmacol 1989; 38: 555–61.

[85] Da Prada M. New approaches to the treatment of age-related brain disorders. Can J Neurol Sci 1991; 18: 384–6.

[86] Danielczyk W, Streifler M, Konradi C, Riederer P, Moll G. Platelet MAO-B activity and the psychopathology of Parkinson's disease, senile dementia and multiinfarction dementia. Acta Psychiatr Scand 1988; 78: 730–6.

[87] Knoll J. Striatal dopamine, aging and deprenyl. In: Borsy J, Kerecsen L, György L, editors. Proc 4th Cong Hung Pharmacol Soc Budapest 1985; 3: 7–25.

[88] Langston JW. Selegiline as neuroprotective therapy in Parkinson's disease: concepts and controversies. Neurology Suppl 3 1980; 40: 61–6.

[89] Knoll J. The striatal dopamine dependency of life span in male rats. Longevity study with (−)-deprenyl. Mech Aging Dev 1988; 46: 237–62.

[90] Carrillo MC, Kanai S, Nokubo M, Kitani K. (−) Deprenyl induces activities of both superoxide dismutase and catalase but not of glutathione peroxidase in the striatum of young male rats. Life Sciences 1991; 48: 517–21.

[91] Blackwell B, Marley E. Interaction of cheese and its constituents with monoamine oxidase inhibitors. Br J Pharmacol Chemother 1966; 26: 120–41.

[92] Murphy DL, Sunderland T, Cohen RM. Monoamine oxidase-inhibiting antidepres-sants. Psychiat Clin North Amer 1984; 7: 549–62.

[93] Youdim MBH, Finberg JPM. Monoamine oxidase B inhibition and the "cheese effect". J Neural Transm Suppl 1987; 25: 27–33.

[94] Palfreyman MG, McDonald IA, Bey P, Schechter PJ, Sjoersma A. Design and early clinical evaluation of selective inhibitors of monoamine oxidase. Prog Neuropsy-chopharmacol Biol Psychiatry 1988; 12: 967–87.

[95]   Jarrott B, Vajda FJE. The current status of monoamine oxidase and its inhibitors. Med J Aust 1987; 146: 634–8.

[96]   Murphy DL, Lipper S, Slatter S, Shilling D. Selectivity of clorgyline and pargyline as inhibitors of monoamine oxidases A and B *in vivo* in man. Psychopharmacology 1979; 62: 129–32.

[97]   Sandler M. Monoamine oxidase inhibitor efficacy in depression and the "cheese effect". Psychol Med 1981; 11: 455–8.

[98]   Blackwell B. Monoamine oxidase inhibitor interactions with other durgs. J Clin Psychopharmacol 1991; 11: 55–59.

[99]   Pickar D, Cohen RM, Jimerson DC, Murphy DL. Tyramine infusions and selective MAO inhibitor treatment. I. Changes in pressor sensitivity. Psychopharmacology 1981; 74: 4–7.

[100] Cooper AJ. Tyramine and irreversible monoamine oxidase inhibitors in clinical practive. Br J Psychiatry 1989; Suppl. 6, 1989; 155: 38–45.

[101] Delini-Stula A, Radeke E, Waldmeier PC. Basic and clinical aspects of the activity of the new monoamine oxidase inhibitors. Psychopharmacol Ser 1988; 5: 147–58.

[102] Da Prada M, Keller HH, Kettler R. Comparison of the new MAO-A inhibitors moclobemide, brofaromine and toloxatone with tranylcypromine in an animal experiment: significance for clinical practice. Psychiatr Prax Suppl 1, 1989; 16: 18–24.

[103] Strolin-Benedetti SM, Dostert P. Overview of the present state of MAO inhibitors. J Neural Transm Suppl 1 1987; 23: 103–19.

[104] Robinson DS, Kurtz NM. Monoamine oxidase inhibiting drugs: pharmacologic and therapeutic issues. In: Meltzer HY, editor. Psychopharmacology: The third generation of progress. New York: Raven Press, 1987: 1297–1304.

[105] Knoll J, Vizi ES, Somogyi G. Phenylisopropyl-methyl-propinylamine (E-250), a new monoamine oxidase inhibitor antagonizing effects of tyramine. Arzneim-Forsch 1968; 18: 109–12.

[106] Sandler M, Glover V, Ashford A, Stern GM, Absence of "cheese effect" during deprenyl therapy, some recent studies. J Neural Transm 1978; 43: 209–15.

[107] Varga E, Tringer L. Clinical trial of a new type of promptly acting psychoenergetic agent (phenyl-isopropylmethyl-propinylamine HCl, E-250). Acta Med Acad Sci Hung 1967; 23: 289–95.

[108] Mendis N, Pare CMB, Sandler M, Glover V, Stern G. (−)-Deprenyl in treatment of depression. In: Youdim MBH, Paykel ES, editors. Monoamine oxidase inhibitors – The state of the art. Chichester: Wiley 1981; 171–6.

[109] Braestrup C, Andersen H, Randrup A. The monoamine oxidase B inhibitor, (−)deprenyl potentiates phenylethylamine behaviour in rats without inhibition of catecholamine metabolite formation. Eur J Pharm 1975; 34: 181–7.

[110] Simpson LK. Evidence that (−)deprenyl, a type B monoamine oxidase inhibitor, is an indirectly acting sympathomimetic amine. Biochem Pharmacol 1978; 27: 1591–5.

[111] Abdorubo A, Knoll J. The effect of various MAO-B inhibitors on the rabbit arterial strip response to tyramine. Pol J Pharmacol Pharm 1988; 40: 673–83.

[112] Abdorubo A. The effect of various monoamine oxidase (MAO) inhibitors on the response of blood pressure of rats and cats to tyramine. Acta Physiol Hung 1990; 75: 321–46.

Inhibitors of Monoamine Oxidase B
Pharmacology and Clinical Use in Neurodegenerative Disorders
ed. by I. Szelenyi
© 1993 Birkhäuser Verlag Basel/Switzerland

CHAPTER 7
The Pharmacological Basis of the Therapeutic Effect of (−)-Deprenyl in Age-Related Neurological Diseases

J. Knoll

1   Introduction
2   The Pharmacological Profile of (−)-Deprenyl
2.1   Single Dose Effects
2.1.1 Selective Inhibition of B-Type MAO
2.1.2 Inhibition of the Uptake of Catecholamines and Indirectly Acting Amines
2.2   Multiple Dose Effects
2.2.1 Facilitation of Scavenger Function in the Striatum
2.2.2 Facilitation of the Activity of the Nigrostriatal Dopaminergic Neurons
3   The Consequences of Long-Term, Small-Dose Administration of (−)-Deprenyl in Rats
3.1   Effect on Sexual Behavior
3.2   Effect on Learning Capacity
3.3   Effect on Longevity
4   The Consequences of Long-Term Administration of (−)-Deprenyl in Parkinson's Disease and Alzheimer's Disease
4.1   Parkinson's Disease
4.2   Alzheimer's Disease
5   Morphological Evidence that Long-Term, Small-Dose (−)-Deprenyl Treatment Counters Age-Related Changes in the Neurocytes of the Substantia Nigra
6   Strategy to Counter the Age-Related Decline of the Striatal Dopaminergic System by (−)-Deprenyl-Administration
7   Outlook
       Summary
       References

1. Introduction

In human, striatal dopamine content and number of nigrostriatal neurons are known to decline rapidly beyond the age of 45 years [1]. According to our present knowledge, the nigrostriatal dopaminergic neurons are the most rapidly aging neurons in the human brain. The dopamine content of the human caudate nucleus decreases enormously, by 13% per decade, over age 45. We know that symptoms of Parkinson's disease (PD) appear if the dopamine content of the caudate sinks below 30% of the normal level. Thus, the normal aging of the system is slow enough so that the appearance of parkinsonian symptoms is not evident within the average lifespan. This is true for 99.9% of the human

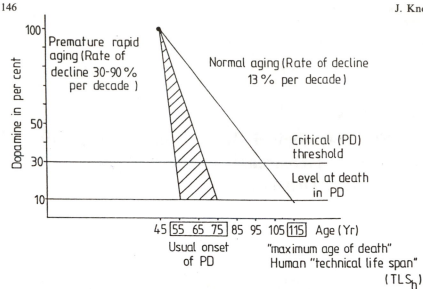

Figure 1. Illustration of the concept that Parkinson's disease (PD) constitutes rapid, premature aging of the striatal dopaminergic system.

population. In 0.1%, however, the striatal dopaminergic system deteriorates rapidly. This small percentage of the population (see Figure 1) crosses the critical threshold and manifests the classical symptoms described by James Parkinson in 1817 in his famous book "Essay on the Shaking Palsy". Parkinson's disease (PD) may be regarded as a premature, rapid aging (of unknown origin) of the striatal dopaminergic machinery.

The onset of PD is extremely rare in the first decades of life. Only about 10% of patients exhibit symptoms of the disease before the age of 50 years. The prevalence increases sharply with age. For example, in Finland [2] the prevalence rate is 22.7 per 100 000 in the age group 40–44 years, whereas 796.9 per 100 000 of the population between the ages of 70 and 74 years have the disease.

Parkinson's disease is the best example of an age-related neurological disease, and the only one for which the biochemical pathology (i.e. striatal dopamine deficiency) is firmly established. Viral infection, immunological abnormality, enzyme defects, and toxins have been proposed as the causes of PD, but the fundamental cause of the illness is still unknown. Is PD necessarily an ordinary disease caused by special pathogenic factor(s)? Based on the well established nature of age-related deterioration of the striatal dopaminergic system, the answer to this question is not necessarily affirmative. Because of the lack of a general factor of physiological age, we know that the variance within a particular age-group for any measurable parameter is large. In cross-sectional studies no single age emerges as the point of sharp decline in function. Any individual may show different levels of performance, and the careful observer finds many dissociations between "chronological" and "physiological" age. A 70-year-old man, for example, may continue his physiological, psychological and sexual performance equal to a 40-year-old, and vice-versa. Therefore, maybe those who display the "shaking palsy" represent that 0.1% of the normal population with the most rapidly aging variants of nigrostriatal dopaminergic neurons and live long enough to pass the critical threshold for exhibiting the symptoms. The argument that those who possess the most rapidly aging striatal system (i.e. they are part of the normal population and no special pathogenic factor is needed to explain the symptoms) may also be valid for the neurodegenerative characteristic of Alzheimer's disease. In this case, a small percentage of the population displays a premature rapid intellectual decline of a kind which develops at a slower rate in all those who live long enough. Unfortunately, in the case of Alzheimer's disease (AD), the morphological and biochemical targets are, for the time being, not as well established as in the case of PD. With regard to the striatal system, dopamine itself might play a main role in the unusually drastic age-related changes of the nigrostriatal dopaminergic neurons. Eighty percent of the brain dopamine is localized in this system. The complex auto-oxidation of the high amounts of dopa and dopamine in the striatum, continuously generating substantial quantities of toxic free radicals and highly reactive quinones, creates a permanent danger for the nigrostriatal dopaminergic neuron, which has to mobilize its natural defense measures against these toxic metabolites.

Neuromelanin, which is generated via the polymerization of oxidative products of dopamine with the evident aim of finally depositing waste products, is in the substantia nigra the visible sign of successful self-defense by the neuron against free radicals and quinones originating from dopamine metabolism. The sluggish depositing of neuromelanin in the human substantia nigra is in excellent agreement with this view. Graham [3] noticed that, until a patient is at least 6 years old, there is too insufficient an amount of neuromelanin in the substantia nigra to see it with the naked eye. With cytophotometry, Mann et al. [4] showed a linear increase in the pigmentation of the substantia nigra in man from 18 months to 60 years. Graham [5] calculated by morphometry that the volume of intraneuronal pigment increased linearly in direct relation to age. He found that the amount of pigment present in the eighth decade was twice that recorded in the fourth decade. Even if the accumulation of neuromelanin in the nigrostriatal dopaminergic neuron is only a corollary of age, and not a pathogenic factor in the process of aging, an excessive depositing of pigment granules with the passing of time may enhance the functional deterioration of the system.

Increasing amounts of data support the view that pigmentation is a real marker for physiological age. Munnel and Getty [6] found that the rate of lipofuscin accumulation in the heart of dogs is about 5.5 times faster than in man, which is proportional to the differences in their respective mean lifespan.

Sohal and Donato [7] analyzed the content of lipofuscin granules and the concentration of fluorescent material in the brain cells in two groups of houseflies kept in different temperatures. As metabolic rate and activity is temperature dependent, they compared low- and high-activity groups. The low-activity flies lived twice as long as the high-activity ones, and the rate of accumulation of lipofuscin was significantly slower in this group as compared to the short-lived, high-activity flies, but the maximal concentration of fluorescent material was similar in both groups, i.e. the short-lived, high-activity flies reached the maximal level much sooner than did the long-lived, low-activity group.

All these data seem to support Fridovich's [8] hypothesis which postulates that, in organisms with aerobic metabolism, oxygen is a source of incessant cellular damage because of the production of $^{\cdot}O_2^-$ and radicals derived of it, and the organisms survive only because of their ability to counteract the free radicals by the aid of superoxide dismutase (SOD) in the cells. The SOD activity of a previously described protein containing copper and zinc named erythrocuprein (hemocuprein) was discovered by McCord and Fridovich [9].

Be that as it may, conspicuous differences in the aging rates of different organs may depend on the balance between the activity-related generation of endogenous toxic products and the cellular mechanism which counters their damaging effect. Each system may have its own characteristic aging process which, when understood in detail, may suggest special pharmacological intervention in helping the system to maintain full activity for a longer duration. In the case of nigrostriatal dopaminergic neurons, the common view about special cytotoxic dopamine metabolites and free radicals being generally due to aerobic metabolism might be helpful for understanding the rapid aging of this system.

The aim of this chapter is to present an overview of the unique, complex pharmacological spectrum of (−)-deprenyl, and to explain 1) the basis for special uses of this drug in the therapy of PD and AD, and 2) why prophylactic maintenance with (−)-deprenyl (*l*-deprenyl, selegiline) from age 45 holds promises of a longer lifespan and an improved quality of life in the later decades.

2. The Pharmacological Profile of (−)-Deprenyl

2.1. Single Dose Effects

2.1.1. Selective inhibition of B-type MAO: B-type MAO is a predominantly glial enzyme found in the brain. The age-related loss of neurons and substitution by glial cells leads to significant increase in MAO-B activity and substantially contributes to the decline of brain dopaminergic activity with age. Thus, inhibition of MAO-B activity essentially works against this corollary of brain aging.

(−)-Deprenyl was the first selective inhibitor of B-type MAO to be described [10]. It is the internationally used reference substance for this purpose, and is still the only selective MAO-B inhibitor in clinical use. It also has a remarkably wide safety margin. In various species 0.17%− 0.36% of the subcutaneous LD_{50} irreversibly blocks MAO-B in the brain. Only very high doses of (−)-deprenyl block MAO-A [11]. In the rat, 0.25 mg/kg (−)-deprenyl s.c. is the standard dose for inhibiting MAO-B completely. In long-term experiments, this dose is administered three times a week for continuous maintenance of the blockade. In humans 10 mg (−)-deprenyl p.o. daily is the most widely used dosage to block MAO-B selectively; proof of effectiveness is the complete inhibition of platelet MAO, which is B-type.

(−)-Deprenyl, due entirely to the MAO-B inhibitory potency of the drug, protects the striatum of monkeys from the neurotoxic effect of MPTP [12].

The proposition that MAO-B should be inhibited in the aging brain from age 45 and, especially, in patients suffering from age-related neurodegenerative diseases, like PD and AD [13−17] is supported by two weighty physiological arguments:

1) The physiological role of dopamine in the striatum is the continuous inhibition of the firing rate of cholinergic interneurons in the caudate. This can be easily demonstrated in the rat striatum [18]. It is a peculiar anatomical situation that there is no synaptical contact between the end organs of the nigrostriatal dopaminergic neuron and the cholinergic interneurons. As a result, dopamine molecules flowing steadily from the nigrostriatal dopaminergic neurons slowly reach (by diffusion) their target. The chances of meeting glial MAO-B and being metabolized are good. The catalytic activity of MAO-B in the brain significantly increases with age, due to the loss of neurons and their substitution by glial cells (cf. 17). Thus, the less dopamine produced in the aging brain, the higher the risk of being metabolized by MAO-B prior to reaching the target. Hence, it follows that, with aging the dopamine-sparing effect of MAO-B inhibition is very necessary.

2) As phenylethylamine (PEA) is the most specific substrate for the enzyme MAO-B, inhibition of the latter increases the former, an endogenous amine (which is probably the most potent physiological psychostimulant in the human brain (cf. [19]) to its highest possible level.

2.1.2. Inhibition of the uptake of catecholamines and indirectly acting amines: (−)-Deprenyl inhibits the uptake of monoamines into the nerve endings of catecholaminergic neurons [10, 11, 19–23]. It interferes with the uptake of the catecholamine transmitters and the indirectly acting sympathomimetics, because it is handled by the catecholaminergic neurons similarly to the physiological substances transported through the axonal end organ and vesicular membranes. *The uniqueness of (−)-deprenyl lies in the fact that, in striking contrast to the indirectly acting amines, it does not displace the transmitter from the storage sites, i.e., it is not a releaser.* The net result is that (−)-deprenyl inhibits the releasing effect of tyramine. This most uncommon property for a MAO inhibitor (hence, its safe therapeutic use) explains why (−)-deprenyl, the first selective inhibitor of B-type MAO, is still the only such drug in clinical use.

It is of great practical importance that, in contrast to other MAO inhibitors in clinical use, (−)-deprenyl inhibits the uptake of tyramine. It is well known that the "cheese effect" [24] is the most serious potential side-effect of the MAO inhibitors in clinical use. This has limited the therapeutic use of MAO inhibitors, whose use requires rigorous dietary restrictions and careful monitoring. The pharmacological profile of (−)-deprenyl [11, 20, 22, 25] has clearly indicated that it is free of the "cheese effect". This claim was substantially supported by studies with tyramine in humans [26, 27] and later justified in Parkinson patients maintained on (−)-deprenyl for years (cf. [28]). Up to now, (−)-deprenyl is the only MAO inhibitor which has proved to be completely free of the "cheese effect" in clinical practice (see Chapters 6, 13).

It was demonstrated that not only non-selective and A-selective MAO inhibitors potentiated the effect of tyramine on vascular smooth muscle (as expected), but also selective inhibitors of MAO-B other than (−)-deprenyl exerted this effect [29–31].

2.2. Multiple-Dose Effects

2.2.1. Facilitation of scavenger function in the striatum: Regarding the production of toxic free radicals, the striatal system is an extremely (maybe the most) endangered part of the brain, for the following reasons: Dopamine cell bodies dominant in the A9 and A10 areas and, in the pars compacta of the substantia nigra, produce such large amounts of dopamine that the striatum, in which the neurons terminate, contains the highest amount of dopamine in the brain. The primary metabolic pathways by which dopamine is inactivated are through oxidative deamination and O-methylation catalyzed by MAO and catechol-O-methyltransferase (COMT), respectively. However from the point of view of age-related deterioration of the nigrostriatal dopaminergic neurons metabolites originating from catabolic pathways other than oxidative deamination and O-methylation might be of prime importance, because of their cytotoxic nature.

A minor catabolic pathway for dopa that leads to an indole derivative, dopachrom, was detected about 60 years ago. Among the intermediates leading to the indole-derivatives, the ringhydroxylated species
6-OH-dopa and 6-hydroxydopamine (6-OHDA), both generated *in vivo*,
are the most potent neurotoxins. The auto-oxidation of 6-OH-dopa and
6-OHDA leads to the genesis of the toxic free radicals, the superoxide
($\cdot O_2^-$) radical, the hydroxyl radical ($\cdot OH$), and to hydrogen peroxide
(H_2O_2). Conversely, dopa and dopamine are oxidized to quinones
which readily react with nucleophiles within the neuron and bind
irreversibly to proteins.

Studies with (−)-deprenyl showing the protection of the nigrostriatal
dopaminergic neurons from the toxic effects of 6-OHDA led to the
assumption that (−)-deprenyl may enhance the scavenger function in
these neurons [32]. To find direct evidence, we measured SOD activity
in the rat striatum. This enzyme is known to play a key role in the
detoxification of free radicals resulting from auto-oxidation of the
endogenous metabolites of dopamine. It has been demonstrated that the
daily administration of (−)-deprenyl for 3 weeks enhanced the activity
of SOD in the striatum of both male and female CFY rats in proportion
to the dose given [33, 34].

(−)-Deprenyl has no direct effect on brain SOD activity in general.
Using the cerebellum as a reference tissue, it was shown that the SOD
activity in this area did not change in a statistically significant manner
in (−)-deprenyl-treated male and female CFY rats [34].

The (−)-deprenyl-induced enhancement of the SOD activity in the
striatum of CFY rats was found to be unrelated to the MAO inhibitory
effects of the drug. Clorgyline, one of the most potent inhibitors of
MAO, inhibited rather than enhanced striatal SOD activity in rats
[33, 35].

The finding that (−)-deprenyl-treatment increases SOD activity in
the striatum of rats was recently confirmed by Carrillo et al. [36]; they
also found a significant increase in the catalase activity. Carrillo et al.
(unpublished observations) also corroborated our finding that (−)-
deprenyl selectively enhances scavenger function in the striatum. No
significant change in the SOD and catalase activity could be detected in
the hippocampus, which they used as a reference tissue.

To demonstrate the peculiar effect of (−)-deprenyl on SOD and
catalase activity in the striatum of rats the results of a new series of
experiments are shown in Tables 1 and 2.

Table 1 demonstrates that both a single 2 mg/kg dose of (−)-
deprenyl and the extremely large 10 mg/kg dose left the activity of SOD
and catalase in the striatum of male rats unchanged.

Table 2 shows that (in agreement with our earlier findings) the
administration of 2 mg/kg (−)-deprenyl daily for 21 days significantly
enhanced SOD activity in the striatum of the rats. In this series of

Table 1. The ineffectiveness of a single dose of (−)-deprenyl on SOD and catalase activity in the striatum of male rats.

Treatment	SOD activity (mean:units/mg protein ±S.E.M.)	Catalase activity ($\times 10^{-3}$) (mean: units/mg protein)
Saline 0.1 ml/100 g single injections s.c.	6.9±0.8	12.7±0.8
(−)-Deprenyl 2 mg/kg single injection s.c.; measurement of enzyme activity 1 h after injection	6.6±0.7	13.4±0.9
Saline 0.1 ml/100 g single injection s.c.	6.4±0.6	15.6 ± 0.8
(−)-Deprenyl 2 mg/kg single injection s.c.; measurement of enzyme activity 24 h after injection	6.1 ± 0.8	11.3 ± 0.7

SOD activity was measured according to Misra and Fridovich [37] and catalase activity according to Beers and Sizers [38] and expressed in Bergmeyer units.

Table 2. Significant enhancement of SOD and catalase activity in the striatum of (−)-deprenyl treated male rats and lack of a significant change in the activity of these enzymes in the Tuberculum olfactorium of the same animals.

Treatment	Tissue	SOD activity (mean:units/mg protein)	Catalase activity ($\times 10^{-3}$) (mean:units/mg protein)
Saline 0.1 ml/100 g injected s.c. daily for 21 days	Striatum Tuberculum olfactorium	15.5±0.3 12.8±0.4	16.0±0.6 18.1±0.7
(−)-Deprenyl 2 mg/kg injected s.c. daily for 21 days	Striatum Tuberculum olfactorium	29.3±0.2* 13.7±0.3	29.2±0.8* 22.3 ± 0.9

Brain samples were prepared 24 h after the last injection.
*$p < 0.01$ (Student's t-test for two means).
SOD activity was measured according to Misra and Fridovich [37] and catalase activity according to Beers and Sizers [38] and expressed in Bergmeyer units.

experiments also the catalase activity in the striatum was significantly higher than in the salt-solution-treated rats.

In contrast to the striatum, (−)-deprenyl treatment had no effect on the SOD activity in the tuberculum olfactorium, a component in the mesolimbic dopaminergic system. Even catalase activity did not change significantly in the tuberculum olfactorium, although the undeniable tendency of an enhanced catalase activity indicates the need for further analysis in this direction (see Chapter 9).

We may conclude that maintenance on (−)-deprenyl unequivocally enhances scavenger function in the striatum. The exact molecular mechanism of this peculiar effect, the development of which requires repeated administration of the drug for at least a few weeks, and which is obviously independent from the MAO and uptake inhibitory effect of (−)-deprenyl, awaits clarification.

2.2.2. Facilitation of the activity of the nigrostriatal dopaminergic neurons: Many years of continuous analysis of functional and biochemical changes in the brain of rats maintained on daily 0.25 mg/kg (−)-deprenyl for at least 21-day periods has furnished convincing evidence that this treatment facilitates the activity of the nigrostriatal dopaminergic neurons with high selectivity [15, 32–34]. This effect proved to be unrelated to both the MAO and dopamine uptake inhibitory effects of this drug. To illustrate the crucial importance of this component within the complex pharmacological spectrum of (−)-deprenyl, the following summarizes some conclusive experimental data.

1) The striata of rats treated with 0.25 mg-kg (−)-deprenyl daily for 3 weeks released significantly higher amounts of dopamine in the resting state and in response to stimulation than did the striata removed from rats treated daily with saline [39–41]. The striata were removed 24 h after the last injection of saline or (−)-deprenyl, respectively.

2) In complete agreement with the findings that (−)-deprenyl increases the firing rate of the nigrostriatal dopaminergic neurons are data proving the increased rate of utilization of dopamine in striatum of (−)-deprenyl-treated rats [14, 42]. According to these experiments (−)-deprenyl treatment induces a significant increase in the turnover rate of dopamine, due to the enhancement of the fractional rate constant of dopamine efflux and to the significant increase in the dopamine content. The facilitation of striatal dopaminergic neurotransmission by long-term treatment was found to be highly specific. With regard to noradrenaline, a significant decrease turnover rate and unchanged level of this amine in the brain stem was found [14, 42]. No change in the turnover rate of serotonin was detected in the raphe of rats treated daily with 0.25 mg/kg (−)-deprenyl for 2 weeks [43].

3) The physiological role of the nigrostriatal dopaminergic neurons in the striatum is the continuous inhibition of the firing rate of the

cholinergic interneurons in the caudate. It was shown by us (using the bioassay technique for measuring acetylcholine release from the caudate) that (−)-deprenyl inhibits the activity of the cholinergic interneurons in the striatum [11, 18]. This was clear evidence for an enhanced dopaminergic tone in the striatum of rats treated with (−)-deprenyl. A further support of this finding was given by turnover experiments showing that the outflow of acetylcholine is significantly decreased in the striata removed from rats pretreated with 0.25 mg/kg (−)-deprenyl daily for 2 weeks [32].

In the striatum taken from rats treated three times a week 0.25 mg/kg, s.c. (−)-deprenyl for weeks or months, a highly significant increase in stimulated release of dopamine was detected. This phenomenon deserves serious attention, as it is completely independent of the effects of (−)-deprenyl on MAO and monoamine uptake.

The nigrostriatal dopaminergic neuron in rats contain mainly MAO-A [11], which means that 0.25 mg/kg (−)-deprenyl cannot facilitate the activity of the nigrostriatal dopaminergic neurons via the inhibition of MAO. This is clearly shown by the data in Table 3. In these experiments we measured dopamine-release from the striatum in the presence of (−)-deprenyl or clorgyline in the bathing fluid. Clorgyline significantly increased the amount of dopamine released to stimulation, whereas (−)-deprenyl acted only in very high concentrations, at which it loses selectivity and starts to inhibit MAO-A.

In an other series of experiments we pretreated the rats with 0.25 mg/kg clorgyline and (−)-deprenyl, respectively, daily for 21 days and excised the striatum 24 h after the last injection. Table 4 shows the conspicuous difference in the effect of the two drugs. In the striatum taken from the clorgyline-treated rats the increase in the release of dopamine from the tissue to stimulation was the same as in the *in vitro* experiments, whereas (−)-deprenyl, which was ineffective *in vitro*, was much more potent *in vivo* than clorgyline.

Table 3. Dopamine release from isolated rat striata under the influence of (−)-deprenyl or clorgyline (*in vitro* drug effect).

Treatment µM		Resting release	20mM KCl-induced release
		pmol/g within 10 min (mean ± S.E.M.)	
Control		103 ± 8	188 ± 28
(−)-Deprenyl	5.0	102 ± 9	242 ± 31
	50.0	121 ± 7	$263 \pm 26^*$
Clorgyline	0.5	$135 \pm 16^*$	$305 \pm 34^*$
	2.5	$202 \pm 18^*$	$498 \pm 43^*$
	5.0	$216 \pm 24^*$	$607 \pm 64^*$

$n = 5$ $^*p < 0.05$ For methodological details see ref. [41]

Table 4. Dopamine release from isolated rat striata under the influence of (−)-deprenyl or clorgyline (*in vivo* drug effect).

	Resting release	20 mM KCl-induced release
Treatment	pmol/g within 10 min (mean ±S.E.M.)	
Control	112 ± 9	218 ± 29
(−)-Deprenyl	$494 \pm 51*$	$1588 \pm 123*$
Clorgyline	$416 \pm 47*$	$604 \pm 63*$

$n = 5$ *$p < 0.05$;
Drug treatment: 0.25 mg/kg s.c. daily for 21 days. Striata were removed 4 h after the last injection. For methodological details see ref. [41].

It is evident that the effect of clorgyline is due completely to the inhibition of MAO-A; the (−)-deprenyl-induced facilitation of the nigrostriatal dopaminergic neurons to stimulation, however, is independent of MAO inhibition. As the substantial increase in dopamine-release to stimulation in the striatum of a rat pretreated with (−)-deprenyl cannot be explained with MAO inhibition or with the inhibition of the uptake of dopamine, the conclusion is compelling that (−)-deprenyl exerts this physiologically most significant effect via an unknown mechanism, the elucidation of which is now in progress.

3. The Consequences of Long-Term, Small-Dose Administration of (−)-Deprenyl in Rats

From the analysis of the complex pharmacological spectrum of (−)-deprenyl, the conclusion can be drawn that the continuous administration of this drug works against the inevitable age-related decline of the activation mechanisms related to mesencephalic dopaminergic systems [34]. Experimental evidence to illustrate the essential consequences of long-term, small-dose (−)-deprenyl administration will be given in the following.

3.1. Effect on Sexual Behavior

Sexual activity of male rats is the subject of conspicuous age-related decline. We selected sexually active males, 25 weeks old, and followed their sexual performance in weekly mating tests. We measure quantitatively three patterns in the test: mounting, intromission, and ejaculation (for methodological details see [44]). To express in an exact manner the rate of the age-related decline of this function, we take, as an "end point", the total inability to ejaculate. According to our experiences, if

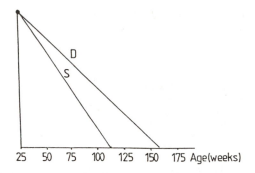

Figure 2. The graph shows the age-related decline of sexual potency in male CFY rats treated with saline or ($-$)-deprenyl, respectively, until they lost the ability to ejaculate. S = Saline-treated group (n = 45); D = ($-$)-deprenyl-treated group (n = 45); Mating test: once a week (each Tuesday); Saline (0.1 ml/100 g) or ($-$)-deprenyl (0.25 mg/kg) were administered subcutaneously each Monday, Wednesday, and Friday. Treatment started at the 25th week of age. "End point" was defined as loss of ability to ejaculate. The average was 112 ± 9 weeks in the saline-treated group (S), and 150 ± 12 weeks (p < 0.001) in the ($-$)-deprenyl-treated group (D).

this function is absent during 12 consecutive weeks, we may take it as the final loss of the ability to ejaculate. Figure 2 shows that long-term, small-dose ($-$)-deprenyl treatment significantly slows down age-related decline of sexual function in male rats. Whereas the saline-treated rats lost their ability to ejaculate within 112 ± 9 weeks, the ($-$)-deprenyl-treated animals did not reach that point of decline until 150 ± 12 weeks (p < 0.001).

3.2. Effect on Learning Capacity

In a series of experiments we followed the age-related changes in the learning ability of selected low performer rats (cf. [33]) testing them every three months in the shuttle box for 12 months. Performance was checked once daily during 5 consecutive days. Table 5 shows that remarkable difference between the salt-solution- and ($-$)-deprenyl-treated groups. ($-$)-Deprenyl treatment substantially improved the performance of the rats during the whole experiment. The effect of the drug in this test became increasingly accentuated with time. A significant improvement in the performance of the ($-$)-deprenyl-treated rats was only detectable after 6 months from the start.

In the salt-solution-treated rats there is an obvious tendency of an age-related decline in performance. In contrast, the ($-$)-deprenyl treated group did not show such a tendency and they performed better at the end than at the beginning of the experiment. The improvement in the performance of rats in the shuttle box (as shown in Table 5 and in previous papers [34, 45]) is further proof of the value of appropriate

Table 5. The effect of long-term (−)-deprenyl-treatment on the learning performance of male rats, selected as sexually inactive ones ("low performers") at an age of 8 months.

| | Total number of conditioned avoidance responses (CAR) (mean ± S.E.M.) | | | | |
| | Before treatment | After treatment for | | | |
		3 months	6 months	9 months	12 months
Saline-treated rats (n = 46)	6.53 ± 1.41	6.68 ± 1.32	6.02 ± 1.38	5.98 ± 1.15	5.05 ± 1.20
(−)-Deprenyl-treated rats (n = 48)	5.57 ± 0.56	6.12 ± 0.78	15.48 ± 1.02	20.73 ± 1.39	20.18 ± 1.29
Statistics: Student's t-test for two means	$p > 0.05$	$p > 0.05$	$p < 0.001$	$p < 0.001$	$p < 0.001$

Male rats which proved to be sexually inactive in four consecutive mating tests, when tested for the first time after completing their 8th month of age, were selected (n = 94). The rats were treated subcutaneously either with 0.1 ml/100 g saline or with 0.25 mg/kg (−)-deprenyl, three times a week for 12 months.
Performance in the shuttle box was tested every three months. Each rat was trained at 20 trials daily for 5 days. Unconditioned stimulus (US) = electric shock via the grid of the floor; conditioned stimulus (CS) = buzzer + light. Unconditioned avoidance response: the rat escapes US within 5 s; conditioned avoidance response (CAR): the rat escapes CS within 10 s. The rat's performance was rated according to the total number of CARs produced during the 5 days of training. Note: sexually "low performer" young rats were found to be low performers in the shuttle box (see ref. [33]).

learning tests in the rat for predicting the usefulness of (−)-deprenyl in humans. The results of the rat experiments are in harmony with the increasing amount of clinical data in Alzheimer's disease and prove the efficiency of (−)-deprenyl-treatment in improving the performance of patients [46–52].

3.3. Effect on Longevity

In long-term studies with male rats [33], it was demonstrated that high performer rats live longer than their low performer peers, and it was concluded that the performance of rats in behavioral tests, as well as the lifespan itself, are, to a large extent, a striatal dopamine-dependent function. Figure 3 shows that male rats treated with (−)-deprenyl lived significantly longer than their saline-treated peers, evidently because of the drug-induced protection against the age-related decline of brain functions. Milgram et al. [53], using the short-living Fischer 344 strain, confirmed recently that maintenance on (−)-deprenyl prolongs life in aged male rats. The (−)-deprenyl-treated animals showed a significant increase in both mean and maximum survival. They also

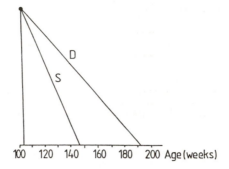

Figure 3. Mortality of male rats treated with saline and ($-$)-deprenyl, respectively. Sexually inexperienced male albino rate (first generation Wistar males × Logan females) were used. S = saline-treated group (n = 66); D = ($-$)-deprenyl-treated group (n = 66). Saline (0.1 ml/ 100 g) or ($-$)-deprenyl (0.25 mg/kg) were administered subcutaneously on Monday, Wednesday, and Friday. Treatment started after rats completed their 2nd year of age. "End point" was death, and was, on average, at 147 ± 0.56 weeks in the saline-treated (S) group, and 198 ± 2.36 weeks in the ($-$)-deprenyl-treated (D) group, (p < 0.001). (For details see ref. [33].)

analyzed the body weights and ruled out ($-$)-deprenyl-induced dietary restriction as an explanation for the group differences in survival. On the contrary, after about 4 months of treatment, the animals on ($-$)-deprenyl showed a slower rate of decrease in body weight than did controls.

4. The Consequences of Long-Term Administration of ($-$)-Deprenyl in Parkinson's Disease and Alzheimer's Disease

From the analysis of the complex pharmacological spectrum of ($-$)-deprenyl the conclusion can be drawn that the continuous administration of this drug works against the inevitable age-related decline of the activation mechanisms related to mesencephalic systems.

4.1. Parkinson's Disease

The remarkable specificity of ($-$)-deprenyl to the striatal system predicts the special value of this drug in PD. The effectiveness of ($-$)-deprenyl treatment in PD is convincing proof that the effects of ($-$)-deprenyl in humans are essentially similar to the ones found in our rat experiments. In support of this view, clinical studies of remarkable importance were published [54–57].

Tetrud and Langston [56] followed 51 patients from first diagnosis of PD and determined the average elapsed time until these patients needed levodopa. Figure 4A shows that, in comparison to the placebo-treated

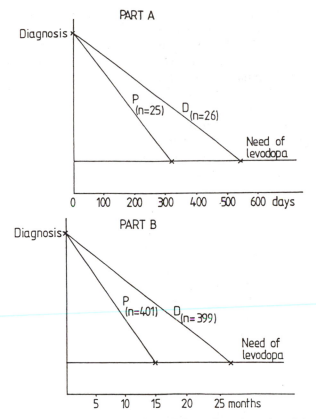

Figure 4. The rate of deterioration from time of diagnosis to time of need for levodopa in placebo (P)- and in (−)-deprenyl (D)-treated patients with PD. Part A: Based on the study performed by Tetrud and Langston [56]. Part B: Based on the Parkinson Study Group's findings [57].

patients (n = 25), (−)-deprenyl administration (n = 26) significantly delayed the start of the necessary levodopa therapy.

The Parkinson Study Group [57] made a similar analysis of 800 recently diagnosed patients and found that patients on (−)-deprenyl (n = 339) needed levodopa significantly later than did their placebo-treated peers (n = 401). The results are illustrated in a synoptical manner in Figure 4B (see Chapters 13, 15).

It is evident that, for technical reasons, it is an almost impossible task to measure exactly in humans the (−)-deprenyl-induced putative shift in the time of death due to natural causes. The age-related deterioration of the striatal dopaminergic system is, however, a continuum; any precisely determinable short period of the process would be sufficient to measure the rate of the functional decline in the system. Such an opportunity presents itself in those individuals who develop PD. A reasonably short period elapses from the appearance of the symptoms (diagnosis) to the need for levodopa; this can be measured with considerable accuracy. The difference in the rate of deterioration of the nigrostriatal dopaminergic neurons between placebo- and (−)-deprenyl-treated humans is therefore comparable in freshly diagnosed patients. Thus, the outcome of the two studies [56, 57] indicates that (−)-deprenyl treatment is capable of slowing down the rate of deterioration of the striatal dopaminergic system in humans. These findings are in perfect agreement with the result of our retrospective analysis regarding the survival of patients treated with Madopar® alone (n = 377) and with Madopar plus (−)-deprenyl (n = 564). Combined treatment prolonged the survival of patients [54, 55] (see Chapter 13).

4.2. Alzheimer's Disease

(−)-Deprenyl-treatment also exerts a significant beneficial effect in AD, which was first reported by Tariot et al. [46] and Martini et al. [49], and confirmed in a number of papers [47, 48, 50–53]. This very important clinical effect of (−)-deprenyl is further proof of the great value of rat experiments in predicting the usefulness of (−)-deprenyl in humans (see Chapter 16).

5. Morphological Evidence that Long-Term, Small-Dose (−)-Deprenyl Treatment Counters Age-Related Changes in the Neurocytes of the Substantia Nigra

The previously summarized data furnished evidence that maintenance on (−)-deprenyl enhances the activity of the nigrostriatal dopaminergic neurons in rats, protects against the age-related decline of striatal dopamine-dependent behavioral functions, and extends life span. The beneficial effect of (−)-deprenyl-treatment in PD and AD proved to be in harmony with the animal data.

It remained to be proved morphologically, however, that (−)-deprenyl protects against the aging of the nigrostriatal dopaminergic neurons. We developed a method, using a TV-image analyzer, to compare different morphological parameters in the substantia nigra of young and old male rats [58].

Twelve untreated male rats (6 aged 3 months and 6 aged 3 years) were used. Their substantia nigra was removed, fixed in buffered formalin, and embedded in paraffin. Two-micro-thick serial sections were cut and stained with combined Ag-Fe-cyan reaction. Sections were studied by a Robotron TV-image analyzer. The image from a Jenaval light microscope (100× magnification; 1, 3, 5 projective; orange filter) was digitalized by a videocamera and stored as points (512 × 512 pixels) by a PDP11 microcomputer. In this system 1 pixel corresponded to 1 mμ. The TV-image analyzer was able to differentiate 64 gray levels and 20 object features.

In the AMBA/R-med system the light microscopic picture was projected by the videocamera onto the display. After fixation, the gray points relative to background were measured row by row. In our program the neurocytes were framed by blue color using a trackball. Within the framed area the system searched for the darkest points, which we accepted by pressing a key. The system covered the selected object with red color. This guaranteed that the selected area had been measured and its area (ACON), sum of the gray values (SEXT), Nm (number of neuromelanin granules in the neurocyte), COMP (compactivity), HEXT (relative hole area within a circumscribed object) had been stored in the data files.

From each animal three sections with the same area were selected; a total of 3477 cells was measured. Cells with and without melanin content were marked by different symbols.

In neurocytes with melanin content our computer program measured the area of melanin granules (ACON), the sum of their gray values (SEXT), the relative hole area within the framed area (HEXT), and compactness (COMP). The latter two served for characterization controls. Sections showing 50% of the cells to contain HEXT values higher than 0 and COMP values less than 500 were excluded from the evaluation. However, neurocytes with COMP values under 500 and HEXT values higher than 0 were considered to be "empty" cells. The computer program recorded the number of melanin granules (Nm). Table 6 shows the measured and calculated features. Results were analyzed by Kolmogorov-Smirnow 2-sample test (SPSS package, SPSS Inc., Chicago).

In contrast to our expectations, the analysis of our data revealed that, with regard to the cell numbers, the identical areas did not differ significantly from each other in the sections of young and old animals. Also unexpectedly, the difference in the proportions of neurocytes with and without melanin did not differ statistically significantly in the two age cohorts (although the tendency of the presence of higher percentage of melanin-containing neurocytes in the old animals was obvious). In the substantia nigra of 3-year-old rats 65.1% of neurocytes (1219) contained melanin and 34.8% (652) showed "empty" cytoplasm. In the 3-month-old rats a total of 1606 neurocytes was measured, of which 773 (48.1%) contained melanin and 833 (51.8%) were empty.

The Kolmogorov-Smirnow 2-sample test revealed the homogeneity of measured features of the young and old animals. Table 6 demonstrates the highly significant differences in the measured and calculated features of the two age cohorts. In the neurocytes of 3-year-old animals melanin granules were less in number, mean: 1.763, compared to the young ones,

Table 6. Comparison of the morphological characteristics of neuromelanin in 3-month-old and 3-year-old male rats by TV-image analyzer. Results were analyzed by the Kolmogorov-Smirnow (K-S Z) 2-sample test.

N	Young rats 773		Old rats 652			
	Mean	SD	Mean	SD	K-S Z	P
Nm	2.621	1.461	1.763	0.861	5.608	0.0001
ACON	130.169	93.994	193.441	81.590	7.843	0.0001
SEXT	154.132	102.984	193.135	91.503	6.242	0.0001
MACON	49.180	18.758	116.306	29.508	13.872	0.0001
MSEXT	1.268	0.332	0.992	0.161	9.966	0.0001
ASEXT	0.709	0.535	0.693	0.317	4.304	0.0001

Measured features:
Nm: number of granules in a neurocyte; ACON area of the granules; SEXT: sum of gray values.
Calculated features:
MACON: area of one granule in a neurocyte; MSEXT: average of gray values; ASEXT: average gray value of one granule; SD: standard deviation.

mean: 2.621 (p < 0.0001). When the area of one melanin granule (MA-CON) was considered the two groups showed a significant difference; the area in the old animals was found to be 116.306 and that of the young males 49.180 mμ^2 (p < 0.0001).

SEXT, MSEXT, ASEXT, i.e. density features, showed fairly similar changes to the total area and area of one granule in the neurocyte.

Thus, we may conclude that aging of nigrostriatal dopaminergic neurons in male rats is not characterized by a significant loss of cells, but there is a highly significant age-related change in the morphological features of neuromelanin granules within the neurocytes. The majority of the neurocytes in the young rats contains a high number of small sized, evenly distributed pigment granules. The majority of the neurocytes of the old rats, however, contains a lower number of large sized, rough, unevenly distributed neuromelanin granules.

The statistically significant age-related morphological differences disclosed by the TV-image analyzer allowed us to check how long-term, small-dose administration of (−)-deprenyl influences the age-related morphological changes of the pigment granules in the neurocytes of the substantia nigra [59].

Experiments were carried out with 9 rats divided into 3 groups, 3 in each. There were two control groups, a young one and an old one. The young animals were 3-month-old naive males. The old males were treated with saline (0.1 ml/100 g), subcutaneously, three times a week; and served as controls to drug-treated males. (−)-Deprenyl was administered similarly in a dose of 0.25 mg/kg. Treatments started with 3-month-old males and the animals were treated continuously for 18 months before the substantia nigra was removed for our morphological studies. A total of 3828 cells was measured and the results were analyzed by the Kolmogorov-Smirnow 2-sample test.

This test proved the homogeneity of the measured features within the young and old control and treated groups [59]. The drug-treated group did not show statistically significant differences in cell number and in the ratio of pigmented and "empty" cells. In the young control rats 52.2% of the neurocytes were empty. The corresponding values in the treated groups were 51.1% and 49.8%.

A comparison of young and old control groups also revealed significant differences in this series of experiments in number, area (total area of granules and area of one granule) and density features: sum and

Table 7. Comparison of the morphological characteristics of neuromelanin in untreated 3-month-old (young control) and 21-month-old male rats, treated with saline (old control) or 0.25 mg/kg (−)-deprenyl, three times a week for 18 months

Results of Kolmogorov-Smirnow 2-sample test (K-S Z)

	Young control rats (n = 473)		Old control rats (n = 481)		K-S Z	P
	Mean	SD	Mean	SD		
Nm	1.994	1.104	1.696	0.924	1.896	0.002
ACON	77.973	60.027	133.909	105.118	5.164	0.0001
SEXT	82.233	63.076	134.075	102.893	5.099	0.0001
MACON	39.632	24.966	74.932	30.602	9.395	0.0001
MSEXT	1.071	0.172	1.016	0.093	4.252	0.0001
ASEXT	0.696	0.354	0.744	0.312	2.782	0.0001

	Young control (n = 473)		(−)-Deprenyl treated group rats (n = 503)		K-S Z	P
	Mean	SD	Mean	SD		
Nm	1.994	1.104	2.032	1.123	0.540	0.932
ACON	77.973	60.027	81.964	63.542	0.992	0.278
SEXT	82.233	63.076	82.761	57.326	1.103	0.175
MACON	39.632	24.966	39.820	19.617	1.267	0.081
MSEXT	1.071	0.172	1.095	0.280	1.728	0.005
ASEXT	0.696	0.354	0.718	0.418	1.026	0.243

	Old control (n = 481)		(−)-Deprenyl treated group rats (n = 503)		K-S Z	P
	Mean	SD	Mean	SD		
Nm	1.696	0.924	2.032	1.123	2.121	0.0001
ACON	133.909	105.118	81.964	63.542	4.728	0.0001
SEXT	134.075	102.893	82.761	57.326	4.390	0.0001
MACON	74.932	30.602	39.820	19.617	8.789	0.0001
MSEXT	1.016	0.093	1.095	0.280	4.548	0.0001
ASEXT	0.744	0.312	0.718	0.418	2.813	0.0001

For abbreviation of measured and calculated features see Table 6.

average of the gray values and average gray value of one pigment granule (p < 0.002). For example, the mean area of the pigment granule changed from 39.63 in the young animals to 74.93 mμ² in the old ones. *(−)-Deprenyl treatment completely prevented age-related morphological change (Table 7).* The mean area of one granule (MACON) in the deprenyl-treated group was found to be 39.83, whereas in the saline-treated group it increased to 74.93 mμ². *This is the first morphological evidence that long-term, small-dose (−)-deprenyl treatment prevents age-related changes in the nigrostriatal dopaminergic neurons.*

Rinne et al. [60] recently found that the number of medial nigral neurons was greater and the number of Lewy bodies fewer in those PD patients who had been treated with (−)-deprenyl in combination with levodopa, as compared with patients who had received levodopa alone. To attribute this change to the reduction of levodopa dosage in deprenyl-treated patients is, in light of our morphological studies, highly improbable. The most plausible explanation is that (−)-deprenyl treatment retards death of nigral neurons in patients.

6. Strategy to Counter Age-Related Decline of the Striatal Dopaminergic System by (−)-Deprenyl-Administration

The proposal (based on animal studies [13–17]) to use in humans, from age 45, small amounts of (−)-deprenyl (2–3 tablets per week) for slowing down the normal rate of decline of the striatal dopaminergic system seems to be substantially supported by experiments with (−)-deprenyl during the last decade. Regarding the consequences of the

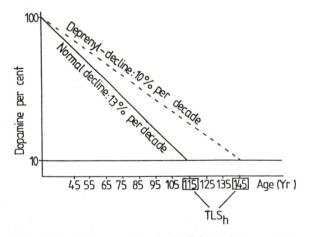

Figure 5. Graph illustrating that even undervalued, slight, (−)-deprenyl-induced changes in the rate of deterioration of the striatal dopaminergic system might considerably delay natural death and increase human "technical life span" (TLS$_h$).

protective effect of (−)-deprenyl in healthy humans against the age-related deterioration of the striatal dopaminergic system it is worth considering that just a small change in the rate of decline, e.g., from 13% per decade to 10% per decade, anticipates (as visualized in Figure 5) at least a 15-year extension in average lifespan (TLS$_h$), which is now estimated to be 115–120 years. Preventive (−)-deprenyl medication may also retard the precipitation of PD and AD in the endangered population. Considering the safeness of (−)-deprenyl and the advantageous risk-benefit ratio, we can only gain by trying to fight against the natural aging process of our striatal dopaminergic system with prophylactic (−)-deprenyl medication. In addition, in the case of the slightest signs of PD or AD, it is advisable to administer 10 mg (−)-deprenyl per day until death, irrespective of other therapies.

7. Outlook

Regarding the future of (−)-deprenyl research, it is hoped that elucidation of the molecular mechanisms of those selective actions of the drug on the nigrostriatal dopaminergic neurons (i.e. those that require long-term administration of the compound) will be useful to counteract brain aging thereby improving quality of life in the later decades of life and delaying natural death.

Summary

The drug (−)-deprenyl, a close structural relative to phenylethylamine, exhibits a unique pharmacological spectrum. Regarding its single-dose effects: 1) it is a highly potent and selective inhibitor of MAO-B, and 2) in striking contrast to MAO inhibitors, (−)-deprenyl inhibits the effect of tyramine, thus, it is free of the "cheese effect". Regarding its multiple-dose effects: 1) it facilitates, with considerable selectivity, the activity of the nigrostriatal dopaminergic neurons; 2) it selectively enhances superoxide dismutase and catalase activity in the striatum; and 3) it prevents age-related neuromelanin changes in the neurocytes of the substantia nigra.

References

[1] Birkmayer W, Riederer P. Parkinson's disease: Biochemistry, clinical pathology and treatment. Wien: Springer Verlag, 1983: 194.
[2] Martilla R. Epidemiological, clinical and virus-serological studies of Parkinson's disease [thesis]. Reports from the Dept. of Neurology. Univ. of Turku, Finland 1974.
[3] Graham DG. Oxidative pathways for catecholamines in the genesis of neuromelanin and cytotoxic quinones. Molec. Pharmacol. 1978; 14: 333–343.

[4] Mann DMA, Yates PO, Barton CM. Neuromelanin and RNA in cells of substantia nigra. J. Neuropathol. Exp. Neurol. 1977; 36: 379–83.

[5] Graham DG. On the origin and significance of neuromelanin. Arch. Pathol. Lab. Med. 1979; 103: 359–62.

[6] Munnel JF, Getty R. Rate of accumulation of cardiac lipofuscin in the aging canine. J. Gerontol. 1968; 23: 145–58.

[7] Sohal RS, Donato H. Effect of experimental prolongation of life span on lipofuscin content and lyposomal enzyme activity in the brain of the housefly, Musca domestica. J. Gerontol. 1979; 34: 489–96.

[8] Fridovich I. Superoxide dismutase. Advanc. Enzymol. 1974; 41: 35–97.

[9] McCord JA, Fridovich I. Superoxide dismutase. An enzymic action of erythrocuprein (heamocuprein). J. Biol. Chem. 1969; 224: 6049–55.

[10] Knoll J, Magyar K. Some puzzling pharmacological effects of monoamine oxidase inhibitors. Adv. Biochem. Psychopharmacol. 1972; 5: 393–08.

[11] Knoll J. The possible mechanism of action of (−)-deprenyl in Parkinson's disease. J. Neural Transm. 1978; 43: 177–98.

[12] Cohen G, Pasik P, Cohen B, Leist A, Mytilineou G, Jahr MD. Pargyline and (−)-deprenyl prevent the neurotoxicity of 1-methyl-4-phenyl-1,2,3,6-tetrahydropyridine (MPTP) in monkeys. Eur. J. Pharmacol. 1984; 106: 209–10.

[13] Knoll J. The pharmacology of selective MAO inhibitors. In: Youdim MBH, Paykel ES, editors. Monoamine oxidase inhibitors. The state of the art. London: Wiley J, 1981: 45–61.

[14] Knoll J. Selective inhibition of B-type monoamine oxidase in the brain: A drug strategy to improve the quality of life in senescence. In: Keverling-Buismann JA, editor. Strategy in drug research. Amsterdam: Elsevier, 1982: 107–35.

[15] Knoll J. (−)-Deprenyl (selegiline): the history of its development and pharmacological action. Acta Neurol. Scand. Suppl. 1983; 95: 57–80.

[16] Knoll J. The facilitation of dopaminergic activity in the aged brain by (−)-deprenyl. A proposal for a strategy to improve the quality of life in senescence. Mech. Ageing. Dev. 1985; 30: 109–22.

[17] Knoll J. Striatal dopamine, aging and (−)-deprenyl. In: Borsy J, Kerecsen L, György L, editors. Dopamine, ageing and diseases. Budapest: Akadémiai Kiadó, New York: Pergamon Press 1986: 7–26.

[18] Harsing LG Jr, Magyar K, Tekes K, Vizi ES, Knoll J. Inhibition by (−)-deprenyl of dopamine uptake in rat striatum: a possible correlation between dopamine uptake and acetylcholine release inhibition. Pol. J. Pharmacol. Pharm. 1979; 31: 297–07.

[19] Knoll J. Analysis of the pharmacological effects of selective monoamine oxidase inhibitors. In: Wolstenholme GES, Knight J, editors. Monoamine oxidase and its inhibition. Ciba foundation Symposium 39 (new series). Amsterdam: Elsevier 1976: 135–61.

[20] Knoll J, Vizi ES, Somogyi G. Phenylisopropylmethylpropylamine (E-250), a monoamine oxidase inhibitor antagonizing the effects of tyramine. Arzneimittel-Forschung 1968; 18: 109–12.

[21] Knoll J. On the dual nature of monoamine oxidase. Horizons Biochem. Biophys. 1978; 5: 37–64.

[22] Knoll J. The pharmacology of selective irreversible monoamine oxidase inhibitors. In: Seiler N, Jung M, Koch-Weser J, editors. Enzyme-activated irreversible inhibitors. Amsterdam: Elsevier 1978: 253–69.

[23] Knoll J. Monoamine oxidase inhibitors: chemistry and pharmacology. In: Sandler M, editor. Enzyme inhibitors as drugs. London: McMillan Press Ltd 1980: 151–71.

[24] Blackwell B. Hypertensive crisis due to monoamine oxidase inhibitors. Lancet 1963; ii: 849–51.

[25] Harsing LG Ir, Tekes K, Magyar K, Vizi ES, Knoll J. Deprenyl inhibits dopamine uptake in the rat striatum in vivo. In: Magyar K, editor. Monoamine oxidase and their selective inhibition. Budapest: Akadémiai Kiadó, New York: Pergamon Press 1979: 45–56.

[26] Elsworth JD, Glover V, Reynolds GP, Sandler M, Lees AJ, Phuapradit P, et al. (−)-Deprenyl administration in man: A selective monoamine oxidase B inhibitor without the "cheese effect". Psychopharmacology 1978; 57: 33–78.

[27] Sandler M, Glover V, Ashford A, Stern G. Absence of "cheese effect" during (−)-deprenyl therapy: some recent studies. J Neurol. Transm. 1978; 43: 209–14.
[28] Knoll J. Critical role of MAO inhibition of Parkinson's disease. Advances in Neurology 1986; 45: 107–10.
[29] Knoll J. The pharmacology of (−)-deprenyl. J. Neurol. Transm. Suppl. 1986; 22: 75–89.
[30] Abdorubo A, Knoll J. The effect of various MAO-B inhibitors on rabbit arterial strip response to tyramine. Pol. J. Pharmacol. Pharm. 1988; 40: 673–83.
[31] Abdorubo A. The effect of various monoamine oxidase (MAO) inhibitors on the response of blood pressure of rats and cats to tyramine. Acta Physiol. Hung. 1990; 75: 321–346.
[32] Knoll J. R-(−)-Deprenyl (Selegiline, Movergan[R]) facilitates the activity of the nigrostriatal dopaminergic neuron. J. Neural. Transm., Suppl. 1987; 25: 45–66.
[33] Knoll J. The striatal dopamine dependency of life span in male rats. Longevity study with (−)-deprenyl. Mech. Ageing Dev. 1988; 46: 237–62.
[34] Knoll J. The pharmacology of selegiline ((−)-deprenyl). New aspects. Acta Neurol. Scand. 1989; 126: 83–91.
[35] Knoll J. Nigrostriatal dopaminergic activity, (−)-deprenyl treatment, and longevity. Adv. Neurology 1990; 53: 425–9.
[36] Carrillo MC, Kanai S, Nokubo M, Kitani K. (−)-Deprenyl induced activities of both superoxide dismutase and catalase but not of glutathione peroxidase in the striatum of young male rats. Life Sci. 1991; 48: 517–21.
[37] Misra HP, Fridovich J. The role of superoxide anion in the autooxidation of epinephrine and a simple assay for superoxide dismutase. J. Biol. Chem. 1972; 247: 3170–75.
[38] Beers RF Jr, Sizer IW. Spectrophotometry for measuring the breakdown of hydrogen peroxidase by catalase. J. Biol. Chem. 1952; 195: 133–40.
[39] Knoll J. Medikamentöse Strategie zur Verbesserung der Lebensqualität in der Seneszenz. Wiener Med. Wschr. 1986; 136: [Suppl.] 3–18.
[40] Knoll J. Role of B-type monoamine oxidase inhibition in the treatment of Parkinson's disease. An uptake. In: Shah NS, Donald AG, editors. Movement disorders. New York: Plenum Press 1986: 53–81.
[41] Kerecsen L, Kalász H, Knoll J. (−)-Deprenyl enhanced dopamine release from isolated striatal preparations of the rat following chronic treatment. In: Borsy J, Kerecsen L, György L, editors. Dopamine, ageing and diseases. Budapest: Akadémiai Kiadó, New York: Pergamon Press 1986: 27–33.
[42] Zsilla G, Knoll J. The action of (−)-deprenyl on monoamine turnover rate in rat brain. Adv. Biochem. Psychopharmacol. 1982; 31: 211–17.
[43] Zsilla G, Földi P, Held Gy, Székely AM, Knoll J. The effect of repeated doses of (−)-deprenyl on the dynamics of monoaminergic transmission. Comparison with clorgyline. Pol. J. Pharmacol. Pharm. 1986; 38: 57–67.
[44] Knoll J, Yen TT, Dalló J. Long-lasting, true aphrodisiac effect of (−)-deprenyl in sexually sluggish old male rats. Mod. Probl. Pharmacopsychiat. 1983; 19: 135–53.
[45] Knoll J. Some clinical implications of MAO-B inhibition. In: Yasuhara H, Parvez SH, Sandler M, Oguchi K, Nagatsu T, editors. Monoamine Oxidase: Basic and clinical aspects. Holland: VPS Press. In press.
[46] Tariot PN, Cohen RM, Sunderland T. Newhouse PA, Yount D, Mellow AM, et at. l-Deprenyl in Alzheimer's disease. Arch. Gen. Psychiatry 1987; 44: 427–433.
[47] Tariot PN, Sunderland T, Weingartner H, Murphy DL, Welkovitz JA, Thompson K, et al. Cognitive effect of l-deprenyl in Alzheimer disease. Psychopharmacology 1987; 91: 489–95.
[48] Tariot PN, Sunderland T, Cohen RM, Newhouse PA, Mueller EA, Murphy DL. Tranylcypromine compared with l-deprenyl in Alzheimer disease. J. Clin. Pschopharmacol. 1988; 8: 23–7.
[49] Martini E, Pataky J, Szilágyi K, Venter V. Brief information on an early phase-II study with (−)-deprenyl in demented patients. Pharmacopsychiatry 1987; 20: 256–7.
[50] Piccinin GL, Finali GC, Piccirilli M. Neuropsychological effects of l-deprenyl in Alzheimer's type dementia. Clin. Neuropharmacol. 1990; 13: 147–63.
[51] Mangoni A, Grassi MP, Frattola L, Piolti R, Bassi S, Motta A, et al. Effects of MAO-B inhibitor in the treatment of Alzheimer disease. Eur. Neurol. 1991; 31: 100–7.
[52] Goad DL, Davis CM, Leim P, Fuselier CC, McCormack JR, Olsen KM. The use of selegiline in Alzheimer's patients with behavior problems. J. Clin. Psychiatry 1991; 53: 342–45.

[53] Milgram NW, Racine RJ, Nellis P, Mendoca A, Ivy G. Maintenance on *l*-deprenyl prolongs life in aged male rats. Life Sci. 1990; 47: 415–20.

[54] Birkmayer W, Knoll J, Riederer P, Youdim MBH. (−)-Deprenyl leads to prolongation of L-dopa efficacy in Parkinson's disease. Mod. Probl. Pharmacopsychiatry 1983; 19: 170–6.

[55] Birkmayer W, Knoll J, Riederer P, Youdim MBH, Hars V, Marton J. Increased life expectancy resulting from addition of *l*-deprenyl to Madopar® treatment in Parkinson's disease: a long-term study. J. Neural Transm. 1985; 64: 133–137.

[56] Tetrud JW, Langston JW. The effect of (−)-deprenyl (selegiline) on the natural history of Parkinson's disease. Science 1989; 245: 519–22.

[57] Parkinson Study Group. Effect of (−)-deprenyl in the progression of disability in early Parkinson's disease. New England Journal of Medicine 1989; 321: 1364–71.

[58] Tóth V, Kummert M, Sugár J, Knoll J. A procedure for measuring neuromelanin in neurocytes by a TV-image analyser. Mech. Ageing Dev. 1992; 63: 215–221.

[59] Knoll J, Tóth V, Kummert M, Sugár J. (−)-Deprenyl and (−)-parafluorodeprenyl-treatment prevents age-related pigment changes in substantia nigra. A TV-image analysis of neuromelanin. Mech. Ageing Dev. 1992; 63: 157–163.

[60] Rinne JO, Röyttä M, Paljärvi L, Rummukainen J, Rinne UK. Selegiline (deprenyl) treatment and death of nigral neurons in Parkinson's disease. Neurology 1991; 41: 859–61.

Inhibitors of Monoamine Oxidase B
Pharmacology and Clinical Use in Neurodegenerative Disorders
ed. by I. Szelenyi
© 1993 Birkhäuser Verlag Basel/Switzerland

CHAPTER 8
Neurotoxins and Monoamine Oxidase B Inhibitors: Possible Mechanisms for the Neuroprotective Effect of (−)-Deprenyl

V. Glover and M. Sandler

1   Introduction
2   Neuroprotective Effects of (−)-Deprenyl
3   How Might (−)-Deprenyl Effect Neuroprotection?
3.1   Inhibition of MAO B: Effect on Substrates
3.2   Inhibition of MAO B: Effect on Toxins
3.3   Inhibition of MAO B: Effect on H_2O_2 Generation
3.4   Other Direct Actions of (−)-Deprenyl
3.5   Effect of (−)-Deprenyl on SOD Induction
4   Conclusion
        Summary
        References

1. Introduction

The 1-methyl-4-phenyl-1,2,3,6-tetrahydropyridine (MPTP) [1–3] model of Parkinson's disease, which came to light by the accidental self-administration of this protoxin by a group of American drug addicts, has stimulated an enormous amount of research and speculation into the cause of this disorder and the possible role of endo- or exotoxins in its pathogenesis. The fact that (−)-deprenyl (selegiline), the selective monoamine oxidase (MAO) B inhibitor, both prevents the development of MPTP toxicity [4, 5] and appears to slow degeneration of the nigrostriatal tract in human idiopathic paralysis agitans has lent support to the idea that analogous toxins may be responsible for Parkinson's disease (PD). They may well be, although there is no convincing evidence for this conclusion at the present time. However, other explanations for the putative neuroprotective effects of (−)-deprenyl are also possible and will be discussed in this chapter.

2. Neuroprotective Effects of (−)-Deprenyl

The first indication that (−)-deprenyl might be neuroprotective came from Birkmayer and colleagues [6]. In a retrospective study, they evaluated the effect of 9 years of treatment in patients receiving Madopar® plus (−)-deprenyl, compared with those taking Madopar alone. The former lived significantly longer. More recently, Tetrud and Langston [7] carried out a small, prospective, double-blind trial on early parkinsonians, comparing (−)-deprenyl with placebo. (−)-Deprenyl delayed the need for L-dopa therapy, and appeared to slow down the disease's progression, as judged from assessments after a 1-month wash-out period.

The largest human study to date has been the DATATOP trial [8], in which 400 patients were given 10 mg of (−)-deprenyl per day and were compared in double-blind fashion with matched controls on placebo. The (−)-deprenyl group reached a predetermined end-point, the need to begin L-dopa therapy, significantly more slowly than patients on placebo. This study has been criticized, predominantly on the grounds that the 1-month wash-out period employed may have been insufficient so that the symptomatic effects of (−)-deprenyl itself may still have been apparent [9]. However, available evidence suggests that the bio-chemical effects of (−)-deprenyl disappear rapidly after cessation of the drug: a 10-mg dose resulted in a 20- to 90-fold rise in output of urinary phenylethylamine (a specific MAO B substrate), which dropped to normal excretion values within a few days of drug withdrawal, and did so more rapidly than the reestablishment of platelet MAO activity [10]. This observation suggests that 1 month should be more than adequate as a wash-out period. The question of whether (−)-deprenyl truly confers neuroprotection might well be settled by employing longitudinal Gompertzian analysis, a relatively "simple method of detecting and distinguishing between symptomatic (competitive) and protective (in-trinsic and environmental) influences on disease mortality at the popula-tion level after the introduction of new therapies" [11].

Rinne and coworkers [12] have studied the effect of (−)-deprenyl treatment on postmortem neuroanatomy of the nigrostriatal tract. The number of medial nigral neurons was greater and the number of Lewy bodies smaller in patients taking (−)-deprenyl in addition to L-dopa, compared with an L-dopa-alone group. This finding would be com-patible with (−)-deprenyl having a neuroprotective action on nigral neurons. Consequently, the patients treated with (−)-deprenyl also received less L-dopa, so that the results might be interpreted in terms of a reduction in the toxic effects of L-dopa or its metabolites. This study also had the disadvantage of being retrospective.

Other evidence supporting a possible neuroprotective effect of (−)-deprenyl comes from animal studies. Knoll and colleagues [13] reported that (−)-deprenyl (0.25 mg/kg s.c., three times weekly) extends the mean lifespan of rats from 147 weeks to 192. The mean lifespan of treated animals was greater than the longest lived of the untreated group, 182 weeks. It is very rare for a therapeutic regimen to extend lifespan, as opposed to average life expectancy, and this is a remarkable claim. Following this claim, Milgram et al. [14] also examined the effect of the drug on rat longevity and found, similarly, that (−)-deprenyl-treated animals showed a significant increase in both mean and maximum survival time. The findings (in a different rat strain) were less dramatic than in the Knoll study, with a moderate increase in mean survival time from the start of the experiment from 115 to 134 days. This work is clearly of considerable potential significance, but needs further confirmation to establish the findings beyond reasonable doubt.

(−)-Deprenyl is known to provide protection against the dopaminergic neuronal toxin, 6-hydroxydopamine (6-OHDA) [15]. In addition, Finnegan et al. [16] have shown that (−)-deprenyl (10 mg/kg i.p.) protects mice against DSP-4, a neurotoxin which selectively causes degeneration of CNS noradrenergic fibres. This action is independent of MAO B inhibition, because the highly selective MAO B inhibitor, MDL 72974, failed to act in a similar manner. However, it is important to note that both 6-OHDA and DSP-4 are monoamines, whilst an additional property of (−)-deprenyl is to inhibit amine uptake [15]. Thus, the apparent neuroprotective ability of (−)-deprenyl against these particular compounds may lie in its property of preventing access of toxin to neuron. In other studies, (−)-deprenyl seemed to be more truly neuroprotective. Tatton and Greenwood [17] have used the mouse MPTP model to show that (−)-deprenyl (either 0.25 or 10 mg/kg) administered 3 days after the last dose of MPTP still had a highly significant effect on neuronal survival in the substantia nigra after degeneration of the corresponding axons. Thus, (−)-deprenyl appears to protect dopaminergic neurons against MPTP by a mechanism other than that of preventing the conversion of MPTP to MPP^+ by MAO B. More recently, Salo and Tatton [18] have shown that (−)-deprenyl (10 mg/kg i.p.) can similarly slow the degeneration of rat cholinergic facial neurons, after axotomy. The mechanism of this type of action is unclear, although Tatton and his colleagues suggest that some trophic factor from the axonal target may normally preserve neuronal body integrity. In its absence, the cell body may die. Whether (−)-deprenyl substitutes directly or liberates some trophic molecule is still a matter for conjecture. Candidate peptides well able to fulfill this role, e.g. the nerve growth factor (NGF)-related, brain-derived neurotrophic factor (BDNF) [19, 20] or epidermal growth factor (EGF) [21] are well known.

Knoll [22] has very recently been able to show, by a sophisticated television camera technique, that a normal series of ageing changes he has identified in rat substantia nigra melanin granules can be retarded by (−)-deprenyl pretreatment, which is presumably another manifestation of the neuroprotective action of this drug. It is of particular interest, within this context, to note that the dopaminergic agonist, pergolide, also appears to prolong the survival of nigral neurons in the ageing rat, as judged from fluorescence evaluation of cell sections [23]. It may be more than coincidental that two reports in the literature, albeit anecdotal, suggest that pergolide may arrest the pathological process in a small subset of PD patients [24, 25].

3. How Might (−)-Deprenyl Effect Neuroprotection?

The studies summarized in Table 1 make a *prima facie* case for (−)-deprenyl having some neuroprotective actions. However, it is not clear by what mechanism it is acting; indeed, it seems unlikely to act by the same mechanism in each case. In human studies [6–8, 12], the drug was used at low doses, selective for MAO B inhibition. It was also employed in similarly low doses in the rat longevity trials [13, 14]. However, in the DSP-4 [16] experiments and the axotomy study [18], it was used in a much higher amount. As mentioned above, in the DSP-4 experiments amine reuptake inhibition mechanisms are likely to have been important, whilst the more speculative trophic factor substitution has been invoked for the latter. Many different mechanisms are, in fact, possible, as summarized in Table 2.

3.1. Inhibition of MAO B: Effect on Substrates

The most obvious way in which (−)-deprenyl may exert neuroprotective effects is via its inhibition of MAO B. In the human striatum, this will, in turn, increase dopamine concentration [26, 27] and may thus, to some extent, potentiate dopaminergic activity. However, in the rodent

Table 1. Summary of evidence for a neuroprotective effect of (−)-deprenyl*.

Species	Authors	Comment
Human	Birkmayer et al. [6]	Retrospective
	Tetrud and Langston [7]	Small numbers
	DATATOP [8]	Wash-out period questioned
	Rinne et al. [12]	Postmortem, retrospective
Rat or mouse	Knoll et al. [13]	Longevity
	Milgram et al. [14]	Longevity
	Salo and Tatton [18]	Protects motoneurons
	Finnegan et al. [16]	Against DSP-4
	Knoll [15]	Against 6-OHDA
	Tatton and Greenwood [17]	After MPP+
	Knoll [22]	Ageing changes in substantia nigra melanin granules

*for abbreviations see text

Table 2. Possible mechanisms for the neuroprotective effect of (−)-deprenyl.

Inhibition of MAO B	Prevents dopamine oxidation in man [26, 27], not rodents [28]; Prevents phenylethylamine oxidation (in all species) [29]; Prevents exotoxin activation (as with MPTP) [32]; Prevents endotoxin activation (as with TIQ) [36]; Prevents generation of H_2O_2 [42].
Other direct actions	Inhibits *in vivo* uptake of monoamines into catecholaminergic nerve endings [15]; Increases turnover rate of dopamine and rate of efflux of dopamine [15].
Indirect action	Increases SOD activity, especially at higher doses [43–45]; Substitutes for or stimulates production of axonal trophic factor(s) [17, 18].

brain, dopamine is predominantly metabolized by MAO A [28], so that any neuroprotective effects described in these experimental animals, using selective (0.25 mg/kg) inhibitory doses of deprenyl, cannot be ascribed to this particular mechanism. This waiver includes the longevity studies [13, 14], and the Tatton and Greenwood findings [17], in which (−)-deprenyl appeared to prevent degeneration due to MPP^+. In all species, MAO B selectively catalyzes the oxidative deamination of phenylethylamine [29]; this is a trace amine with an amphetamine-like action and may thus indirectly potentiate dopaminergic activity. However, there is little evidence, at present, that it does have such an action at physiological concentrations.

3.2. Inhibition of MAO B: Effect on Toxins

The most obvious and, indeed, well-known way in which (−)-deprenyl may exert its neuroprotective effects is by preventing the conversion of protoxins such as MPTP to their corresponding active neurotoxin. With MPTP the reaction takes place in two stages, with MAO B first catalyzing the production of 1-methyl-4-phenyl-2,3,dihydropyridinium ($MPDP^+$).

$$\text{MPTP} \xrightarrow{\text{MAO B}} \text{MPDP}^+ \longrightarrow \text{MPP}^+$$

The experimental and clinical backgrounds of MPTP have been extensively reviewed (e.g. [30, 31]), so that detailed consideration would be supererogatory.

A wide variety of prodrug neurotoxic analogues of MPTP is now known [32]. In order to be neurotoxic, the MAO B substrate must possess a methyl group on the nitrogen, a 4-5 double bond in the pyridine ring and an additional group attached to this ring [32]. Many

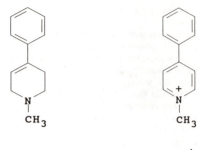

MPTP   MPP$^+$

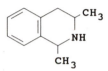   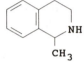

1,3 DiMe TIQ   1 Me TIQ

Trp-P-1   Trp-P-2

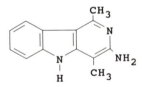   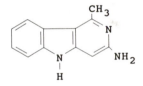

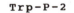

TIQ   NMTIQ   NMIQ$^+$

Figure 1. Structure of MPTP and related analogues. MPTP: 1-methyl-4-phenyl-1,2,3,6-tetrahydropyridine; MPP$^+$: 1-methyl-4-phenylpyridinium; 1,3,DiMe TIQ: 1,3,dimethyltetra-hydroisoquinoline; 1 Me TIQ: 1-methyltetrahydroisoquinoline; TIQ: tetrahydroisoquinoline; NMTIQ: N-methyltetrahydroisoquinoline; NMIQ$^+$: N-methylisoquinolinium; NMT: N-methyltransferase; MAO: monoamine oxidase; Trp-P-1: 3-amino-1,4-dimethyl-5H-pyrido [4,3-b] indole; Trp-P-2: 3-amine-1-methyl-5H-pyrido [4,3-b] indole.

of the analogues of MPTP that have been investigated are also substrates for MAO A [33, 34]. Other analogous toxins, such as paraquat, are active without further chemical modification.

To our knowledge, MPTP does not exist in the natural environment and is unlikely, therefore, to be a cause of the idiopathic disease. In an attempt to identify a possible endogenously-generated neurotoxin, Nagatsu and coworkers [35] have extensively screened compounds with an analogous structure to MPTP and found that tetrahydroisoquinoline (TIQ) is a candidate to produce parkinsonism (see Figure 1). Its long-term administration may give rise to motor disturbances in monkeys and mice that can be reversed by L-dopa [36]. Associated reductions of dopamine and tyrosine hydroxylase in the nigrostriatal tract have been described, although there was no evidence of cell death. Apart from being present in the normal brain [37], TIQ is also found in many foods, such as bananas, cheese and milk. It has also been shown to inhibit mitochondrial respiration in a similar way to MPP^+. In fact, Nagatsu and his colleagues have shown that TIQ can be N-methylated by human brain homogenates, and that the resulting NMTIQ is a substrate for MAO, which catalyzes the formation of $NMIQ^+$, an analogue of MPP^+ [38] (see Figure 1). Both forms of MAO catalyse this activation, having a similar K_m, and somewhat higher V_{max} value for MAO A.

1-Methyl-TIQ has also been found in rat brain. It has been considered by some as a possible protective rather than a toxic agent [39].

Makino et al. [40] have described how a different but related neurotoxin, 1,3-dimethyl-TIQ, can be formed *in vivo* in rats given both ethanol and amphetamine. This compound caused marked behavioural abnormalities, but nothing resembling a PD model.

β-Carbolines have also been suggested as potential endo- or exo-neurotoxins. Takahashi et al. [41] have investigated the properties of Trp-P-1 and Trp-P-2 (see Figure 1 for structures and full names). These two indoles can be produced by the pyrolysis of tryptophan in food. They can be taken up by a specific dopamine transport system, and inhibit the activity of tyrosine hydroxylase and amino acid decarboxylase.

All these studies are of great potential interest. However, in no case has it yet been proved that the potential toxin is present in sufficient quantity *in vivo*, in particular individuals, in order to have a parkinsonian effect. Nor is there yet any convincing epidemiological evidence to implicate any particular dietary factors. Furthermore, in none of the examples discussed above would a selective dose (as used therapeutically) of (−)-deprenyl be expected to prevent toxicity. In the case of TIQ, which is one of the closest analogues of MPTP, even if MAO B were blocked, MAO A would still be available to convert the N-methylated derivative to its toxic form.

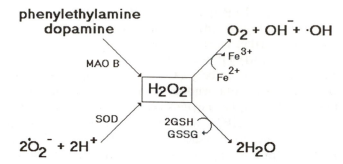

Figure 2. Mechanism for the formation and removal of hydrogen peroxide (H_2O_2). MAO B: monoamine oxidase B; SOD: superoxide dismutase; GSH: reduced glutathione; GSSG: glutathione disulphide; $\cdot O_2^-$: superoxide radical; OH^-: hydroxyl ion; $\cdot OH$: hydroxyl radical.

3.3. Inhibition of MAO B: Effect on H_2O_2 Generation

Cohen and Spina [42] have suggested that the H_2O_2 generated by the action of MAO may itself be toxic; thus, blocking the action of MAO may be neuroprotective (see Figure 2). They showed that the concentration of glutathione disulphide in the mouse striatum is tripled by the injection of haloperidol, which increases dopamine turnover. $(-)$-Deprenyl (2.5 mg/kg i.p.) suppresses this rise. They concluded that $(-)$-deprenyl suppresses oxidant stress associated with increased dopamine turnover. However, as discussed above, in the rodent brain at least, dopamine is predominantly oxidized by MAO A, so that selective inhibition of MAO B is unlikely to have a significant effect on H_2O_2 production in the nigrostriatal tract. Cohen and Spina [42] stated that the dose of drug they used would have resulted in selective inhibition of MAO B. However, they provided no direct evidence for this conclusion; Knoll [15] recommends a dose ten times smaller for selective inhibition. It is thus unclear whether the former's results are meaningful. Moreover, if the induction of superoxide dismutase (SOD) is instrumental in promoting the neuroprotective effects of $(-)$-deprenyl, as discussed below, then it is unlikely that H_2O_2 is harmful, as this chemical compound is actually produced by SOD.

3.4. Other Direct Actions of $(-)$-Deprenyl

$(-)$-Deprenyl, however, has other actions apart from the inhibition of MAO. It reportedly protects against the toxic effects of 6-hydroxydopamine in the rat brain, whereas clorgyline has no such effect (both used at 5 mg/kg i.p.) [15]. As discussed earlier, it presumably achieved this effect by blockade of amine uptake. It also increases the "dopaminergic tone" of the brain. Knoll [15] has described how the drug can sensitize dopaminergic neurons to physiological and pharmacological influences without eliciting any acute increase in dopaminergic activity. Repeated administration of small daily doses of (−)-deprenyl (0.25 mg/kg s.c.) significantly increases the turnover of dopamine in the rat striatum, but only after sufficient time has elapsed, because this phenomenon is not detectable after as short a period as 24 h. The effect is due to a significant increase in dopamine efflux.

3.5. Effect of (−)-Deprenyl on SOD Induction

Knoll [43] originally reported that (−)-deprenyl injected s.c. for 3 weeks at doses ranging from 0.25 to 2.0 mg/kg causes an induction of SOD activity in rat striata which is significant at higher doses. Clorgyline, the selective MAO A inhibitor, actually resulted in a significant decrease in SOD activity. These two findings argue strongly against the inhibition of MAO being the mechanism via which SOD is induced. Carillo et al. [44] have also reported that (−)-deprenyl causes a significant increase in activity of both cytosolic and particulate forms of SOD in rat striata, but not elsewhere in the brain. We have repeated this experiment [45] and confirmed that (−)-deprenyl at 2 but not 0.25 mg/ kg causes a significant increase in SOD activity. However, we have found repeatedly that the effect is confined to the soluble, cytosolic form of the enzyme (Cu-Zn dependent), with the level of the particulate, mitochondrial form (Mn-dependent) being quite unchanged.

We have also examined the effects of pergolide, a dopamine receptor agonist used in the treatment of Parkinson's disease, and have shown that it also induces a significant increase in activity of soluble SOD, while leaving the particulate form unaffected (in preparation). This finding confirms that the inhibition of MAO is not in itself necessary for the SOD induction effect, but is consistent with the hypothesis that it is due to an increase in "dopaminergic tone". We have also noted that isatin, an endogenously generated MAO B inhibitor [46, 47], is similarly able to promote an increase in striatal SOD activity.

These findings with SOD may well be relevant to the apparent neuroprotective ability of (−)-deprenyl. These is a considerable literature linking SOD activity with longevity in different species [48], and in different strains of the same species [49, 50]. SOD has also been shown to protect against MPTP toxicity [51], as well as preventing sympathetic denervation caused by 6-hydroxydopamine [52].

The mechanisms of ageing in general, and of the nigrostriatal tract in particular, are still unknown, but several of the most plausible hypotheses have focussed on the role of free radicals and toxic oxygen. The complex oxidation of L-dopa and dopamine can generate free radicals and quinones; it is thought that these, in turn, can lead to the formation of neuromelanin. It is the cells richest in neuromelanin that are most likely to degenerate in Parkinson's disease, and it may be no coincidence that these cells are most rich in SOD mRNA [53]. Thus, it is not inconceivable that, by induction of this enzyme, ($-$)-deprenyl brings about at least some of the remarkable effects claimed for it.

4. Conclusion

The causes of Parkinson's disease are still unknown and endo- and exotoxins may or may not play a role in its pathogenesis. ($-$)-Deprenyl, although no "wonder drug" when used clinically, appears to have some remarkable properties, particularly in animal models. It is important that its apparent neuroprotective effects be confirmed in further experiments and, if they exist, that their mode of action be unravelled. It is also important to known when (if at all) it acts as a neuroprotective agent through the inhibition of MAO B; this is easily checked by using other, "cleaner", selective MAO B inhibitors, such as MDL 72974. It is also necessary to establish the dose at which ($-$)-deprenyl is effective: if it works best at higher doses, and clorgyline is ineffective, as with the induction of SOD, then it is unlikely to be acting through the inhibition of MAO A or B. An understanding of these mechanisms may well lead to the development of drugs that are much more effective as neuroprotective agents, and may well open up a new era in the treatment of Parkinson's and perhaps other neurodegenerative diseases.

Summary

The prodrug 1-methyl-4-phenyl-1,2,3,6-tetrahydropyridine (MPTP) is activated to its neurotoxic metabolite 1-methyl-4-phenylpyridinium (MPP$^+$) by monoamine oxidase (MAO) B, and this conversion can be prevented by prior administration of ($-$)-deprenyl (selegiline). ($-$)-Deprenyl also appears to be neuroprotective in a number of different systems, and there is evidence that it prolongs life. In this paper, we discuss possible mechanisms by which the drug manifests such effects in experimental and clinical situations. They include prevention of protoxin activation and inhibition of substrate oxidation by MAO B, increase of dopaminergic tone, and induction of superoxide dismutase (SOD). The latter is of particular interest, because parallel studies have indicated that its activity may correlate directly with longevity in different strains and species and, in certain circumstances, may protect against neurodegeneration.

References

[1] Davis GC, Williams AC, Markey SP, Ebert MH, Caine ED, Reichert C, Kopin IJ. Chronic parkinsonism secondary to intravenous injection of meperidine analogues. Psychiatry Res 1979; 1: 249–254.

[2] Langston JW, Ballard P, Tetrud JW, Irwin I. Chronic parkinsonism in humans due to a product of meperidine-analog synthesis. Science 1983; 219: 979–980.

[3] Langston JW, Langston EB, Irwin I. MPTP-induced parkinsonism in human and non-human primates – clinical and experimental aspects. Acta Neurol Scand 1984; 100 (Suppl.): 49–54.

[4] Heikkila RE, Manzino L, Cabbat FS, Duvoisin RC. Protection against the dopaminergic neurotoxicity of 1-methyl-4-phenyl-1,2,5,6-tetrahydropyridine by monoamine oxidase inhibitors. Nature 1984; 311: 467–469.

[5] Cohen G, Pasik P, Cohen B, Leist A, Mytilineou C, Yahr MD. Pargyline and deprenyl prevent the neurotoxicity of 1-methyl-4-phenyl-1,2,3,6-tetrahydropyridine (MPTP) in monkeys. Europ J Pharmacol 1984; 106: 209–210.

[6] Birkmayer W, Knoll J, Riederer P, Youdim MBH, Hars V, Marton J. Increased life expectancy resulting from addition of l-deprenyl to Madopar treatment in Parkinson's disease: a long term study. J Neural Transm 1985; 64: 113–127.

[7] Tetrud JW, Langston JW. The effect of deprenyl (selegiline) on the natural history of Parkinson's disease. Science 1989; 245: 519–522.

[8] Parkinson Study Group. Effect of deprenyl on the progression of disability in early Parkinson's disease. N Engl J Med 1989; 321: 1364–1371.

[9] Landau WM. Clinical neuromythology IX. Pyramid sale in the bucket shop: DATATOP bottoms out. Neurology 1990; 40: 1337–1339.

[10] Elsworth JD, Glover V, Reynolds GP, Sandler M, Lees AJ, Phuapradit P, Shaw KM, Stern GM, Kumar P. Deprenyl administration in man; a selective monoamine oxidase B inhibitor without the "cheese effect". Psychopharmacology 1978; 57: 33–38.

[11] Riggs JE. Parkinson's disease: an epidemiologic method for distinguishing between symptomatic and neuroprotective treatments. Clin Pharmacol 1991; 14: 489–497.

[12] Rinne JO, Röyttä M, Paljärvi L, Rummukainen J, Rinne UK. Selegiline (deprenyl) treatment and death of nigral neurons in Parkinson's disease. Neurology 1991; 41: 859–861.

[13] Knoll J, Dallo J, Yen TT. Striatal dopamine, sexual activity and lifespan. Longevity of rats treated with (−)deprenyl. Life Sci 1989; 45: 525–531.

[14] Milgram NW, Racine RJ, Nellis P, Mendonca A, Ivy GO. Maintenance on l-deprenyl prolongs life in aged male rats. Life Sci 1990; 47: 415–420.

[15] Knoll J. Striatal dopamine, ageing and (−)deprenyl. Jugoslav Physiol Pharmacol Acta 1986; 22: 261–273.

[16] Finnegan KT, Skratt JJ, Irwin I, DeLanney LE, Langston JW. Protection against DSP-4-induced neurotoxicity by deprenyl is not related to its inhibition of MAO B. Europ J Pharmacol 1990; 184: 119–126.

[17] Tatton WG, Greenwood CE. Rescue of dying neurons: a new action for deprenyl in MPTP parkinsonism. J Neurosci Res 1991; 30: 666–672.

[18] Salo PT, Tatton WG. Deprenyl reduces the death of motoneurons caused by axotomy. J Neurosci Res 1992; 31: 394–400.

[19] Snyder SH. Parkinson's disease. Fresh facts to consider. Nature 1991; 350: 195–196.

[20] Hyman C, Hofer M, Barde Y-A, Juhasz M, Yancopoulos GD, Squinto SP, Lindsay RM. BDNF is a neurotrophic factor for dopaminergic neurons of the substantia nigra. Nature 1991; 350: 230–232.

[21] Pezzoli G, Zecchinelli A, Ricciardi S, Burke RE, Fahn S, Scarlato G, Carenzi A. Intraventricular infusion of epidermal growth factor restores dopaminergic pathway in hemiparkinsonian rats. Movement Disorders 1991; 6: 281–287.

[22] Knoll J. The pharmacological basis of the beneficial effects of (−)deprenyl (selegiline) in Parkinson's and Alzheimer's diseases. J Neural Transm 1992. In press.

[23] Felten DL, Felten SY, Fuller RW, Romano TD, Smalstig EB, Wong DT, Clemens JA. Chronic dietary pergolide preserved nigrostriatal neuronal integrity in aged Fischer 344 rats. Neurology of Ageing 1992; 13: 339–351.

[24] Lichter P, Kurlan R, Miller C, Shoulson I. Does pergolide slow the progression of Parkinson's disease? A 7-year follow-up study. Neurology 1988; 38 (Suppl. 1): 122.

[25] Zimmerman T, Sage JI. Long-term pergolide treatment and progression of Parkinson's disease. Neurology 1989; 39 (Suppl. 1): 200.

[26] Glover V, Elsworth JD, Sandler M. Dopamine oxidation and its inhibition by ($-$)-deprenyl in man. J Neural Transm 1980; 16 (Suppl): 163–172.

[27] Glover V, Sandler M, Owen F, Riley GJ. Dopamine is a monoamine oxidase B substrate in man. Nature 1977; 265: 80–81.

[28] Waldmeier PC, Delini-Stula A, Maitre L. Preferential deamination of dopamine by an A type monoamine oxidase in rat brain. Naunyn-Schmiedeberg's Arch Pharmacol 1976; 292: 9–14.

[29] Neff NH, Garrison CK, Fuentes J. Trace amines and the monoamine oxidases. In: Usdin E, Sandler M, editors. Trace Amines and the Brain. New York: Marcel Dekker 1976; 41–57.

[30] Irwin I. The neurotoxin 1-methyl-4-phenyl-1,2,3,6-tetrahydropyridine (MPTP): a key to Parkinson's disease? Pharm Res 1986; 3: 7–11.

[31] Langston JW. MPTP and Parkinson's disease. Trends Neurosci 1985; 80: 79–83.

[32] Langston JW, Irwin I. Pyridine toxins. In: Calne DB, editor. Drugs for the Treatment of Parkinson's Disease. New York: Springer 1989: 205–226.

[33] Gibb C, Willoughby J, Glover V, Sandler M, Testa B, Jenner P, Marsden CD. Analogues of 1-methyl-4-phenyl-1,2,3,6-tetrahydropyridine as monoamine oxidase substrates: a second ring is not necessary. Neurosci Letters 1987; 76: 316–322.

[34] Basma AN, Heikkila E, Nicklas WJ, Giovanni A, Geller HM. 1-Methyl-4-phenyl-1,2,3,6-tetrahydropyridine- and 1-methyl-4-(2'-ethylphenyl)-1,2,3,6-tetrahydropyridine-induced toxicity in PCl2 cells: role of monoamine oxidase A. J Neurochem 1990; 55: 870–877.

[35] Nagatsu T, Hirata Y. Inhibition of the tyrosine hydroxylase system by MPTP, 1-methyl-4-phenylpyridinium ion (MPP$^+$) and the structurally related compounds in vitro and in vivo. Europ Neurol 1987; 26 (Suppl. 1): 11.

[36] Yoshida M, Niwa T, Nagatsu T. Parkinsonism in monkeys produced by chronic administration of an endogeneous substance of the brain, tetrahydroisoquinoline: the behavioral and biochemical changes. Neurosci Lett 1990; 119: 109–113.

[37] Niwa T, Takeda N, Sasaoka T, Kaneda N, Hashizume Y, Yoshizumi H, Tatematsu A, Nagatsu T. Detection of tetrahydroisoquinoline in parkinsonian brain as an endogenous amine by use of gas chromatography-mass spectrometry. J Chromatogr 1989; 491: 397–403.

[38] Naoi M, Matsuura S, Takahashi T, Nagatsu T. An N-methyltransferase in human brain catalyses N-methylation of 1,2,3,4-tetrahydroisoquinoline into N-methyl-1,2,3,4-tetrahydroisoquinoline, a precursor of a dopaminergic neurotoxin, N-methylisoquinolinium ion. Biochem Biophys Res Commun 1989; 161: 1213–1219.

[39] Makino Y, Tasaki Y, Ohta S, Hirobe M. Confirmation of the enantiomers of 1-methyl-1,2,3,4-tetrahydroisoquinoline in the mouse brain and foods applying gas chromatograph/mass spectrometry with negative ion chemical ionization. Biomed Environ Mass Spectrometry 1990; 19: 415–419.

[40] Makino Y, Tasaki Y, Kashiwasake M, Tachikawa O, Ohta S, Hirobe M. Formation of a novel and neurotoxic tetrahydroisoquinoline derivative, 1,3-dimethyltetrahydroisoquinoline (1,3DiMeTIQ), a condensation product of amphetamines and acetaldehyde in vivo. In: Nagatsu T, Fisher A, Yoshida M, editors. Basic, Clinical, and Therapeutic Aspects of Alzheimer's and Parkinson's Disease. New York: Plenum Press, 1990: 325–328.

[41] Takahashi T, Naoi M, Ichinose H, Kojima T, Nagatsu T. Food-derived heterocyclic amines as potent inhibitors of catecholamine metabolism. In: Nagatsu T, Fisher A, Yoshida M, editors. Basic, Clinical, and Therapeutic Aspects of Alzheimer's and Parkinson's Disease. New York: Plenum Press, 1990: 345–348.

[42] Cohen G, Spina MB. Deprenyl suppresses the oxidant stress associated with increased dopamine turnover. Ann Neurol 1989; 26: 689–690.

[43] Knoll J. The striatal dopamine dependency of life span in male rats. Longevity study with ($-$)deprenyl. Mech Ageing Devel 1988; 46: 237–262.

[44] Carillo M-C, Kanai S, Nokubu M, Kitani K. ($-$)Deprenyl induces activities of both superoxide dismutase and catalase but not of glutathione peroxidase in the striatum of young male rats. Life Sci 1991; 48: 517–521.

[45] Clow A, Hussain T, Glover V, Sandler M, Dexter DT, Walker M. (−)-Deprenyl can induce soluble superoxide dismutase in rat striata. J Neural Transm 1991; 86: 77–80.
[46] Glover V, Halket JM, Watkins PJ, Clow A, Goodwin BL, Sandler M. Isatin: identity with the purified endogeneous monoamine oxidase inhibitor tribulin. J Neurochem 1988; 51: 656–659.
[47] Watkins P, Clow A, Glover V, Halket J, Przyborowska A, Sandler M. Isatin, regional distribution in rat brain and tissues. Neurochem Int 1990; 17: 321–323.
[48] Tolmasoff JM, Ono T, Cutler RG. Superoxide dismutase: correlation with life-span and specific metabolic rate in primate species. Proc Nat Acad Sci USA 1980; 77: 2777–2781.
[49] Sohal RS, Farmer KJ, Allen RG. Correlates of longevity in two strains of the housefly, Musca domestica. Mech Ageing Devel 1987; 40: 171–179.
[50] Kellog EW, Fridovich I. Superoxide dismutase in the rat and mouse as a function of age and longevity. J Gerontol 1976; 4: 405–408.
[51] Przedborski S, Kostic V, Jackson-Lewis V, Carlson E, Epstein CJ, Cadet JL. Transgenic mice expressing the human SOD gene are resistant to MPTP-induced toxicity. Soc Neurosci Abstr 1990; 16: 1260.
[52] Albino-Teixeira A, Azevedo I, Martel F, Osswald W. Superoxide dismutase partially prevents sympathetic denervation by 6-hydroxydopamine. Arch Pharmacol 1991; 344: 36–40.
[53] Ceballos I, Lafon M, Javoy Agid F, Hirsch E, Nicole A, Simet P, Agid Y. Superoxide dismutase and Parkinson's disease. Lancet 1990; i: 1035–1036.

Inhibitors of Monoamine Oxidase B
Pharmacology and Clinical Use in Neurodegenerative Disorders
ed. by I. Szelenyi
© 1993 Birkhäuser Verlag Basel/Switzerland

CHAPTER 9
The Mode of Action of MAO-B Inhibitors

M. Gerlach, P. Riederer and M. B. H. Youdim

1   Introduction
2   Recently Developed MAO-B Inhibitors in the Treatment of Psychiatric and
     Neurological Disorders
3   The Distribution and Localization of the MAO-B in the Brain: The Role of
     Intraneural and Glial Inhibition
4   MAO-B-Relevant Substrates: The Significance of Dopamine, β-Phenylethylamine
     and Polyamines for the Clinical Action of MAO-B Inhibitors
5   The Neuroprotective Action of MAO-inhibitors: Attempts at a Pharmacological
     Explanation
5.1 The "Oxidative Stress" Hypothesis
5.2 The Indirect Effect of MAO-B Inhibitors on the Function of the NMDA Receptor
6   Future Outlook
     Summary
     References

1. Introduction

Monoamine oxidase (EC 1.4.3.4; amine: oxygen oxidoreductase (deaminating; flavin-containing) (MAO) is an enzyme of the outer mitochondrial membrane and catalyzes the oxidative deamination of amines according to the overall equation

$$R-CH_2NH_2 + O_2 + H_2O \longrightarrow R-CHO + NH_3 + H_2O_2. \qquad (1)$$

The enzyme occurs in both the central nervous system (CNS) and peripheral tissues, and metabolizes monoaminergic neurotransmitters or neuromodulators such as dopamine (DA), noradrenaline (NA), serotonin (5-HT), and β-phenylethylamine (PEA), as well as amines such as tyramine which are absorbed from the diet or arise as the result of bacterial transformations. The name "monoamine oxidase" is not entirely appropriate, because the enzyme is also capable of deaminating long-chain diamines such as 1,10-decamethylene diamine [1], compounds such as 2-n-pentylaminoacetamide [2], and even tertiary cyclic amines such as 1-methyl-4-phenyl-1,2,3,6-tetrahydropyridine (MPTP) [3, 4] and 1-methyl-β-carboline, harman [5]. Further particulars, including the molecular structure of the enzyme and the enzymatic reaction mechanism are described in recent review articles [6, 7].

The existence of two forms of MAO was postulated on the basis of differential substrate specificities and inhibition properties in *in vitro* enzyme assays. In 1968, Johnston [8] reported for the first time that the inhibition of rat brain MAO by the acetylenic inhibitor clorgyline was dependent on the substrate used to assay for enzyme activity, and suggested that there were two forms of the enzyme: the A-form being sensitive to inhibition by clorgyline and active towards 5-HT; and the B-form being relatively insensitive to clorgyline-inhibition and active towards benzylamine (BA). This study, together with a number of subsequent ones (e.g., [9–11]) has led to the present definition of the two forms of MAO. MAO-A predominantly deaminates 5-HT and NA and is inhibited by low (around nanomolar) concentrations of clorgyline, whereas MAO-B is not inhibited until micromolar concentrations of this inhibitor are used. MAO-B has a greater affinity for BA and for PEA and is selectively inhibited by low concentrations of l-deprenyl (selegiline). In the brain, as in other tissues, DA and tyramine are substrates for both forms of the enzyme, while DA in human brain has a somewhat higher affinity for MAO-B [12, 13]. The existence of the two subtypes A and B has been confirmed, not only by immuno-histochemical investigations using monoclonal antibodies which specifically bind to either MAO-A or MAO-B [14–16], but also by molecular genetics [17–19]. The two enzymes exhibit approximately 70% sequence homology, and are coded by distinct, but closely related genes [18–19].

   MAO inhibitors inhibit the activity of MAO at physiological concentrations. We can distinguish two main types, corresponding to whether the inhibition is reversible or not [6, 7]:

1) Competitive, reversible inhibitors, and
2) Enzyme-activated, irreversible inhibitors.

Competitive, reversible inhibitors bear a structural resemblance to the natural MAO substrates, but are resistant to oxidation by the enzyme (examples of such inhibitors are β-carbolines, and aryl- or indolylalkyl-amines). Enzyme-activated, irreversible inhibitors, also known as mechanism-based, or K_{cat}, or suicide inhibitors [20–22], also initially form a non-covalent complex in a first, reversible step. However, subsequent oxidation of the MAO inhibitor leads to the formation of a covalent bond within this complex. By definition, the inhibition in this case cannot be reversed by dialysis, gel filtration or dilution, and *in vivo* recovery will depend on *de novo* biosynthesis of fresh enzyme. Examples of this class of inhibitors include hydrazines, cyclopropylamines, and propargylamines. Earlier work on the classification, mechanisms of action, and pharmacological effects of MAO inhibitors has been reviewed in detail [6, 7, 23]. In the present chapter, we are almost exclusively concerned with human brain MAO and MAO-B inhibitors in clinical use or at least in clinical trials, and we present relevant aspects of their modes of action in Parkinson's disease (PD).

2. Recently Developed MAO-B Inhibitors in the Treatment of Psychiatric and Neurological Disorders

Although the antidepressive effect of MAO inhibitors has been confirmed in numerous studies (for a review, see [24]), they have been of only minor significance in the treatment of psychiatric disorders. This was predominantly because treatment of patients with the older generation MAO inhibitors (the non-selective, partially reversible kind) was accompanied by considerable side-effects. For example, iproniazid [25, 26], the first MAO inhibitor to be introduced into clinical practice, had to be recalled because of hepatotoxic side-effects. However, the successor substances (tranylcypromine, phenelzine) were also not free of side-effects. Blackwell et al. [27] were the first to point out the connection between the frequent appearance of hypertensive crises in patients receiving MAO inhibitors and the consumption of tyramine-containing foods, especially cheese or dairy products (known as "cheese effect"). Today, we are aware that these hypertensive crises are elicited by an augmented sympathomimetic effect of dietary tyramine which is caused by a non-selective inhibition of MAO (for a review, see [28]). The diminished enzyme activity (especially that of the A-form in the gastrointestinal tract) permits absorption of large amounts of indirectly-acting sympathomimetic amines (particularly, tyramine) into the circulation, which then release increased amounts of NA from sympathetic nerve endings. This leads to vasoconstriction and a rise in blood pressure (see Chapter 6).

Because of these experiences and the insights gained, new, selective MAO inhibitors were developed [28–36]. Of these substances only *l*-deprenyl has become available for the symptomatic treatment of Parkinson's disease (PD) ([37]; for a review, see [38, 39]) and the treatment of cognitive disturbances in Alzheimer's disease [40, 41]; thus far, it has not exhibited any of the side-effects that appeared with the older generation MAO inhibitors. The other MAO inhibitors, e.g. AGN 1135 (N-propargylamino-indane), Ro 19-6327 (N-[2-aminoethyl]-5-chloro-2-pyridine carboxamide) and MDL 72974 (2-(4-fluoro-phenethyl)-3-fluoroallylamine) are still undergoing clinical trials.

A determination of the IC_{50}-concentrations of MAO inhibitors for selective MAO-A or MAO-B substrates permits an evaluation of their potency and selectivity. Table 1 collects the IC_{50} values of various selective MAO-B inhibitors which have already been tested in clinical trials. It can be seen that *l*-deprenyl is the most potent. If one calculates the ratios of potencies using the IC_{50} values for MAO-A and MAO-B, one recognizes that Ro 19-6327 is a more selective MAO-B inhibitor than *l*-deprenyl or AGN 1135 (Table 1). However, in contrast to the enzyme-activated irreversible inhibitors *l*-deprenyl, AGN 1133 or MDL 72145, the action of the reversible MAO-B inhibitor Ro 19-6327 is

Table 1. *In vitro* selectivity of MAO-B inhibitors.

Inhibitor	IC$_{50}$ (µmol/l)		MAO-A/MAO-B	Tissue	Reference
	5-HT (MAO-A)	PEA (MAO-B)			
AGN 1133	0.02	0.05	0.4	human frontal cortex	13
AGN 1135	8	0.02	400	human frontal cortex	13
	2	0.3	67	rat brain	35
l-deprenyl	2	0.005	400	rat brain	35
MDL 72145	40	0.3	133	human frontal cortex	13
	5	0.03	167	rat brain	35
Ro 19-6327	900	0.03	30000	rat brain	35

5-HT, serotonin; PEA, β-phenylethylamine.

relatively short: after 24 h the inhibition of MAO has ceased completely [35].

3. The Distribution and Localization of MAO-B in the Brain: The Role of Intraneural and Glial Inhibition

The highest MAO-specific activity in almost all human brain regions is found with the substrate kynuramine (Table 2), which is a substrate for both MAO-A and MAO-B [42]. The rate of deamination of kynuramine, DA, and 5-HT by the enzyme was found to exhibit considerable differences in the various regions of the brain (Table 2). The highest specific activity was in the hypothalamus and in the nigro-striatal system (caudate nucleus, putamen, and substantia nigra), including the globus pallidus; the lowest specific activity was in the thalamus, hippocampus, and frontal cortex. Similar results were obtained with ^{11}C-labeled *l*-deprenyl in *in vitro* autoradiography, which was used to study the regional distribution of MAO-B in the human brain [43].

What is the distribution of MAO in the brains of patients with PD who have been treated with MAO-B inhibitors? Table 3 shows this distribution in respect to the substrates DA and 5-HT in the post mortem brain of PD patients who had been treated with a daily dose of 10 mg *l*-deprenyl. According to these results, the deamination of DA in all the brain areas investigated was completely inhibited; the moderate degree of inhibition of 5-HT metabolism by MAO leads to the conclusion that there is only an insubstantial effect on the activity of MAO-A.

Table 2. The activity of human brain MAO in different brain regions (according to [13]).

Brain area	Substrate Kynuramine (mitochondrial preparations)	DA (homogenate)	5-HT (homogenate)
Caudate nucleus	5.80 ± 0.38	1.55 ± 0.82	0.64 ± 0.25
Putamen	5.50 ± 2.13	1.36 ± 0.45	0.59 ± 0.05
Globus pallidus	6.00 ± 3.03	1.83 ± 0.72	0.86 ± 0.24
Substantia nigra	3.97 ± 1.35	2.27 ± 0.37	1.08 ± 0.23
Nucleus amygdalae	3.45 ± 0.87	1.67 ± 0.73	1.06 ± 0.28
Gyrus cinguli	0.56 ± 0.15	1.29 ± 0.36	0.82 ± 0.07
Raphe	1.76 ± 0.62	1.80 ± 0.64	0.94 ± 0.20
Red nucleus	2.51 ± 1.07	—	—
Hypothalamus	6.93 ± 1.14	2.74 ± 1.19	1.94 ± 0.44
Thalamus medialis	2.62 ± 0.86	1.07 ± 0.53	0.70 ± 0.32
Corpus mammilare	3.15 ± 0.84	2.42 ± 1.39	1.60 ± 0.42
Substantia pellucidum	3.20 ± 0.65	—	—
Nucleus dentatus	2.42 ± 1.48	—	—
Gyrus dentatus	1.43 ± 0.36	0.92 ± 0.27	1.04 ± 0.10
Pineal gland	2.11 ± 1.60	—	—
Locus ceruleus	—	2.36 ± 0.64	1.24 ± 0.32
Nucleus ruber	—	1.67 ± 0.53	1.05 ± 0.31
Hippocampus	—	1.05 ± 0.26	6.78 ± 0.09
Frontal cortex	—	0.99 ± 0.50	0.46 ± 0.26
Nucleus accumbens	—	1.42 ± 0.62	1.30 ± 0.14

DA, dopamine; 5-HT, serotonin; —, not investigated.

Table 3. MAO activity in brains of parkinsonian subjects treated with *l*-deprenyl (according to [13]).

Brain area	Percent inhibition DA	5-HT
Caudate nucleus	89 ± 2	64 ± 12
Putamen	88 ± 3	38 ± 2
Globus pallidus	93 ± 3	64 ± 16
Thalamus	86 ± 8	70 ± 16
Hypothalamus	90 ± 5	84 ± 8
Corpus mammilare	94 ± 3	58 ± 22
Substantia nigra	94 ± 2	67 ± 10
Locus ceruleus	95 ± 2	67 ± 17
Nucleus ruber	94 ± 2	70 ± 13
Raphe	93 ± 4	83 ± 10
Gyrus cinguli	93 ± 6	65 ± 19
Nucleus amygdalae	95 ± 4	77 ± 12
Hippocampus	94 ± 3	66 ± 24
Gyrus dentatus	94 ± 2	65 ± 25
Nucleus accumbens	93 ± 3	65 ± 12
Frontal cortex	94 ± 2	60 ± 20

DA, dopamine; 5-HT, serotonin.

Indeed, in post mortem brains from patients with PD who had been treated with *l*-deprenyl at a daily dose of 10 mg, the concentrations of DA [13] and of PEA [44] in the nigro-striatal system are substantially higher (by 350–545%, depending on the brain region, and 1192% in the striatum) than values from parkinsonian patients not on *l*-deprenyl treatment, while those of 5-HT and of 5-hydroxyindole acetic acid (the major metabolite of 5-HT) are not altered.

Table 2 also shows that the activities towards the substrates DA and 5-HT do not show a 1:1 relationship, but that, with the exception of activities within the hippocampus, they are clearly displaced in favor of a greater turnover of DA. This does not, however, unequivocally indicate that the DA-rich regions of the nigro-striatal system necessarily contain increased proportions of MAO-B. Further evidence concerning this is provided by investigations using monoclonal antibodies which specifically recognize either MAO-A or MAO-B [16]. Table 4 summarizes the results of these investigations. It shows that the glia contain both forms in roughly equal proportions, but that in the various brain regions the distribution is variable: thus, for example, the striatum has an excess of MAO-B (about 60% of the total MAO activity). While the nerve cells of the locus ceruleus contain only MAO-A activity, the enzyme activity of the neurons of the dorsal raphe nucleus is almost exclusively MAO-B. It is therefore valid to assume that, because NA is primarily a substrate for MAO-A (it is deaminated by MAO-B only at high substrate concentrations), then the corresponding intraneuronal form of the enzyme in noradrenergic cell bodies must be MAO-A. This does not, however, hold for the serotonergic dorsal raphe nucleus,

Table 4. Intensity of specific MAO-A and MAO-B antibody staining in different brain areas (according to [16]).

Brain area	MAO-A	MAO-B	TH
Central tegmental tract	−	−	+
Dorsal efferent nucleus of vagus	+++	−	+++
Dorsal nucleus of raphe	±	+++	−
Locus ceruleus	+++	−	+++
Midbrain reticular formation	+	+	++
Oculomotor nucleus	++	−	−
Putamen	±	±	+++
Reticular formation of mesencephalon	+	+	++
Reticular formation, nucleus gigantocellularis	++	++	+++
Substantia nigra	−	−	+++
Ventral tegmental area	+	+	+++
Astroglia	+++	+++	−

TH, Tyrosine hydroxylase; +++, high density of neurons stained; ++, medium density of neurons stained; +, moderate density of neurons stained; ±, staining uncertain (glial staining too dark or cross-reaction of antibodies possible); −, no staining of neurons observed.

because 5-HT is primarily a substrate for MAO-A. Surprisingly, no antibody activity against either MAO-A or MAO-B could be detected in the neurons of the substantia nigra; however, both enzyme subtypes were present there in the glia. However, other immunocytochemical studies using fluorescence techniques have shown that, among the neurons of the substantia nigra, only 10% MAO-A-containing cells can be demonstrated [45, 46].

The latest histochemical investigations by Konradi et al. [15], using various substrates and inhibitors, have confirmed the results obtained with the antibodies as presented above. Thus, the noradrenergic locus ceruleus is positively stained with the MAO-A substrate 5-HT and the non-selective substrate tyramine (Table 5), while no staining can be demonstrated in the presence of the irreversible MAO-A inhibitor LY 51641 [47] or of clorgyline [8]; on the other hand, the presence of the irreversible MAO-B inhibitor *l*-deprenyl is without effect on the staining density. The serotonergic neurons of the dorsal raphe nucleus predominantly show MAO-B, as evidenced by staining with PEA and tyramine (Table 5) and by inhibitor studies. Although the glial cells of the substantia nigra and some fibers showed MAO-B-related staining, the perikarya of this area were not stained by any of the three substrates (Table 5). Glial cell staining was more pronounced in the brain of neonates, showing that there is a preponderance of MAO-B in all the sections examined (Table 5). Here, 5-HT stained only a few astroglial cells, primarily around and within in the locus ceruleus.

Hence, it is reasonable to conclude that the selective inhibition of MAO-B – particularly and predominantly in the glia – leads to diminished catabolism of DA in the nigro-striatal system and to a significant increase in the concentration of the neurotransmitter at the synapses (Figure 1). Since PD is basically characterized by a DA loss in the striatum (see Chapter 2), this is the most plausible mechanism to be responsible for the observed clinical effects of the combination therapy of L-dopa and *l*-deprenyl ([37]; for review, see [38, 39]). The predomi-

Table 5. Histochemical staining of the main monoaminergic areas in the human brainstem (according to [15]).

Brain area	5-HT (MAO-A)	Tyramine (MAO-A/MAO-B)	PEA (MAO-B)
Raphe nuclei	−	+++	+++
Locus ceruleus	+++	+++	−
Substantia nigra	−	−	−
Astroglia	+	+++	+++

5-HT, serotonin; PEA, β-phenylethylamine; +++, high density of neurons stained; +, moderate density of neurons stained; −, no staining of neurons observed.

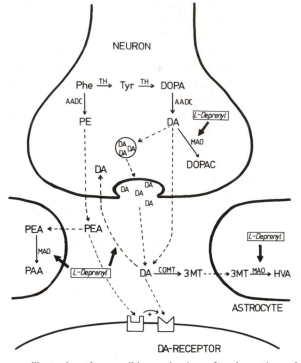

Figure 1. Diagram illustrating the possible mechanisms for the action of *l*-deprenyl in Parkinson's disease. DA is synthesized in the neuron and stored in vesicles until it is released in a calcium-dependent manner. The action of the released DA will be terminated largely by reuptake into the neuron where it is metabolized by MAO, but some will be catabolized by extraneuronal COMT. PEA is also synthesized by dopaminergic neurons, but it is not stored and is released by diffusion. PEA potentiates the effects of DA and is selectively metabolized by MAO-B. For the sake of clarity only postsynaptic receptors were drawn. AADC, aromatic L-amino acid decarboxylase; COMT, catechol-O-methyl transferase; DA, dopamine; DOPA, 3,4-dihydroxy-phenylalanine; DOPAC, 3,4-dihydroxyphenylacetic acid; HVA, homovanillic acid; MAO, monoamine oxidase; MT, methoxytyramine; PAA, phenylacetic acid; PEA, β-phenylethylamine; Phe, phenylalanine; TH, tyrosine hydroxylase; Tyr, tyrosine.

nant features of such a regime lie in the beneficial effect on fluctuations in mobility (which are such a troublesome feature of long-term treatment with L-dopa (3-hydroxy-L-tyrosine or 3,4-dihydroxy-phenylalanine) on its own), and in its ability to reduce the dose of L-dopa. It is not clear (though this is highly probable), whether the glia become enriched with DA which might then have a hormone-like influence on dopaminergic neurotransmission. This hormone-like action and the catabolism of extraneuronal DA by catechol-O-methyl transferase (COMT) might explain why *l*-deprenyl alone is a less potent antiparkinson drug than are L-dopa or DA agonists.

4. MAO-B-Relevant Substrates: The Significance of Dopamine, β-Phenylethylamine, and Polyamines for the Clinical Action of MAO-B Inhibitors

Many substrates, even those described as specific for one or the other form of MAO, are metabolized by both subtypes of the enzyme *in vivo*. The deamination of a substrate by MAO-A and/or MAO-B within the tissues depends on three parameters: the K_m and the molecular turnover number (k_{cat}) (values which are characteristics of the enzyme forms and their substrates), and the amount of each form of MAO present in the tissues.

The relative concentrations of active centers of the two forms of MAO can vary considerably from brain region to brain region (see Tables 3 and 4), and this may result in apparent differences being found in the substrate specificities of the two forms. DA, which is the neurotransmitter fundamentally involved in the pathophysiology of PD, is an example. Tipton et al. [48] classify DA as a pure MAO-A substrate, but other authors [49] have described how it is a specific MAO-B substrate in the brain. More recent and more detailed studies have shown that DA is a substrate for both MAO subtypes [12, 50–52]. Our results (Table 1) do, however, indicate that in the human nigro-striatal system DA shows a higher affinity for MAO-B.

The K_m-value of each form of MAO for a substrate is representative of its interaction with the enzyme, whereas V_{max}, the maximum velocity, depends on both k_{cat} and the amount of enzyme present ($V = k_{cat} \times$ enzyme). Table 6 summarizes some kinetic parameters of the two forms of MAO towards different substrates. K_m-values of 10^{-4}–10^{-6} M indicate that the endogenous substrate of MAO are only weakly bound. The considerably higher K_m-value for the MAO-A subtype toward PEA in the human brain (Table 6) suggests that the B-form would predominate in the oxidation of PEA at low substrate concentrations. This difference in the K_m-value is reinforced by the B-form having a higher maximum velocity. One would therefore assume that selective inhibition of MAO-B by low doses of MAO-B inhibitors would lead to an accumulation of PEA in the brain. In fact, Riederer et al. [44] found up to 12 times higher PEA concentrations in the striatum of PD patients who had been on *l*-deprenyl treatment, and up to 35 times higher PEA levels in limbic areas. Since PEA acts as a DA-releasing agent (for review, see [54]) and, in this way, stimulates dopaminergic neurons (Figure 1), an endogenous "amphetamine-like" activity of *l*-deprenyl could contribute to its overall tonic action.

Beside DA and PEA, N-acetylated polyamines such as N-acetyl-putrescine [55] are among the most important endogenous MAO-B substrates in the brain. The mono-acetylation of polyamines and subsequent oxidation of these N-acetylated derivatives are the most impor-

Table 6. Kinetic parameters of the two forms of MAO in homogenates from human cerebral cortex (according to [53]).

Substrate	MAO-A		MAO-B	
	K_m	V_{max}	K_m	V_{max}
(+), (—)-Adrenaline	208 ± 56	379 ± 54	226 ± 16	465 ± 61
Dopamine	212 ± 33	680 ± 123	229 ± 33	702 ± 158
Serotonin	137 ± 24	228 ± 31	1093 ± 20	7 ± 1
(—)-Noradrenaline	284 ± 17	561 ± 42	238 ± 30	321 ± 13
2-Phenylethylamine	140 ± 22	20 ± 8	4 ± 3	309 ± 24
Tyramine	427 ± 18	182 ± 26	107 ± 21	343 ± 48

The activity of each form of MAO was determined at 37°C and pH 7.2 after inhibition of one of the forms by treatment with 0.3 μM clogyline or 0.1 μM l-deprenyl. K_m-values are expressed in μM and maximum velocities (V_{max}) as pmol/mg protein/min^{-1} (means $\pm$ SEM).

tant catabolic reactions in the brain for the inactivation of these bioactive compounds (for review, see [56]). According to current thinking, polyamines such as putrescine, spermine, and spermidine have a multifunctional role, not only within the machinery that is involved in cell growth and replication, but also in differential cells with specialized function (for review, see [57]). Furthermore, they are precursors for the neurotransmitter γ-aminobutyric acid (GABA), and preliminary evidence suggests structural roles in membranes and a modulatory function in certain neuronal systems [56]. Because of the high activity of MAO-B, N-acetylated polyamines are normally detectable in brain in only minute amounts [58]. However, regarding inhibition of MAO-B, as is the case in patients with PD on l-deprenyl, it is conceivable that one might be able to show increased values for N-acetylated polyamines alongside reduced values for the free polyamines. But, because of the methodological difficulties associated with the method for the determination and the instability of such compounds, direct experimental evidence is lacking.

5. The Neuroprotective Action of MAO-B Inhibitors: Attempts at a Pharmacological Explanation

Evidence from a number of studies in experimental animals has shown that selective inhibition of MAO-B confers protection against the damaging effects of several neurotoxins, including the dopaminergic agents MPTP [3, 4, 59–61] and 6-hydroxydopamine (6-OHDA) [62], and the noradrenergic neurotoxin N-(2-chloroethyl)-N-ethyl-2-bromo-benzyl-amine (DSP-4) [63]. Recent findings, however, suggest that the ability of l-deprenyl to protect against MPTP- and DSP-4-induced neuronal degeneration may not depend on its MAO-B-inhibiting properties

[62, 64, 65]. The possible mechanisms responsible for the observed neuro-protective effects of MAO-B inhibitors are discussed in the following.

5.1. The "Oxidative Stress" Hypothesis

6-OHDA is thought to induce nigro-striatal dopaminergic neuronal lesions via generation of hydrogen peroxide and oxygen free radicals derived from it, such as superoxide and hydroxyl radicals [66–68], which are presumably initiated by a transition metal (Figure 2). 6-OHDA releases iron from ferritin [69] and the prototype selective iron-chelator desferrioxamine ("desferal") protects against the production of lesions in rat nigro-striatal dopaminergic neurones [70]. Furthermore, intranigral injections of iron produce lesions similar to those observed with 6-OHDA [71]. One of the two main hypotheses for the ultimate cause of the destruction of dopaminergic neurons by MPTP (for review, see [72]) also suggests that the damage may result from intraneuronal generation of superoxides and other cytotoxic free radicals during intracellular reduction and reoxidation of MPP$^+$ (Figure 2), the ultimate metabolite of MPTP. MAO-B inhibitors can only prevent this neurotoxic action by blocking the metabolism of MPTP which is itself non-toxic [3, 4, 59–61]. However, in addition to these MAO-B-inhibiting components there appear to be (particularly for l-deprenyl) other mechanisms which contribute to its neuroprotective action. Tatton and Greenwood [65] briefly reported that l-deprenyl protects neurons against the neurotoxic action of MPTP, even when it is given 3 days after MPTP-treatment (i.e., at a time when all the MPTP had been metabolized or excreted).

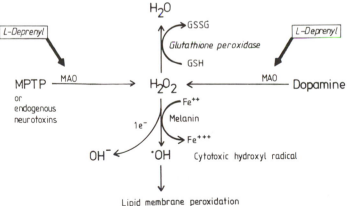

Figure 2. Hydrogen peroxide and MPTP and 6-OHDA neurotoxicity. GSH, reduced glu-tathione; GSSG, oxidized glutathione; MAO, monoamine oxidase; MPTP, 1-methyl-4-phenyl-1,2,3,6-tetrahydropyridine; 6-OHDA, 6-hydroxydopamine.

Since the toxic action of 6-OHDA does not involve any processes that are catalyzed by MAO-B, Knoll [62, 73] concluded that the protective effect of l-deprenyl is due to its increased scavenger function. Although there is as yet no direct evidence for a neuroprotective effect of l-deprenyl in the 6-OHDA model, more recent investigations into the mechanisms for the removal of free radicals (Table 7) do indicate such a function for l-deprenyl. When oxidative stress was provoked by injection of haloperidol (1 mg/kg), the concentration of oxidized glutathione (GSSG), as an index of glutathione peroxidase (glutathione: hydrogen peroxide oxidoreductase; E.C. 1.11.1.9.) activity, tripled [75]. Treatment with l-deprenyl (2.5 mg/kg) 18 h before the haloperidol injection suppressed this rise in GSSG by 71.9%. A 3-week course of daily l-deprenyl injections (2.0 mg/kg subcutaneously) leads to an increased activity of superoxide dismutase (SOD; superoxide: superoxide oxidoreductase; E.C. 1.15.1.1) in the striatum of rats, to a 10-fold level compared to controls [76]. A 3-fold increase in the soluble form of SOD was found by Carrillo et al. [77], but only two times of the control values for the Cu/Zn-form of SOD was found by Clow et al. [78]. There was also an increase in the activity of catalase (hydrogen peroxide: hydrogen peroxide oxidoreductase; E.C. 1.11.1.6) to 1.7 times of the control values [77], but not of glutathione peroxidase [77]. In contrast to these findings with l-deprenyl, injection of 6-OHDA resulted in significant decreases in the activity of SOD and catalase in the striatum of the rat [79]. SOD catalyzes the dismutation of two molecules of superoxide to form a molecule of hydrogen peroxide and a molecule of molecular oxygen (Table 7). The role of SOD is to protect cells from the deleterious effects of the superoxide free radical. However, the radical-scavenging effect of SOD, in order to be effective, has to be followed by the actions of catalase or of glutathione peroxidase (Table 7), because

Table 7. Detoxification of peroxide and superoxide within neurons (according to [74]).

1. Glutathione peroxidase and associated enzymes:

   a) $2GSH + H_2O_2 \longrightarrow GSSG + 2H_2O$
   b) $2GSH + ROOH \longrightarrow GSSG + ROH + H_2O$
   c) $GSSG + NADPH + H^+ \xrightarrow{\text{GSSG Reductase}} 2GSH + NADP^+$
   d) $NADP^+ + G\text{-}6\text{-}P \xrightarrow{\text{G-6-P Dehydrogenase}} NADPH + 6\text{-}PG$

2. Catalase:

   a) $H_2O_2 + H_2O_2 \longrightarrow O_2 + 2H_2O$
   b) $H_2O + RH_2 \longrightarrow R + 2H_2O$

3. Superoxide dismutase:

   $^\cdot O_2^- + {}^\cdot O_2^- + 2H^+ \longrightarrow O_2 + H_2O_2$

G-6-P, glucose-6-phosphate; GSH, reduced glutathione; GSSG, oxidized glutathione; $^\cdot O_2^-$, superoxide free radical; 6-PG, 6-phosphogluconate; ROOH, lipid peroxide.

SOD generates hydrogen peroxide which, in the presence of transition metals, is also capable of forming highly reactive radicals (Figure 2).

5.2. The Indirect Effect of MAO-B Inhibitors on the Function of the NMDA Receptor

The cationic polyamines spermidine and spermine enhance the binding of agonists to the N-methyl-D-aspartate (NMDA) receptor, above that induced by glutamate and glycine, via an increase in binding affinity (for review, see [80]). Structure-affinity relationship studies suggest that this positive modulation is receptor mediated, and studies with competitive antagonists suggest that occupation of this receptor is obligatory for NMDA receptor function. According to current thinking, this subtype of the glutamate receptor is involved in the neurotoxic effects of excitatory toxins and in synaptic plasticity (for review, see [80]). As mentioned above, polyamines were mainly catabolized via mono-acetylation and oxidation. Since N-acetylated polyamines are good substrates of MAO-B, it is likely that, under treatment with MAO-B inhibitors, these compounds will be present in the brain in increased concentrations. It therefore seems possible that they will exert a neuroprotective effect via an antagonistic modulation of the polyamine binding site of the NMDA receptor (Figure 3). On the other hand, it is also possible that polyamines will be present in the brain in decreased amounts because of the inhibition of the metabolism of the N-acetylated derivatives. Hence, the

NMDA - RECEPTOR

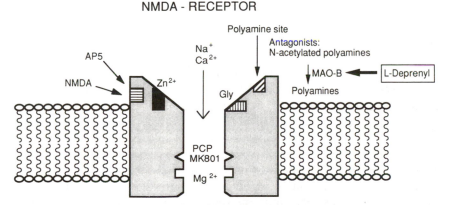

Figure 3. Diagram illustrating the indirect effect of *l*-deprenyl on the function of the NMDA receptor. The NMDA-receptor gates a cation channel that is permeable to Ca^{2+} and Na^+ and is gated by Mg^{2+} in a voltage-dependent fashion; K^+ is the counterion. The NMDA-receptor channel is blocked by PCP and MK801 and the complex is regulated at three modulatory sites by glycine, Zn^{2+} and polyamines. Gly, glycine; MK801, (+)-5-methyl-10,11-dihydro-5H-dibenzo[a,d]cyclohepten-5,10-imine maleate; NMDA, N-methyl-D-aspartate; PCP, phencylidine.

neuroprotective effect of MAO-B inhibition may also receive a contribution from the diminished modulation of the NMDA receptor by the polyamine binding site.

6. Future Outlook

It is possible that MAO-B inhibitors do not have any specific neuroprotective activity in PD, but if they do have such activity, it may be a generalized feature of both MAO-A and MAO-B inhibitors. Thus, moclobemide (p-chloro-N-[2-morpholino-ethyl]benzamide), the selective, reversible MAO-A inhibitor, has been reported to have antihypoxic and neuroprotective effects due to the inhibition of the generation of hydrogen peroxide via MAO-A reactions [81]. At the present time, we cannot draw too many conclusions from the action of l-deprenyl on the brain in patients with PD and its effect on DA metabolism and its neuroprotective properties. It has to be remembered that DA is a substrate for both MAO-A and MAO-B in the striatum [12, 13], and not (as envisaged by Glover et al. [49]) a selective MAO-B substrate in this region. Thus, the contribution of MAO-A to the metabolism of DA is also important and calls for further examination. However, because of the side-effects associated with MAO-A inhibitors, this problem has not been as fully examined in man. Furthermore, a comparison with other selective MAO-B inhibitors such as AGN 1135, Ro 19-6327, and MDL 72974, etc. is required, to establish whether there is some intrinsic property of l-deprenyl which is not shared with other MAO-B inhibitors (see Chapters 6, 7, 13).

Summary

Relevant aspects of the mode of action of selective monoamine oxidase type B (MAO-B) inhibitors in the treatment of Parkinson's disease have been evaluated, with special reference to the possible mechanisms responsible for the observed neuroprotective effects of the MAO-B inhibitor l-deprenyl (selegiline). MAO types A and B play important roles in the metabolism of biogenic amines. The existence of the two forms of MAO was originally postulated on the basis of differential substrate and inhibitor sensitivities in *in vitro* assays and has been confirmed by molecular genetics and immunological approaches. MAO-B has a greater affinity for benzylamine and for β-phenylethylamine and is selectively and irreversibly inhibited by low concentrations of l-deprenyl. In the brain, dopamine – the essential neurotransmitter in the basal ganglia – is metabolized by the two forms of MAO. However, recent studies with human brain tissue show that dopamine has a higher affinity for MAO-B. Since Parkinson's disease is basically characterized by a diminished dopaminergic neurotransmission in the basal ganglia, it is reasonable to suppose that the selective inhibition of MAO-B – particularly and predominantly in the glia – should lead to diminished catabolism of dopamine in the nigro-striatal system and to a significant increase in the concentration of the neurotransmitter at the synapses. It is not clear (although it is highly probable) whether the glia become enriched with dopamine, which might then have a hormone-like influence on dopaminergic neurotransmission. Beside MAO-B inhibition, which above all explains the clinical effectiveness of MAO-B inhibitors in the treatment of Parkinson's disease, *l*-deprenyl in particular appears to exhibit other mechanisms of action that are independent of its action on MAO-B. These mechanisms have been discussed above in connection with two hypotheses of the neuroprotective mode of action of MAO-B inhibitors: the inhibition of oxidative stress, and an indirect influence on the N-methyl-D-aspartate receptor by MAO-B inhibitors.

References

[1] Blaschko H. Amine oxidase and amine metabolism. Pharmac Rev 1952; 4: 415–53.
[2] De Varebeke PJ, Cavalier R, David-Remacle M, Youdim MBH. Formation of the neurotransmitter glycine from the anticonvulsant milacemide is mediated by brain monoamine oxidase B. J Neurochem 1988; 50: 1011–16.
[3] Chiba K, Trevor A, Castagnoli Jr N. Metabolism of the neurotoxic tertiary amine, MPTP, by brain monoamine oxidase. Biochem Biophys Res Commun 1984; 120: 574–78.
[4] Heikkila RE, Manzino L, Cabbat FS, Duvoisin RS. Protection against the dopaminergic neurotoxicity of 1-methyl-4-phenyl-1,2,3,6-tetrahydropyridine by monoamine oxidase inhibitors. Nature 1984; 311: 467–9.
[5] May T, Strauss S, Rommelspacher H. [³H]Harman labels selectively and with high affinity the active site of monoamine oxidase (EC 1.4.3.4) subtype A (MAO-A) in rat, marmoset, and pig. J Neural Transm [Supplement] 1990; 32: 93–102.
[6] Dostert PL, Strolin-Benedetti M, Tipton KF. Interactions of monoamine oxidase with substrates and inhibitors. Med Res Rev 1990; 9: 45–89.
[7] Youdim MBH, Finberg JPM, Tipton KF. Monoamine oxidase. In: Trendelenburg U, Weiner N, editors. Catecholamines I, handbook of experimental pharmacology, Vol 90/I. Berlin Heidelberg New York: Springer-Verlag, 1988: 119–92.
[8] Johnston JP. Some observations upon a new inhibitor of monoamine oxidase in brain tissue. Biochem Pharmacol 1968; 17: 1285–97.
[9] Fowler CJ, Callingham BA, Mantle TJ, Tipton KF. Monoamine oxidase A and B: a useful concept? Biochem Pharmacol 1978; 27: 97–101.
[10] Tipton KF, Fowler CJ, Houslay MD. Specifities of the two forms of monoamine oxidase. In: Kamijo K, Usdin E, Nagatsu T, editors. Monoamine oxidase. Amsterdam: Oxford, Princeton: Excerpta Medica, 1982: 87–99.
[11] Kinemuchi H, Fowler CJ, Tipton KF. Substrate specifities of the two forms of monoamine oxidase. In: Tipton KF, Dostert PL, Strolin-Benedetti M, editors. Monoamine oxidase and disease. London New York: Academic Press, 1984: 53–62.
[12] O'Carroll AM, Fowler CJ, Phillips JP, Tobia I, Tipton KF. The deamination of dopamine by human brain monoamine oxidase: specificity for the two enzyme forms in seven brain regions. Naunyn-Schmiedeberg's Arch Pharmacol 1983; 322: 198–202.
[13] Riederer P, Youdim MBH. Monoamine oxidase activity and monoamine metabolism in brains of parkinsonian patients treated with *l*-deprenyl. J Neurochem 1986; 46: 1359–65.

[14] Denney RM, Patel NT, Fritz RR, Abell CW. A monoclonal antibody elicited to human platelet monoamine oxidase, isolation and specificity for human monoamine oxidase B but not A. Mol Pharmacol 1982; 22: 500–8.

[15] Konradi C, Kornhuber J, Froelich L, Fritze J, Heinsen H, Beckmann H et al. Demonstration of monoamine oxidase-A and -B in the human brainstem by a histochemical technique. Neuroscience 1989; 33: 383–400.

[16] Konradi C, Svoma E, Jellinger K, Riederer P, Denney RM, Thibault J. Topographic immunocytochemical mapping of monoamine oxidase-A, monoamine oxidase-B and tyrosine hydroxylase in human post mortem brain stem. Neuroscience 1988; 26: 791–802.

[17] Bach AWJ, Lan NC, Johnson DL, Abell CW, Bembenek ME, Kwan SW et al. cDNA cloning of human liver monoamine oxidase A and B: molecular basis of differences in enzymatic properties. Proc Natl Acad Sci USA 1988; 85: 4934–8.

[18] Bach AWJ, Lan NC, Johnson DL, Abell CW, Bembenek ME, Kwan SW et al. cDNA cloning of human liver monoamine oxidase A and B: molecular basis of differences in enzymatic properties. Neurobiology 1988; 85: 4934–38.

[19] Lan NC, Chan C, Shih J. Expression of functional human monoamine oxidase A and B cDNAs in mammalian cells. J Neurochem 1989; 52: 1652–54.

[20] Rando RR. Chemistry and enzymology of k_{cat} inhibitors. Science 1974; 185: 320–4.

[21] Singer TP. Active site-directed irreversible inhibitors of monoamine oxidase. In: Singer TP, von Korf, RW, Murphy DL, editors. Monoamine oxidase: structure, function, and altered functions. New York: Academic Press, 1979: 7–24.

[22] Tipton KF, Fowler CJ. The kinetics of monoamine oxidase inhibitors in relation to their clinical behaviour. In: Tipton KF, Dostert PL, Strolin-Benedetti M, editors. Monoamine oxidase and disease. London New York: Academic Press, 1984: 27–40.

[23] Gerlach M, Riederer P, Youdim MBH. The molecular pharmacology of l-deprenyl. European J Pharmacol [Molec Pharamacol Sect.] 1992; 226: 97–108.

[24] Schmauss M, Erfurth A. Indikationen für eine Therapie mit MAO-Hemmern. Psychiat Prax [Sonderheft] 1989; 16: 2–6.

[25] Crane GE. Iproniazid (Marsilid) phosphate, a therapeutic agent for mental disorders and debilitating disease. Psychiat Res Rep 1957; 8: 142–52.

[26] Kline DF. Clinical experience with iproniazid (Marsilid). J Clin Exp Psychopathol [Supplement] 1958; 1: 72–8.

[27] Blackwell B, Marley E, Price J, Taylor D. Interactions with cheese and its constituents with monoamine oxidase inhibitors. Br J Psychiat 1967; 113: 349–65.

[28] Youdim MBH, Finberg JPM. MAO type-B inhibitors as adjunct to L-dopa therapy. In: Yahr MD, Bergmann KJ, editors. Advances in Neurology, Vol 45. New York: Raven Press, 1986: 127–36.

[29] Kalir A, Sabbagh A, Youdim MBH. Selective acetylenic 'suicide' and reversible inhibitors of monoamine oxidase types A and B. Br J Pharmacol 1981; 73: 55–64.

[30] Dollery CT, Davies DS, Strolin-Benedetti M. Clinical pharmacology of MD 780515, a selective and reversible MAO-A inhibitor. In: Kamijo K, Usdin E, Nagatsu T, editors. Monoamine oxidase, basic and clinical frontiers. Amsterdam: Excerpta Medica, 1982: 221–9.

[31] Knoll J. The pharmacology of (−)-deprenyl. J Neural Transm [Supplement] 1986; 22: 75–89.

[32] Palfreyman MG, Zreika M, McDonald I, Fozard J, Bey P. MDL 72,145, an irreversible inhibitor of MAO-B. In: Tipton KF, Dostert P, Strolin-Benedetti M, editors. Monoamine oxidase and disease. London: Academic Press, 1986: 563–4.

[33] Keller HH, Kettler R, Keller G, Da Prada M. Short-acting novel MAO inhibitors: in vitro evidence for the reversibility of MAO inhibition by moclobemide and Ro 16-6491. Naunyn-Schmiedeberg's Arch Pharmacol 1987; 335: 15–20.

[34] Da Prada M, Kettler R, Keller HH, Burkard WP. Ro 19-6327, a reversible, highly selective inhibitor of type-B monoamine oxidase, completely devoid of tyramine-potentiating effects: comparison with selegiline. Neurol Neurobiol 1988; 42B: 359–63.

[35] Da Prada M, Kettler R, Zürcher G, Kettler HH. Hemmer der MAO-B und COMT: Möglichkeiten ihrer Anwendung bei der Parkinson-Therapie aus heutiger Sicht. In: Fischer P-A, editor. Modifizierende Faktoren bei der Parkinson-Therapie. Basel: Editiones (Roche), 1988: 309–22.

[36] Zreika M, Fozard JR, Dudley MW, Bey Ph, McDonald IA, Palfreyman MG. MDL 72,974: a potent and selective enzyme-activated irreversible inhibitor of monoamine oxidase type B with potential for use in Parkinson's disease. J Neural Transm [P-D Sect.] 1989; 1: 243–54.

[37] Birkmayer W, Riederer P, Youdim MBH, Linauer W. The potentiation of the anti-akinetic effect after L-dopa-treatment by an inhibitor of MAO-B, deprenyl. J Neural Transm 1975; 36: 303–26.

[38] Riederer P, Przuntek H, editors. MAO-B-inhibitor selegiline (R-(−)-deprenyl). A new therapeutic concept in the treatment of Parkinson's disease. Vienna New York: Springer-Verlag, 1987.

[39] Golbe LI. Deprenyl as symptomatic therapy in Parkinson's disease. Clinical Neuropharmacology 1988; 11: 387–400.

[40] Tariot PN, Sunderland T, Weingartner H, Murphy DL, Welkowitz JA, Thompson K et al. Cognitive effects of l-deprenyl in Alzheimer's disease. Psychopharmacology 1987; 91: 489–95.

[41] Mangoni A, Grassi MP, Frattola L, Piolti R, Bassi S, Motta A et al. Effects of a MAO-B inhibitor in the treatment of Alzheimer disease. Eur Neurol 1991; 31: 100–7.

[42] Youdim MBH, Finberg JPM. Monoamine oxidase inhibitor antidepressants. In: Grahame-Smith DG, Hippius H, Winokur G, editors. Psychopharmacology 1/1. Amsterdam: Excerpta Medica, 1982: 37–51.

[43] Jossan SS, d'Argy R, Gillberg PG, Aquilonius SM, Långström B, Halldin C et al. Localization of monoamine oxidase B in human brain by autoradiographical use of ^{11}C-labelled l-deprenyl. J Neural Transm 1989; 77: 55–64.

[44] Riederer P, Jellinger K, Seemann D. Monoamine oxidase and parkinsonism. In: Tipton KF, Dostert P, Strolin-Benedetti M, editors. Monoamine oxidase and disease. London New York: Academic Press, 1984: 403–15.

[45] Moll G, Moll R, Riederer P, Heinsen H, Denney RM. Distribution pattern of MAO-A and MAO-B in human substantia nigra shown by immunofluorescence cytochemistry on thin frozen section. Pharm Res Comm [Supplement 4] 1988; 20: 80–90.

[46] Moll G, Moll R, Riederer P, Gsell W, Heinsen H, Denney RM. Immunofluorescence cytochemistry on thin sections of human substantia nigra for staining of monoamine oxidase A and monoamine oxidase B: a pilot study. J Neural Transm [Supplement] 1990; 32: 67–77.

[47] Tipton KF, Dostert P, Strolin-Benedetti M, editors. Monoamine oxidase and disease: prospects for therapy with reversible inhibitors. London: Academic Press, 1984.

[48] Tipton KF, Houslay MD, Garrett N. Allotropic properties of human brain monoamine oxidase. Nature 1973; 246: 213–4.

[49] Glover V, Sandler M, Owen F, Riley GJ. Dopamine is a monoamine oxidase-B substrate in man. Nature 1977; 265: 80–1.

[50] Roth JA, Feor K. Deamination of dopamine and its 3-O-methylated derivative by human brain monoamine oxidase. Biochem Pharmacol 1978; 27: 1616–23.

[51] Glover V, Elsworth JD, Sandler M. Dopamine oxidation and its inhibition by (−)-deprenyl. J Neural Transm [Supplement] 1980; 16: 163–71.

[52] Garrick NA, Murphy DL. Differences in the preferential deamination of L-norepinephrine, dopamine and serotonin by MAO in rodent and primate brain. In: Usdin E, Weiner N, Youdim MBH, editors. Function and regulation of monoamine enzymes. London: Macmillan, 1981: 517–28.

[53] O'Carroll A-M, Bardsley ME, Tipton KF. The oxidation of adrenaline and noradrenaline by the two forms of monoamine oxidase from human and rat brain. Neurochem Int 1986; 8: 493–500.

[54] Paterson IA, Juorio AV, Boulton AA. 2-Phenylethylamine: a modulator of catecholamine transmission in the mammalian central nervous system? J Neurochem 1990; 55: 1827–37.

[55] Seiler N, Al-Therib MJ. Putrescine catabolism in mammalian brain. Biochem J 1974; 144: 29–35.

[56] Seiler N. Polyamine metabolism and function in brain. Neurochem Int 1981; 3: 95–110.

[57] Zappia V, Pegg AE, editors. Progress in polyamine research. New York: Plenum Press, 1988.

[58] Seiler N, Knödgen B. High-performance liquid chromatographic procedure for the simultaneous determination of the natural polyamines and their monoacetyl derivatives. J Chromatogr 1980; 221: 227–35.

[59] Cohen G, Pasik P, Cohen B, Leist A, Mytilineou C, Yahr MD. Pargyline and deprenyl prevent the neurotoxicity of 1-methyl-4-phenyl-1,2,3,6-tetrahydropyridine (MPTP) in monkeys. European J Pharmacol 1984; 106: 209–10.

[60] Langston JW, Irwin I, Langston EB, Forno LS. Pargyline prevents MPTP-induced parkinsonism in primates. Science 1984; 225: 1480–82.

[61] Markey JP, Johannessen JN, Chiueh CC, Burns RS, Herkenham MA. Intraneuronal generation of a pyridinium metabolite may cause drug-induced parkinsonsim. Nature 1984; 311: 464–7.

[62] Knoll J. R-(−)-deprenyl (Selegiline, Movergan^R) facilitates the activity of the nigrostriatal dopaminergic neuron. J Neural Transm [Supplement] 1987; 25: 45–66.

[63] Gibson C. Inhibition of MAO B, but not MAO A, blocks DSP-4 toxicity on central NE neurons. European J Pharmacol 1987; 141: 135–8.

[64] Finnegan KT, Skratt JJ, Irwin I, DeLanney LE, Langston JW. Protection against DSP-4-induced neurotoxicity by deprenyl is not related to its inhibition of MAO B. European J Pharmacol 1990; 184: 119–26.

[65] Tatton WG, Greenwood CE. Rescue of dying neurons: a new action for deprenyl in MPTP parkinsonism. J Neurosci Res 1991; 30: 666–72.

[66] Heikkila RE, Cohen G. Further studies on generation of hydrogen peroxide by 6-hydroxydopamine: potentiation by ascorbic acid. Mol Pharmacol 1972; 8: 241–8.

[67] Sachs CH, Johnsson G. Mechanism of action of 6-hydroxydopamine. Pharmacology 1975; 24: 1–25.

[68] Graham DG, Tiffany SM, Bell WR, Gutknecht WF. Autooxidation versus covalent binding quinones as the mechanism of toxicity of dopamine, 6-hydroxydopamine and related compounds towards C1300 neuroblastoma cells in vitro. Mol Pharmacol 1978; 14: 644–53.

[69] Monterio HP, Winterbourn CC. 6-Hydroxydopamine releases iron from ferritin and promotes ferritin-dependent lipid peroxidation. Biochem Pharmacol 1989; 38: 4177–82.

[70] Ben-Shachar D, Eshel G, Finberg JPM, Youdim MBH. The iron chelator desferrioxamine (Desferal) retards 6-hydroxydopamine-induced degeneration of nigrostriatal dopamine neurons. J Neurochem 1991; 56: 1441–5.

[71] Ben-Shachar D, Youdim MBH. Intranigral iron injection induces behavioural and biochemical "parkinsonism" in the rat. J Neurochem 1991; 57: 2133–5.

[72] Gerlach M, Riederer P, Przuntek H, Youdim MBH. MPTP mechanisms of neurotoxicity and their implications for Parkinson's disease. European J Pharmacol [Molec Pharmacol Sect.] 1991; 208: 273–86.

[73] Knoll J. The pharmacology of (−)-deprenyl. J Neural Transm [Supplement] 1986; 22: 75–89.

[74] Cohen G. The pathobiology of Parkinson's disease: biochemical aspects of dopamine neuron senescence. J Neural Transm [Supplement] 1983; 19: 89–103.

[75] Cohen G, Spina MB. Deprenyl suppresses the oxidant stress associated with increased dopamine turnover. Ann Neurol 1989; 26: 689–90.

[76] Knoll J. The striatal dopamine dependency of life span in male rats, longevity study with (−)deprenyl. Mech Ageing Dev 1988; 46: 237–62.

[77] Carrillo M-C, Kanai S, Nokubo M, Kitani K. (−)-Deprenyl induces activities of both superoxide dismutase and catalase but not of glutathione peroxidase in the striatum of young male rats. Life Sci 1991; 48: 517–21.

[78] Clow A, Hussain T, Glover V, Sandler M, Dexter DT, Walker M. (−)-Deprenyl can induce soluble superoxide dismutase in rat striata. J. Neural Transm [Gen Sect.] 1991; 86: 77–80.

[79] Perumal AS, Tordzro WK, Katz M, Jackson-Lewis V, Cooper TB, Fahn S et al. Regional effects of 6-hydroxydopamine (6-OHDA) on free radical scavengers in rat brain. Brain Res 1989; 504: 139–44.

[80] Lodge D, Collingridge GL. The pharmacology of excitatory amino acids. Trends in Pharmacological Sciences, a special report. Cambridge: Elsevier, 1991.

[81] Da Prada M, Kettler R, Burkhard WP, Lore HP, Haefely W. Some basic aspects of reversible inhibitors of monoamine oxidase-A. Acta Psychiatr Scand [Supplement] 1990; 360: 7–12.

Inhibitors of Monoamine Oxidase B
Pharmacology and Clinical Use in Neurodegenerative Disorders
ed. by I. Szelenyi
© 1993 Birkhäuser Verlag Basel/Switzerland

CHAPTER 10
Pharmacokinetics and Clinical Pharmacology of Selegiline

E. H. Heinonen, M. I. Anttila and R. A. S. Lammintausta

1 Introduction
2 Absorption and Distribution of Selegiline
3 MAO Inhibition by Selegiline
4 Phenylethylamine
5 Metabolism and Excretion of Selegiline
6 Interactions of Selegiline and Other Drugs
  Summary
  References

1. Introduction

Selegiline (formerly called l-($-$)-deprenyl) is a selective, irreversible inhibitor of monoamine oxidase (MAO) type B. In the human brain dopamine is metabolized via MAO-B [1]. By inhibiting this enzyme the dopamine concentration in the brain is increased [2]. Selegiline has also been shown to inhibit the uptake of dopamine and noradrenaline [3]. Due to these properties, selegiline is widely used in the treatment of Parkinson's disease (PD) as either an adjuvant to levodopa therapy or alone in the early phase of the disease [4–6]. Preliminary results have suggested that selegiline may also alleviate the symptoms of Alzheimer's disease [7, 8]. High dosages (up to 50 mg daily) have been successfully used in the treatment of depression [9]. In the following the pharmacokinetics, metabolism, and interactions of selegiline will be reviewed.

2. Absorption and Distribution of Selegiline

Selegiline is rapidly absorbed from the gastrointestinal tract. This has been demonstrated by use of the ^{14}C-labeled drug, both in animals and in humans [10, 11]. In mice, the highest level of radioactivity in the blood was reached 0.5 h following subcutaneous administration and 1 h after oral administration [10]. Within 30 s after intravenous injection, high concentrations of radiolabeled selegiline were detected in the brain and spinal cord of mice [10]. Retention of selegiline occurs also in the heart and, similarly, in the lung, although to a lesser degree [12]. In man, the maximum plasma concentrations of radiolabeled selegiline (0.033–0.045 μg/ml) after a 5-mg dose of ^{14}C-selegiline were attained within 0.5–2 h [11]. The kinetics of ^{14}C-selegiline were fitted to a two-compartment model. The parent drug was not separated from its metabolites in this study. Using the analytical methods currently available, it has not been possible to measure the parent compound reliably subsequent to a 10-mg oral dose of selegiline. After intravenous injection the observed half-life of selegiline is around 0.15 h. Selegiline is thus distributed and metabolized very rapidly.

Selegiline is lipophilic and it therefore penetrates quickly into the tissues; the median apparent volume of distribution at steady state (V_{ss}) after an intravenous 10-mg dose is approximately 130 L. Selegiline is moderately bound to proteins (75–85%). The binding takes place especially to macroglobulins, but, to a lesser extent, also to albumin [13, 14]. Positron emission tomography (PET) studies have shown that ^{11}C-labeled selegiline enters the brain within seconds after injection, and that the radioactivity stays constant throughout the 90 min of the PET session [15]. This is in contrast to d-($+$)-deprenyl, which does not offer a strong MAO-inhibitory capacity. d-Deprenyl is rapidly washed away from the brain. These results reflect the irreversible binding of selegiline and provide a means to assess the distribution of MAO-B in the human brain. The uptake of selegiline in the PET study was higher in the thalamus and striatum than in the cortex. The magnitude of uptake of ^{11}C-selegiline was over two times higher than that of clorgyline in the thalamus, striatum, cortex, and brainstem [15]. This may reflect the higher concentration of MAO-B compared to that of MAO-A in the human brain [16].

In autoradiographic studies carried out with post-mortem human brain, high binding of ^{3}H-labeled selegiline can be detected in the caudate nucleus, putamen, cingulate gyrus, insula cortex, anterior and dorsomedial nuclei of the thalamus, pulvinar, hippocampus, substantia nigra, and periaqueductal gray matter [17, 18]. White matter indicated the lowest binding [18]. These results are in line with PET results and the earlier biochemical determination of the ratio of MAO-A/B in various parts of the brain [16]. Within the cerebral cortex, cingulate gyrus demonstrated the highest, and the occipital cortex the lowest selegiline binding. In all cortical regions, lamina I showed the highest density of binding. In the parietal cortex and cingulate gyrus, laminae II and III showed moderate and laminae IV and V the lowest binding of ^{3}H-selegiline. In the hippocampus, the highest density was found in the ependymal cell layer and the dentate gyrus [18].

3. MAO Inhibition by Selegiline

In tissues, selegiline binds specifically to MAO. The reaction between the enzyme and selegiline is assumed to take place in two steps in which the initial reaction is competitive and reversible; this step is followed by an irreversible reaction. Selegiline binds to the flavine part of MAO, forming a covalent adduct [19]. After this irreversible adduct has been formed, the enzyme can not be activated by extensive dialysis or gelfiltration. It has been suggested that the MAO-B selectivity of selegiline in lower concentrations is determined by reversible rather than by irreversible inhibition. The IC_{50} value for selegiline to inhibit human brain MAO was approximately 0.05–0.95 nM in various brain regions, whereas that of clorgyline was approximately 500–3000 nM [2]. *In vitro*, the highest degree (80–83%) of inhibition of dopamine (a substrate of both MAO-A and MAO-B) with a concentration of 1 μM of selegiline in the human brain takes place in the striatum and nucleus accumbens [1].

In the post-mortem human brain, MAO activity towards dopamine has been demonstrated to be inhibited by about 90%, and towards serotonin by about 65%, when the patients were treated with 10 mg daily about 6 days prior to death [2], It is clear that the remaining MAO-A is sufficient to take care of the metabolism of serotonin, as the concentrations of this monoamine were not increased. The proportion of inhibition, MAO-A/B, seems to remain quite stable during long-term therapy [20]. With higher dosages of selegiline (over 20 mg daily), the MAO-A is also significantly inhibited, as shown by increased sensitivity towards tyramine and decrease in plasma concentrations of MHPG (3-methoxy-4-hydroxyphenylglycol), a metabolite of noradrenaline [21].

The intestinal MAO is almost entirely of type A, which is only partially inhibited by means of those concentrations of selegiline that completely inhibit type B [22]. The intestinal MAO is approximately 1000 times less sensitive to inhibition by selegiline than the platelet MAO. Therefore, the metabolism of tyramine and many other biogenic amines can still occur in the intestines, despite the complete inhibition of MAO-B in the body. This partly explains the lack of the so-called "cheese effect" during selegiline treatment. The cheese effect received its name when increases of blood pressure – even hypertensive crises – were occasionally observed during treatment with nonspecific MAO-inhibitors as a result of the patients eating food that contained large quantities of tyramine, e.g., aged cheese [23]. With specific concentration (μM) of selegiline inhibiting about 60–80% of dopamine breakdown in the brain, the dopamine oxidizing activity in jejunum is inhibited by only about 34%, compared to 60% in the liver [1] (for details see Chapter 6).

Platelet MAO is almost totally of type B [24]. In man, the platelet MAO-B is completely inhibited with a 5–10 mg daily dosage of selegiline. Four hours after oral administration of 5 mg of selegiline, the platelet MAO-B activity was inhibited by 86% [25]. After 2–4 h, greater than 96% inhibition was achieved, and this degree of inhibition was maintained during continuous selegiline administration [25, 26]. A typical pattern of inhibition of platelet MAO-B after a single oral, 5-mg dose of selegiline given to healthy volunteers is shown in Figure 1. According to Lee et al. [25] 50% platelet MAO-B inhibition was attained in about 0.7 h after a 10-mg oral dose [25] and after 3 h the inhibition was about 90%. With a 10-mg daily dose over a 1-week period, the platelet MAO-B is usually inhibited by 99.9% [26, 27]. The rate and degree of platelet MAO-B-inhibition is similar after a 10-mg single dose in the morning, and a divided dosage of two 5-mg tablets daily (morning and noon) [25]. Platelet MAO-B is actually inhibited by rather small doses of selegiline. After repeated doses of 1 mg daily a complete inhibition of the platelet MAO-B can be achieved occasionally [28]. Data are not available regarding the inhibition of brain MAO-B after administration of such very low doses of selegiline. It has, however, been demonstrated that most of the patients with advanced Parkinson's disease treated with levodopa do require a dosage of 10 mg daily [29]. Furthermore, it is probable that the degree of platelet MAO-B inhibition does not directly reflect inhibition in the brain, at least not with lower doses.

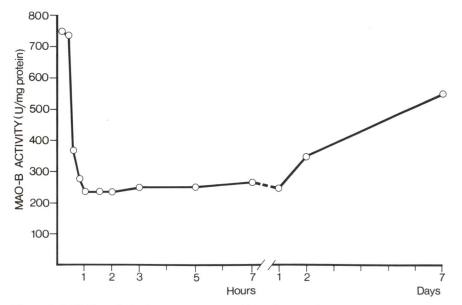

Figure 1. Inhibition of platelet MAO-B in a healthy volunteer after a single, 5-mg oral dose of selegiline.

The recovery of MAO-B activity after selegiline treatment depends on the dosage, the organ, and the species in question. In the rat brain, 50% of MAO-B activity is recovered in approximately 8–12 days, even after an extremely high dose (5–10 mg/kg s.c. or i.p.) of selegiline [30–32], Using PET techniques, it has been calculated that the half-life for the recovery of MAO-B activity in the pig brain is about 6.5 days after a single selegiline dose [33]. In contrast, a PET study carried out on a baboon suggested that the half-life of recovery could be as long as 30 days [34]. Human studies using the same technique are underway (Oreland, personal communications). The recovery of MAO-B activity in the liver is substantially faster, requiring only approximately 1–3 days in rodents [16, 26, 35]. The differences are at least partly due to the organ-specific variability in the rate of synthesis of MAO. The recovery of the platelet MAO-B in humans takes place at a rate of approximately 10% daily. Therefore, 50% is recovered over a 5–7-day period, total recovery being reached in 10–14 days. These recovery times relevant to platelet MAO-B in humans parallel those found in respect to brain enzyme recovery in rodents and pigs.

The clinical effect of selegiline is lost after approximately 2–3 days subsequent to terminating treatment [27]. It is conceivable that, in addition to the irreversible inhibition of MAO-B, the reversible mechanisms such as the inhibition in the uptake of catecholamines may also play an important role in regard to the clinical action of selegiline.

4. Phenylethylamine

An alternative method for assessing the degree of MAO-B inhibition is through measuring the concentrations of phenylethylamine (PEA). PEA is the substrate for MAO-B and, consequently, the PEA excretion increases significantly during selegiline treatment. PEA is normally present in the brain, serum, and urine in trace amounts only. In the human brain the highest concentrations of PEA are found in the putamen, hippocampus, hypothalamus, and cerebellum [36]. During selegiline treatment the concentrations of PEA in the human brain increase up to 6 ng/g [37]. Urinary excretion of PEA increases following the 10-mg dose of selegiline, which is the ordinarily used effective daily dose in the treatment of PD [22]. An increase in urinary excretion rate of PEA after a single oral 10-mg dose of selegiline in a healthy volunteer is shown in Figure 2. PEA has been shown to release catecholamines from a presynaptic, extragranular pool; it may also have some direct, postsynaptic, dopamine-receptor-stimulating effect [38–40]. Therefore, increased concentrations of PEA may play some role in the treatment of PD.

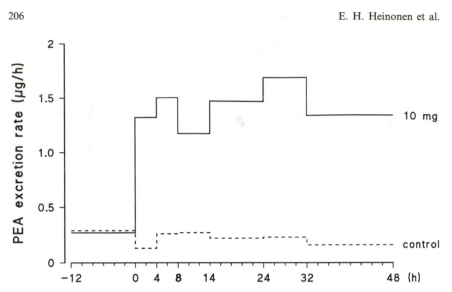

Figure 2. An increase in the rate of excretion of phenylethylamine (PEA) during 24 h in a healthy volunteer after a single, 10 mg dose of selegiline as compared to the excretion without the drug (control).

5. Metabolism and Excretion of Selegiline

In rodents, selegiline is metabolized to desmethylselegiline (DES) and l-(−)-methamphetamine (l-MA), which can be further converted to l-(−)-amphetamine (l-A) and corresponding p-hydroxylated metabolites [10, 14, 41], The hydroxylation is followed by conjugation with glucuronic acid. Metabolism takes place mainly in the liver and is dependent on the microsomal cytochrome P-450. The formation of l-A is partially catalyzed by mono-oxygenase containing FAD. Liver and kidney microsomes are also able to metabolize selegiline, although to a much less significant degree [42]. Some sex and strain differences in the rate of the metabolism of selegiline have been described in rodent studies [42]. The stereoisomeric configuration is maintained during metabolism (see above), the metabolites are of *levo* form, and no racemic transformation occurs [43, 44].

Only the concentrations of l-A have been studied in the post-mortem human brain. The highest concentration, 56 ng/g, was found in the thalamus, and l-A was also found in the striatum, red nucleus, hypothalamus, raphe nuclei, and nucleus accumbens [37]. The three main metabolites, DES, l-MA, and l-A, have been identified in human plasma, CSF and urine (for review see [45]). The pharmacokinetic parameters in plasma after single and multiple 10 mg daily doses of selegiline in 12 healthy volunteers are shown in Table 1. There are no significant differences in the pharmacokinetic parameters of the metabolites after single and multiple dosing of the drug, i.e., no metabolite

Table 1. The serum pharmacokinetics of metabolites of selegiline after single and multiple (7 days) dose administration of selegiline 10 mg daily in 12 healthy volunteers (mean ± SD).

	Single dose			Multiple dose		
	C_{max} (ng/ml)	T_{max} (h)	$T_{1/2}$ (h)	C_{max} (ng/ml)	T_{max} (h)	$T_{1/2}$ (h)
Desmethylselegiline	19.0 ± 8.8	0.9 ± 0.6	2.1	23.6 ± 15.4	0.7 ± 0.4	5.6
l-Methamphetamine	40.0 ± 17.0	3.1 ± 1.9	20.5	37.0 ± 12.1	2.7 ± 2.2	19.7
l-Amphetamine	28.4 ± 16.5	4.6 ± 2.1	17.7	20.1 ± 11.1	3.7 ± 2.6	18.1

Table 2. Concentration (ng/ml) of the three major metabolites of selegiline in cerebrospinal fluid (CSF) during long-term continuous therapy with 10 mg selegiline daily (mean ± SD).

Patients				
Type	No.	*l*-A	*l*-MA	DES
AD	12	7.0 ± 3.0	15.0 ± 6.0	1.1 ± 0.8
PD	9	6.3 ± 2.1	14.2 ± 7.0	0.7 ± 0.4

Abbreviations: AD = Alzheimer's disease, PD = Parkinson's disease, *l*-A = *l*-(−)-amphetamine, *l*-MA = *l*-(−)-methamphetamine, DES = desmethylselegiline.

accumulation takes place. The morning through values of *l*-A, *l*-MA, and DES were 5.8, 9.0, and 1.3 ng/ml, respectively, in four parkinsonian patients who had been receiving 10 mg doses of selegiline for 22 months [45]. The CSF concentrations of metabolites in patients with Alzheimer's or Parkinson's disease were, to a high degree, parallel with the serum concentrations (Table 2).

The median total body clearance of the drug from plasma is approximately 500 L/h. The metabolites are mainly excreted via urine, with approximately 15% also discharged in feces. The 24-h urinary recovery of the given drug dose as metabolites has varied considerably (30–90%) between different clinical trials, with *l*-MA accounting for most of the metabolite pool (Table 3). The pH of urine has a significant effect on excretion of the amphetamine metabolites. Acidification of the urine enhances excretion, whereas alkalinization can cause retention of the metabolites. Elsworth et al. [46] have studied whether modification in exretion of the metabolites of selegiline would alter the clinical response to the drug. The pH of urine in parkinsonian patients was manipulated by administering either ammonium chloride or sodium bicarbonate to the patients. By rendering the urine alkaline, a clear reduction in exretion of the amphetamine metabolites was detected, thus, accumulation in the body had occurred. However, no changes in clinical disability were noted, despite the accumulation of the metabolites. Furthermore, two patients showed marked deterioration

Table 3. The 24-h excretion of metabolites of selegiline in urine after multiple dosing, 10 mg daily (values expressed as mean ± SD, range in brackets, % = mean recovery of the parent drug).

Study	Subject		l-A		l-MA		DES	
	Type	No.	(mg)	(%)	(mg)	(%)	(mg)	(%)
Reynolds et al. 1978 [61]	Healthy volunteers	6	0.5 (0.5–1.1)	15.1 (11–20)	3.4 (1.7–5.0)	63.3 (46–104)	—	—
Schachter et al. 1980 [44]	Parkinsonian	6	1.1 (0.5–1.6)	—	2.5 (1.5–4.0)	—	—	—
Karoum et al. 1982 [62]	Parkinsonian / Depression	5 / 6	0.5 ± 0.1 / 0.7 ± 0.3	— / —	1.1 ± 0.3 / 1.6 ± 0.4	— / —	—	—
Elsworth et al. 1982 [46]	Parkinsonian	5	—	15.1 (5.1–22.3)	—	43.6 (11.4–63.2)	—	—
Liebowitz et al. 1985 [63]	Depression	6	0.6 ± 0.4	8.7	1.6 ± 0.7	20.0	—	—
Heinonen et al. 1989 [45]	Parkinsonian	4	1.6 (0.9–2.4)	26.3 ± 11.8 (15–41)	3.9 (2.3–7.9)	59.2 ± 40.3 (34–119)	0.09 (0.04–0.6)	1.1 ± 0.5 (0.6–1.5)

l-A = l-(−)-amphetamine, l-MA = l-(−)-methamphetamine, DES = l-(−)-desmethylselegiline.

when selegiline was replaced with placebo or methamphetamine-amphetamine. It is important to remember the stereoselectivity of the metabolites: the *levo* form amphetamines are two to three times less active CNS stimulators than the corresponding *dextro* forms [47].

In rats, DES has been shown to be an irreversible inhibitor of MAO-B [48]. Although the concentration of DES during the low-dose selegiline treatment was rather small, DES can be important in regard to the clinical efficacy of selegiline, due to the irreversibility of the inhibition.

6. Interactions of Selegiline and Other Drugs

Selegiline enhances the efficacy of levodopa by prolonging the duration of action of a levodopa dose. The dose of levodopa can be significantly reduced and fluctuations in clinical disability decreased [5]. In order to clarify the effect of selegiline on the peripheral pharmacokinetics of levodopa, we measured levodopa concentrations after 100 mg of levodopa (+25 mg benserazide) with or without 10 mg selegiline in 12 healthy volunteers in a randomized cross-over trial. The pharmacokinetic parameters were not markedly different between the levodopa and the combination (Table 4, Figure 3). These results are in agreement with a study carried out with parkinsonian patients [49]. Selegiline does not exert an effect on plasma COMT activity, either [50]. It may therefore be concluded that the beneficial effects of selegiline in the treatment of PD are not due to peripheral effects, but are rather due to central pharmacological factors (for review, see [51]).

Relatively few interactions between selegiline and other drugs have been described. The hypotension caused by non-selective MAO-inhibitors can be potentiated by selegiline [52] and, therefore, the combined use of these drugs is not recommended. Agitation, shivering, cold sweat, and hypertension have been described when fluoxetine and selegiline have been used at the same time [53]. Fluoxetine is known tointeract with many other CNS drugs, including tricyclic antidepressants and antipsychotics [54].

Table 4. The pharmacokinetic parameters of levodopa after 100 mg (+25 mg of benserazide) oral dose with or without 10 mg of selegiline in 12 healthy volunteers.

	Levodopa	Levodopa + selegiline
C_{max} (mg/ml)	1.7 ± 1.0	1.5 ± 0.8
T_{max} (h)	0.9 ± 0.6	1.0 ± 0.6
AUC (μg h/ml)	2.3 ± 0.6	2.2 ± 0.5
$T_{1/2}$ (h)	1.2 ± 0.1	1.1 ± 0.1

The differences were not statistically significant.

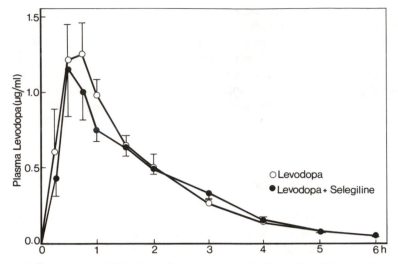

Figure 3. The mean (±SE) plasma levodopa concentrations after 100 mg of levodopa (+25 mg benserazide) with or without selegiline (10 mg orally) in 12 healthy volunteers.

The concomitant use of pethidine (meperidine) and nonspecific MAO-inhibitors like phenelzine may lead to excitation, hyperthermia, convulsions, and severe respiratory depression. According to animal studies, selegiline does not affect pethidine toxicity [55, 56]. Agitation, muscular rigidity, and raised temperature have, however, been reported in only one patient who was simultaneously administered selegiline, dopamine agonists, inhibitors of noradrenaline uptake and pethidine [57]. The causal relationship of the clinical interaction between selegiline and pethidine was unclear in this case, due to polypharmacy. In addition, hyperthermic reactions have been reported after withdrawal or decrease in concentrations of levodopa or dopamine agonists [58, 59], or even due to an "off" period in Parkinson's disease [60]. Because the basic mechanism of the interaction is, at this stage, poorly understood, it is preferable to avoid the concomitant use of selegiline and pethidine.

No pharmacokinetic interactions between selegiline and other drugs have been reported.

Summary

Selegiline is an irreversible, selective inhibitor of monoamine oxidase type B (MAO-B) which has been widely used in the treatment of Parkinson's disease. Selegiline is rapidly absorbed in the intestine and distributed throughout the body. By means of positron emission tomography (PET) studies in man, selegiline has been shown to bind to certain brain areas, such as striatum, which are known to be rich in MAO-B. Selegiline causes irreversible inhibition of MAO-B, which can be monitored by assessing platelet MAO-B activity. With a 10-mg daily dosage, the platelet MAO-B is completely inhibited, the recovery to baseline level taking approximately 10–14 days. Another way to assess MAO-B inhibition is to assess the excretion of phenylethylamine (PEA), a substrate of MAO-B. PEA levels in plasma and urine rise significantly during selegiline therapy. Selegiline is metabolized to desmethylselegiline, *l*-(−)-amphetamine and *l*-(−)-methamphetamine, which are excreted in the urine. The metabolism takes place mainly in the liver and is dependent on microsomal cytochrome P-450. The stereoisomeric configuration is maintained in the metabolism of selegiline, all the metabolites are of *levo* form, and no transformation of the metabolites into *dextro* forms takes place. Selegiline may interact with nonspecific MAO-inhibitors, pethidine and fluoxetine, and, therefore, the concomitant use of selegiline and these drugs is not recommended.

References

[1] Glover V, Eisworth JD, Sandler M. Dopamine oxidation and its inhibition by (−)-deprenyl in man. J Neural Transm 1980; [Supplement] 16: 163–172.
[2] Riederer P, Youdim M. Monoamine oxidase activity and monoamine metabolism in brains of parkinsonian patients treated 5 with *l*-deprenyl. J Neurochemistry 1986; 46: 1359–1365.
[3] Knoll J. The pharmacology of selegiline ((−)-deprenyl). New aspects. Acta Neurol Scand 1989; 126: 83–91.
[4] The Parkinson study group. Effect of deprenyl on the progression of disability in early Parkinson's disease. N Engl J Med 1989; 321: 1364–1371.
[5] Heinonen EH, Rinne UK. Selegiline in the treatment of Parkinson's disease. Acta Neurol Scand 1989; 126: 103–111.
[6] Myllylä W, Sotaniemi KA, Vuorinen JA, Heinonen EH. Selegiline as primary treatment in *de novo* parkinsonian patients. Neurology 1992; 42: 339–343.
[7] Tariot PN, Cohen RM, Sunderland T et al. *l*-Deprenyl in Alzheimer's disease. Preliminary evidence for behavioral change with monoamine oxidase B inhibition. Arch Gen Psychiatry 1987; 44: 427–433.
[8] Mangoni A, Grassi MP, Frattola L et al. Effects of MAO-B inhibitor in the treatment of Alzheimer disease. Eur Neurol 1991; 31: 100–107.
[9] Mann JJ, Aarons SF, Wilner PJ et al. A controlled study of the antidepressant efficacy and side effects of (−)-deprenyl. Arch Gen Psychiatry 1989; 46: 45–50.
[10] Magyar K, Tóthfalusi L. Pharmacokinetic aspects of deprenyl effects. Pol J Pharmacol Pharm 1984; 36: 373–384.
[11] Benakis A. Pharmacokinetic study in man of ^{14}C-Jumex. [A study report.] Turku, Finland: Orion Corporation Farmos, 1981.
[12] MacGregor RR, Halldin C, Fowler JS et al. Selective, irreversible *in vivo* binding of [^{11}C]clorgyline and [^{11}C]-*l*-deprenyl in mice: potential for measurement of functional monoamine oxidase activity in brain using positron emission tomography. Biochem Pharmac 1985; 34(17): 3207–3210.
[13] Szökö É, Kalász H, Kerecsen L, Magyar K. Binding of (−)-deprenyl to serum proteins. Pol J Pharmacol Pharm 1984; 36: 413–421.
[14] Kalász H, Kerecsen L, Knoll J, Pucsok J. Chromatographic studies on the binding, action and metabolism of (−)-deprenyl. J Chromatogr 1990; 499: 589–599.

[15] Fowler JS, MacGregor RR, Wolf AP et al. Mapping human brain monoamine oxidase A and B with ^{11}C-labeled suicide inactivators and PET. Science 1987; 235: 481–485.

[16] Oreland L, Arai Y, Stenström A. The effect of deprenyl (selegiline) on intra- and extraneuronal dopamine oxidation. Acta Neurol Scand 1983; [Supplement] 95: 81–85.

[17] Jossan SS, d'Argy R, Gillberg PG et al. Localization of monoamine oxidase B in human brain by autoradiographical use of ^{11}C-labelled l-deprenyl. J Neural Transm 1989; 77: 55–64.

[18] Jossan SS, Gillberg PG, d'Argy R et al. Quantitative localization of human brain monoamine oxidase B by large section autoradiography using l-[^{3}H]deprenyl. Brain Res 1991; 547: 69–76.

[19] Youdim MBH. The active centers of monoamine oxidase types "A" and "B": binding with (^{14}C)-clorgyline and (^{14}C)-deprenyl. J Neural Transm 1978; 43: 199–208.

[20] Riederer P, Reynolds GP. Deprenyl is a selective inhibitor of brain MAO-B in the long-term treatment of Parkinson's disease. Br J Clin Pharmac 1980; 9: 98–99.

[21] Sunderland T, Mueller A, Cohen RM, Jimerson DC, Pickar D, Murphy DL. Tyramine pressor sensitivity changes during deprenyl treatment. Psychopharmacology 1985; 86: 432–437.

[22] Elsworth JD, Glover V, Reynolds G et al. Deprenyl administration in man: a selective monoamine oxidase B inhibitor without the 'cheese effect'. Psychopharmacology 1978; 57: 33–38.

[23] Blackwell B. Hypertensive crises due to monoamine-oxidase inhibitors. Lancet 1963; 2: 849–850.

[24] Riederer P, Youdim MBH, Rausch WD, Birkmayer W, Jellinger K, Seemann D. On the Mode of Action of l-Deprenyl in the Human Central Nervous System. J Neural Transm 1978; 43: 217–226.

[25] Lee DH, Mendoza M, Dvorozniak MT, Chung E, van Woert MH, Yahr MD. Platelet monoamine oxidase in Parkinson patients: effect of l-deprenyl therapy. J Neural Transm 1989; 1: 189–194.

[26] Simpson GM, Frederickson E, Palmer R, Pi E, Sloane RB, White K. Platelet monoamine oxidase inhibition by deprenyl and tranylcypromine: implications for clinical use. Biol Psychiatry 1985; 20: 680–684.

[27] Birkmayer W, Riederer P, Ambrozi L, Youdim MBH. Implications of combined treatment with 'Madopar' and l-deprenyl J in Parkinson's disease. Lancet 1977; i: 439–443.

[28] Oreland L, Johansson F, Ekstedt J. Dose regimen of deprenyl (selegiline) and platelet MAO activities. Acta Neurol Scand 1983; [Supplement] 95: 87–89.

[29] Teychenne PF, Parker S. Double-blind, crossover, placebo controlled trial of selegiline in Parkinson's disease – an interim analysis. Acta Neurol Scand 1989; 126: 119–125.

[30] Felner AE, Waldmeier PC. Cumulative effects of irreversible MAO inhibitors *in vivo*. Biochem Pharmac 1979; 28: 995–1002.

[31] Turkish S, Yu PH, Greenshaw AJ. Monoamine oxidase-B inhibition: a comparison of *in vivo* and *ex vivo* measures of reversible effects. J Neural Transm 1988; 74: 141–148.

[32] Timár J. Recovery of MAO-B enzyme activity after (−)deprenyl (selegiline) pretreatment, measured *in vivo*. Acta Physiol Hung 1989; 74(3–4): 259–266.

[33] Oreland L, Jossan SS, Hartvig P, Aquilonius SM, Långström B. Turnover of monoamine oxidase B (MAO-B) in pig brain by positron emission tomography using ^{11}C-l-deprenyl. J Neural Transm 1990; [Supplement] 32: 55–59.

[34] Arnett CD, Fowler JS, MacGregor RR et al. Turnover of brain monoamine oxidase measured *in vivo* by positron emission tomography using l-[^{11}C]deprenyl. J Neurochem 1987; 49: 522–527.

[35] Egashira T, Kamijo K. Synthetic rates of monoamine oxidase in rat liver after clorgyline or deprenyl administration. Jpn J Pharmacol 1979; 29: 677–680.

[36] McQuade PS. Analysis and the effects of some drugs on the metabolism of phenylethylamine and phenylacetic acid. Prog Neuropsychopharmacol Biol Psychiatry 1984; 8: 607–614.

[37] Reynolds GP, Riederer P, Sandler M, Jellinger K, Seemann D. Amphetamine and 2-phenylethylamine in post-mortem parkinsonian brain after (−)deprenyl administration. J Neural Transm 1978; 43: 271–277.

[38] Ono H, Ito H, Fukuda H. 2-Phenylethylamine and methamphetamine enhance the spinal monosynaptic reflex by releasing noradrenaline from the terminals of descending fibers. Jpn J Pharmacol 1991; 55: 359–366.

[39] Fuxe K, Grobecker H, Jonsson J. Effect of beta-phenylethylamine on central and peripheral monoamine-containing neurons. Eur J Pharmacol 1967; 2: 203–207.

[40] Boulton AA. Phenylethylaminergic modulation of catecholaminergic neurotransmission. Prog Neuropsychopharmacol Biol Psychiatry 1991; 15: 139–156.

[41] Yoshida T, Yamada Y, Yamamoto T, Kuroiwa Y. Metabolism of deprenyl, a selective monoamine oxidase (MAO) B inhibitor in rat: relationship of metabolism to MAO-B inhibitory potency. Xenobiotica 1986; 16: 129–136.

[42] Yoshida T, Oguro T, Kuroiwa Y. Hepatic and extrahepatic metabolism of deprenyl, a selective monoamine oxidase (MAO) B inhibitor of amphetamines in rats: sex and strain differences. Xenobiotica 1987; 17(8): 957–963.

[43] Meeker JE, Reynolds PC. Postmortem tissue methamphetamine concentrations following selegiline administration. J Anal Toxicol 1990; 14: 330–331.

[44] Schachter M, Marsden CD, Parkes JD, Jenner P, Testa B. Deprenyl in the management of response fluctuations in patients with Parkinson's disease on levodopa. J Neurol Neurosurg Psych 1980; 93: 1016–1021.

[45] Heinonen EH, Myllylä V, Sotaniemi K et al. Pharmacokinetics and metabolism of selegiline. Acta Neurol Scand 1989; 126: 93–99.

[46] Elsworth JD, Sandler M, Lees AJ, Ward C, Stern GM. The contribution of amphetamine metabolites of (−)-deprenyl to its antiparkinsonian properties. J Neural Transm 1982; 54: 105–110.

[47] Ariens EJ. Stereochemistry: A source of problems in medicinal chemistry. Med Res Rev 1986; 6: 451–466.

[48] Borbe HO, Niebch G, Nickel B. Kinetic evaluation of MAO-B-activity following oral administration of selegiline and desmethyl-selegiline in rat. J Neural Transm 1990; [Supplement] 32: 131–137.

[49] Cedarbaum JM, Silvestri M, Clark M, Harts A, Kutt H. l-Deprenyl, levodopa pharmacokinetics, and response fluctuations in Parkinson's disease. Clin Neuropharmacol 1990; 13(1): 29–35.

[50] Russ H, Gerlach M, Dettner O, Kuhn W, Przuntek H. (−)-Deprenyl treatment of patients with Parkinson's disease does not affect erythrocyte catechol-O-methyl transferase activity. J Neural Transm 1991; 3: 215–223.

[51] Heinonen E, Lammintausta R. A review of the pharmacology of selegiline. Acta Neurol Scand 1991; 84 [Supplement] 136: 44–59.

[52] Pare CMB, Mousawi MA, Sandler M, Glover V. Attempts to attenuate the 'cheese effect'. J Affective Disord 1985; 9: 137–141.

[53] Suchowersky O, de Vries J. Possible interactions between deprenyl and prozac. Can J Neurol Sci 1990; 17(3): 352–353.

[54] Ciraulo DA, Shader RI. Fluoxetine drug-drug interactions. II. J Clin Psychopharmacol 1990; 10: 213–217.

[55] Jounela AJ, Mattila MJ, Knoll J. Interaction of selective inhibitors of monoamine oxidase with pethidine in rabbits. Biochem Pharmacol 1977; 26: 806–808.

[56] Boden R, Botting R, Coulson P, Spanswick G. Effect of nonselective and selective inhibitors of monoamine oxidases A and B on pethidine toxicity in mice. Br J Pharmacol 1984; 82: 151–154.

[57] Zornberg GL, Bodkin JA, Cohen BM. Severe adverse interaction between pethidine and selegiline. Lancet 1991; 337: 246.

[58] Sechi G, Tanda F, Mutani R. Fatal hyperpyrexia after withdrawal of levodopa. Neurology 1984; 34: 249–251.

[59] Tojo K, Iizuka K, Honda H, Shimojo S, Miyahara T. A case of neuroleptic malignant syndrome due to levodopa withdrawal. Jikeikai Med J 1989; 36: 195–202.

[60] Pfeiffer RF, Sucha EL. "On-off"-induced lethal hyperthermia. Mov Disord 1989; 4: 338–341.

[61] Reynolds GP, Riederer P, Sandler M, Jellinger K, Seeman D. Amphetamine and 2-phenylethylamine in post-mortem parkinsonian brain after (−)-deprenyl administration. J Neural Transm 1978; 43: 271–277.

[62] Karoum F, Chuang L-W, Eisler T et al. Metabolism of (−)-deprenyl to amphetamine and methamphetamine may be responsible for deprenyl's therapeutic benefit: A biochemical assessment. Neurology 1982; 32: 503–509.

[63] Liebowitz MR, Karoum F, Quitkin FM et al. Biochemical effects of l-deprenyl in atypical depressives. Biol Psychiatry 1985; 20: 558–565.

Inhibitors of Monoamine Oxidase B
Pharmacology and Clinical Use in Neurodegenerative Disorders
ed. by I. Szelenyi

CHAPTER 11
Preclinical Evaluation of *l*-Deprenyl: Lack of Amphetamine-Like Abuse Potential

S. Yasar, G. Winger, B. Nickel, G. Schulze and S. R. Goldberg

1   Introduction
2   Assessment of the EEG Effects of *l*-Deprenyl
3   Assessment of *l*-Deprenyl for Physical Dependence Liability
4   Behavioral Methods for Preclinical Evaluation of Abuse Liability
4.1 Drug-Discrimination Studies
4.2 Pharmacological Modification of Intracranial Self-Stimulation Behavior
4.3 Intravenous Drug Self-Administration Behavior
5   Conclusions
    Summary
    References

1. Introduction

l-Deprenyl is a useful and effective drug in the clinical treatment of parkinsonism and holds promise for treatment of Alzheimer's disease. However, a recurrent concern with its use has been that it is a phenyl-alkylamine derivative which undergoes metabolic transformation to active compounds with its major metabolites *in vivo* being *l*-meth-amphetamine and *l*-amphetamine [1–3]. As the clinical use of am-phetamine-like psychostimulants is limited by their potential for abuse, the question arises as to whether *l*-deprenyl possesses amphetamine-like abuse liability. Also, the reinforcing effects of cocaine may be mediated by inhibition of dopamine reuptake [4]; *l*-deprenyl, in addition to its MAO-B actions, also inhibits dopamine reuptake [5, 6]. Therefore, evaluation of *l*-deprenyl for cocaine-like abuse liability also is a relevant topic of research.

A variety of different experimental procedures have been used to assess the abuse liability of drugs, including electroencephalogram

(EEG) analysis, physical-dependence assessment, drug discrimination procedures, and intravenous self-administration techniques. This chapter will focus on the use of these various procedures for evaluation of the abuse liability of *l*-deprenyl.

2. Assessment of the EEG Effects of *l*-Deprenyl

The EEG is a reliable and sensitive measure of drug effects in both animals and human subjects [7]. The undisturbed, control EEG patterns and values (such as frequency and voltage) for specific electrode sites have been fairly well-mapped for most species, including humans, monkeys, cats, dogs, rabbits, and rats. It is these control patterns to which drug-induced EEG changes are compared. Objective measures for quantifying EEG parameters have been developed that ultimately will provide empirically-derived criteria for classifying drug effects [8–12]. Of all drug classes, psychoactive drugs produce the most pronounced changes in EEG voltage (amplitude components) and frequency. Fink [13] reviewed drug-induced alterations of EEG activity and devised a scheme for classifying psychoactive drugs. He used four principal patterns related to alterations in frequency and five subtypes based on concurrent amplitude changes. Amphetamines were placed in a class called IIb which was characterized by increased fast-wave activity and decreased amplitude [14].

A series of studies was performed by Nickel et al. [15] in order to compare changes in the EEG and in nonlearned behavior of freely moving rats that were induced by *l*-deprenyl, *d*-deprenyl, *d,l*-amphetamine, *d*-amphetamine, and *l*-amphetamine. The effects of each drug on the EEG were recorded continuously over 2.5 hours. The EEG was analyzed by Fourier analysis, as originally suggested by Dietsch [16], and the power spectra were divided into four frequency bands, in accordance with clinical standards [17, 18]. Changes in EEG frequency bands after oral administration of the test compounds are summarized in Figure 1.

Oral doses of the *l*-enantiomers of both deprenyl (5.0 mg/kg, p.o.) and amphetamine (10.0 mg/kg, p.o.) had similar effects, including marked decreases in mean power values in delta bands and increases in theta frequency bands. In marked contrast to the *l*-enantiomers, *d*-deprenyl, *d*-amphetamine, and the racemic form of amphetamine produced increases in mean power values in delta frequency bands and decreases in theta frequency bands. With both the *d*- and *l*-enantiomers of these drugs, onset of EEG changes occurred in the first observation period after oral administration of drug; peak changes were reached 30 to 45 min after drug administration, and EEG changes lasted at least 150 min. Both *d*-deprenyl and *d*-amphetamine also produced a delayed increase in beta activity. All compounds caused only small changes in alpha frequency. In agreement with the EEG studies, the *l*- and *d*-enantiomers of amphetamine and deprenyl had different effects on the behavior of the rats. In comparison to untreated control rats, there was a highly significant increase in exploratory activity and rearing activity

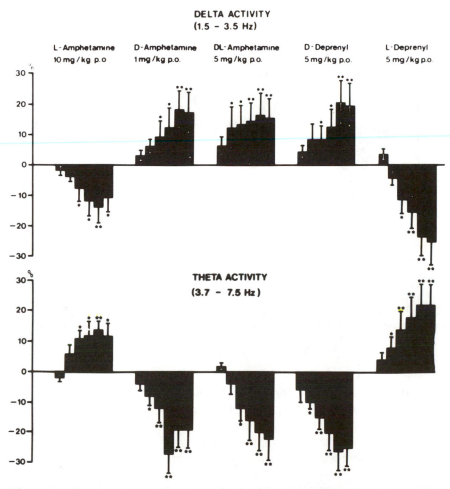

Figure 1A. Time-dependent EEG changes in the delta (1.5–3.5 Hz), theta (3.7–7.5 Hz), frequency bands of freely moving rats after oral administration of *l*-amphetamine (10.0 mg/kg), *d*-amphetamine (1.0 mg/kg), *d,l*-amphetamine (5.0 mg/kg), *d*-deprenyl (5.0 mg/kg) and *l*-deprenyl (5.0 mg/kg) Abscissa: EEG-changes in % after drug administration related to baseline activity. Asterisks indicate that the EEG frequency changes after administration of drug differed significantly from control values of untreated rats (*<0.005, **<0.01) [15].

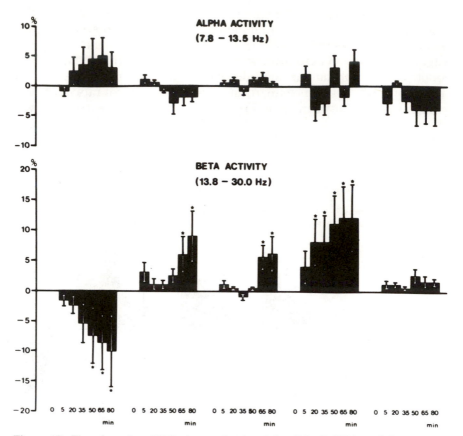

Figure 1B. Time-dependent EEG changes in the alpha (7.8–13.5 Hz), and beta (13.8–30.0 Hz) frequency bands of freely moving rats after oral administration of *l*-amphetamine (10.0 mg/kg), *d*-amphetamine (10. mg/kg), *d,l*-amphetamine (5.0 mg/kg), *d*-deprenyl (5.0 mg/kg) and *l*-deprenyl (5.0 mg/kg) Abscissa: EEG-changes in % after drug administration related to baseline activity. Asterisks indicate that the EEG frequency changes after administration of drug differed significantly from control values of untreated rats ($*<0.005$, $**<0.01$) [15].

of rats treated with *d*-deprenyl and *d*-amphetamine, but not in those treated with *l*-deprenyl or *l*-amphetamine [15]. Thus, the effects of *l*-deprenyl and *l*-amphetamine on electrical activity of the cortex and on behavior in the rat, could be separated from the effects of *d*-deprenyl, *d*-amphetamine or *d,l*-amphetamine.

3. Assessment of *l*-Deprenyl for Physical Dependence Liability

Chronic administration of a drug to small laboratory animals, combined with periodic episodes when drug is withdrawn, allows for preclinical evaluation of possible physical dependence liability of the drug. Nickel et al. [15] modified a procedure developed by Hosoya [19] for assessing physical dependence liability of drugs in order to assess dependence liability of amphetamine-like compounds. Using this procedure, a variety of actions of *d*-amphetamine were demonstrated that indicate physical dependence liability. *l*-Deprenyl, *d*-deprenyl, *l*-amphetamine, and *d,l*-amphetamine were then studied in comparison with *d*-amphetamine in order to characterize physical-dependence liability of *l*-deprenyl. Test drugs were administered orally 6 days a week for 6 weeks. On the seventh day of each week, the test compounds were withdrawn. Since changes in body weight were the most striking indicator of development of physical dependence in the studies by Hosoya [19], the animals were weighed daily. Mean values of changes in body weight of the rats, measured on the 6 withdrawal days, are summarized in Figure 2.

As previously noted by Hosoya, there was a marked decrease in body weight during opiate (codeine) withdrawal. In contrast, during withdrawal of *d,l*-amphetamine, *d*-amphetamine, and *d*-deprenyl there were significant increases in body weight of the rats. However, withdrawal from *l*-amphetamine and *l*-deprenyl did not produce any significant changes in body weight. Thus, the racemic and *d*-enantiomers of amphetamine and deprenyl induced an increase in body weight during withdrawal of drug, and not the usual loss of weight considered to be an indicator of physical dependence development with opioids or benzodiazepines [20]. Simple reversal of anorectic effects of *d*-amphetamine during its withdrawal may explain the increases in weight on days when *d*-amphetamine was withdrawn. There was a reduction in overall body weight with administration of codeine and *d*-amphetamine over the 6-week period, indicating that these two drugs had anorectic effects that were not observed with *l*-amphetamine or *d*- or *l*-deprenyl. Even though no anorectic effect of *d*-deprenyl (5 mg/kg/day, p.o.) was evident, there were increases in body weight on the last 3 days of *d*-deprenyl withdrawal. This was never seen when *l*-deprenyl (5 mg/kg/day, p.o.) was withdrawn.

There also were a number of signs other than body weight increases that occurred during withdrawal of *d*-deprenyl, *d*-amphetamine and *d,l*-amphetamine which indicate physical-dependence development. These signs included increased exploration, stereotypy, and sniffing, as shown in Table 1 from Nickel et al. [15]. None of these signs was seen during withdrawal of *l*-deprenyl or *l*-amphetamine. In summary, in contrast to *d*-deprenyl, *d*-amphetamine, and *d,l*-amphetamine, which produced signs of physical-dependence development, no signs of physical dependence development were noted in rats chronically administered *l*-deprenyl.

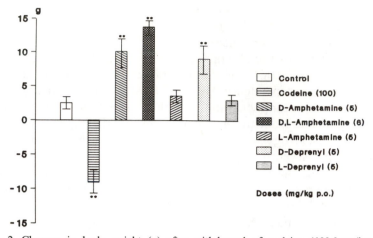

Figure 2. Changes in body weight (g) after withdrawal of codeine (100.0 mg/kg, p.o.), *d,l*-amphetamine (6.0 mg/kg, p.o.), *d*-amphetamine (5.0 mg/kg, p.o.), *l*-amphetamine (5.0 mg/kg, p.o.), *d*-deprenyl (5.0 mg/kg, p.o.) and *l*-deprenyl (5.0 mg/kg, p.o.) in rats. Each bar represents the mean of results from 6 days of drug withdrawal in six rats. Asterisks indicate that changes in weight after withdrawal of drug differed significantly from control values of untreated rats. (**$p < 0.01$) [15].

Table 1. Withdrawal syrnptoms evaluated during chronic oral treatment over 45 days after withdrawal of the test compounds [15].

Compounds	Control	*l*-Deprenyl	*d*-Deprenyl	*l*-Amph.	*d*-Amph.	*d,l*-Amph.	Codeine
Number of animals	12	6	6	6	6	6	12
Diarrhea	—	—	—	—	—	—	10
Convulsions	—	—	—	—	—	—	7
Straub tail	—	—	4	—	3	3	11
Changes in respiration rate	—	—	—	—	—	—	9
Pupil diameter	—	—	—	—	—	—	7
Piloerection	—	—	—	—	—	—	10
Exploration	2	1	5	1	4	5	2
Hyperactivity	—	1	4	—	5	5	2
Grooming	—	—	5	1	5	4	—
Rearing	2	1	6	1	4	6	2
Stereotypy	—	—	5	—	3	5	—
Sniffing	1	1	4	1	2	5	1

4. Behavioral Methods for Preclinical Evaluation of Abuse Liability

Since the 1960s all definitions of drug abuse or drug dependence have had
as a central concept the occurrence of persistent behavior aimed at
obtaining additional amounts of drug for consumption (drug-seeking and
drug self-administration behavior). As a result, over the past 25 years
investigators have developed a range of procedures for preclinically
assessing the abuse liability of a drug (e.g., [21]). Using operant-conditioning methods developed by Skinner [22] and employing schedules of
intermittent reinforcement first comprehensively described by Ferster and
Skinner [23], objective and quantitative techniques for establishment of
reproducible behavioral baselines have been developed which are sensitive
to the effects of drugs of abuse.

Operant behavior can be defined simply as behavior controlled by its
consequences [22, 24]. When an environmental event occurs as a consequence of a specified response by an experimental subject, the frequency
of occurrence of that response may increase, and this increased frequency
may be maintained on subsequent occasions. Thus, food delivery to a
food-deprived rat immediately after it presses a lever may result in an
increased frequency of pressing the lever. In this case, the lever-pressing
response is defined as an operant, and the increased frequency of
occurrence of the response is defined as the process of operant condition-
ing or reinforcement, and delivery of food is defined as a reinforcer. Events
as different as presentation of food or water, electrical stimulation of the
brain, termination of a stimulus associated with occasional electric shock
or the intravenous injection of various drugs can all function as reinforcers
to maintain operant behavior under appropriate conditions.

The most direct means of preclinically assessing abuse liability of
drugs is the use of i.v. drug self-administration procedures in nonhuman
primates. Although acquisition of drug self-administration behavior in
drug-naive subjects is sometimes studied, the most frequent procedure
involves training animals to self-administer a prototype drug from a class
of drugs with abuse potential (e.g., cocaine for psychomotor stimulants)
and then testing the drug in question by substitution. Since i.v. self-administration procedures in primates require long periods of time and can
be very expensive to conduct, a variety of less direct and less costly
procedures are often employed in rodents, particularly during early
development of a drug. These include drug-discrimination procedures,
place-preference procedures, and procedures for assessing drug-induced
changes in intracranial self-stimulation behavior.

4.1. Drug-Discrimination Studies

Laboratory animals can be trained to discriminate between a drug and
its vehicle by requiring them to emit one operant response following the

administration of that drug and another operant response following the administration of the drug vehicle, with the discrimination being made presumably on the basis of drug-induced interoceptive stimuli. Stimuli which set the occasion for differential responding are termed "discriminative stimuli" (e.g., [25]). Reinforcement of responses in the presence of one stimulus increases the tendency to respond, not only in the presence of that stimulus, but also in the presence of similar stimuli. When this occurs the behavior is said to generalize among stimuli. Stimulus generalization is defined functionally. Behavior is said to generalize to those stimuli in whose presence the probability of responding increases after the response has been reinforced in the presence of another stimulus. The probability of occurrence of a response may covary with different values of a stimulus presented along a continuum. The function generated in this way relates responding to stimulus value and is termed a "stimulus-generalization gradient". d-Amphetamine, as a prototype psychomotor stimulant drug, has been studied using drug discrimination procedures.

The discriminative stimulus effects of d-amphetamine have been extensively studied in different laboratories using different species of animals and different schedules of reinforcement [26]. The most commonly used discrimination procedure and species is a two-lever operant choice procedure with rats. During daily experimental sessions, the rat is placed in an operant chamber, as shown in Figure 3, one wall of which contains two levers, stimulus lights and, when food is used as a reinforcer, an

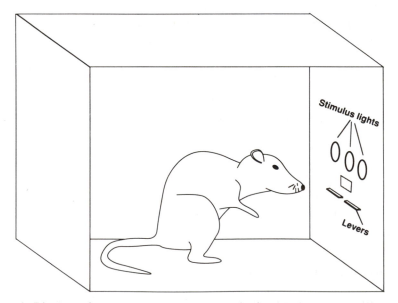

Figure 3. Diagram of an operant chamber for conducting two-lever drug-discrimination studies in rats.

opening to a receptacle for small food pellets. The floor of the chamber consists of metal rods through which electric shock can be delivered.

During training for drug discrimination, in order for lever-pressing responses to be correct the animal must press the lever appropriate (as defined by the investigator) to the presession drug condition. For example, in order for lever presses to produce food pellets, the rat might be required to press the right lever on days when they receive an amphetamine injection, but press the left lever on days when they receive vehicle or no drug. Thus, as illustrated in Table 2 [27], training is accomplished by reinforcing only correct responses and by not reinforcing (extinction) incorrect responses.

As the subject learns to respond appropriately to the injection condition, the complexity of the response required for reinforcement can be increased until a final schedule condition is reached. For example, under a fixed-ratio schedule, the number of responses required to produce each food pellet can be gradually increased to a final value (e.g., [20]). Usually, drug and no-drug days are alternated until the subject reaches a defined criterion of making a certain percentage of responses during the session on the correct lever (e.g., 90%). When this criterion performance is reached, test sessions are then alternated with training sessions. During test sessions, different doses of the training drug are first tested to establish a dose-response curve for the training drug. A range of doses of other compounds is then tested for generalization to the training drug. During these test sessions, responding on either lever is usually considered correct.

The discriminative stimulus effects of *d*-amphetamine have been extensively investigated using the procedures described above, with the most commonly employed training doses in rats being 0.8 or 1.0 mg/kg, i.p.. Usually, acquisition of a criterion level of performance is reached in 4 to 6 weeks. When the optical enantiomers of amphetamine are compared they usually show differences in potency, with *d*-amphetamine being about three-fold more potent than *l*-amphetamine (e.g., [28–30]).

Several groups have investigated the discriminative stimulus properties of MAO-B inhibitors, with the focus generally being on deprenyl

Table 2. Stimulus control of discrete repertoires is established and maintained by differential reinforcement contingencies [27].

		Contingencies	
	Stimuli	Response 1	Response 2
Establishment and maintenance of control	Drug	FR 20: food	Extinction
	Saline	Extinction	FR 20: food
Tests of control Type 1 Type 2	Test drug Test drug	FR 20: food Extinction	FR 20: food Extinction

due to its selective action and its wide clinical use. For comparative purposes, the specific MAO-A inhibitor clorgyline is often concurrently studied. In addition to MAO-B inhibition, *l*-deprenyl has dopamine reuptake blocking effects as well as antagonistic actions at dopamine autoreceptors [5, 6]. Also, the preferred substrate for MAO-B enzyme is β-phenylethylamine [31], with dopamine being another substrate [32]. Since cocaine's action has long been considered to be mediated by dopaminergic mechanisms, the extent to which the stimulus effects of *l*-deprenyl generalize to those of cocaine has been another focus of studies.

In one series of studies by Colpaert et al. [33], rats were trained to discriminate *l*-cocaine (5.0 mg/kg, s.c.) from saline in a two-bar drug discrimination procedure using a fixed-ratio 10 schedule of food presentation. At a dose of 10.0 mg/kg, deprenyl produced complete generalization to the cocaine training dose, while doses of clorgyline as high as 40.0 mg/kg failed to produce any generalization to cocaine. Similarly, Johanson and Barrett [34] reported complete generalization of deprenyl to a training dose of 1.7 mg/kg cocaine in pigeons. Unfortunately, both of these publications fail to specify whether the *l*- or *d*-enantiomer of deprenyl or racemic deprenyl was studied.

In a more recent series of experiments by Yasar et al. (unpublished observation), rats were trained to discriminate *l*-cocaine (10.0 mg/kg, i.p.) from saline in a two-bar discrimination procedure using a fixed-ratio 10 schedule of food presentation. Complete generalization to *l*-cocaine was found with a high dose of 17.0 mg/kg of *l*-deprenyl. Although a higher dose of *l*-deprenyl was needed for generalization in these studies than in those by Colpaert et al. [33], that could be related to the use of a higher training dose of *l*-cocaine (10.0 mg/kg vs 5.0 mg/kg, s.c.).

Since *l*-deprenyl undergoes metabolic transformation to pharmacologically active compounds with the major metabolites *in vivo* being *l*-methamphetamine and *l*-amphetamine [1, 35] there also has been an interest in evaluating its capacity to induce amphetamine-like discriminative stimulus effects. In a series of experiments by Porsolt et al. [36, 37] rats were trained to discriminate between *d*-amphetamine (0.6 mg/kg, i.p.) and saline in a two-lever drug-discrimination procedure using a fixed-ratio 10 schedule of food presentation. Unfortunately, they studied the racemic *d,l* form of deprenyl, rather than the clinically used *l*-deprenyl. At a dose of 4.0 mg/kg, *d,l*-deprenyl generalized completely to the 0.6 mg/kg training dose of *d*-amphetamine. However, other MAO-B inhibitors such as MD 260928 and pargyline and MAO-A inhibitors such as clorgyline and moclobemide failed to generalize to the *d*-amphetamine training stimulus. In other studies reported only in abstract form by Moser [38], *l*-deprenyl was studied in rats trained to discriminate 0.8 mg/kg, i.p., *d*-amphetamine from saline. Moser reported complete generalization of 3.0 and 10.0 mg/kg doses of *l*-deprenyl to *d*-amphetamine. In contrast, MDL 72974, a selective, irreversible MAO-B inhibitor without the sympathomimetic actions of *l*-deprenyl, failed to generalize to *d*-amphetamine in doses as high as 10.0 mg/kg.

The most extensive series of studies of different enantiomers of amphetamine and deprenyl was conducted by Yasar et al. [30]. Rats were trained under a fixed-ratio 5 schedule of stimulus-shock termination or a fixed-ratio 10 schedule of food presentation to discriminate *d*-amphetamine (1.0 mg/kg, i.p.) from saline in two-lever, operant-conditioning chambers. A stimulus-shock termination baseline was studied in addition to the food-presentation baseline in order to control for the potential anorectic effects of amphetamine-like compounds. *d*-Deprenyl and *l*-amphetamine were also studied. The effects of *l*-deprenyl pretreatment on the *d*-amphetamine dose-effect functions were examined to determine whether these compounds might interact when given in combination. Finally, an attempt was made to use *l*-deprenyl as a training stimulus in order to further characterize its discriminative stimulus properties.

l-Deprenyl (2.0–17.0 mg/kg, i.p.) did not show complete generalization to *d*-amphetamine, neither under the stimulus-shock termination nor the food-presentation schedule. In contrast to *l*-deprenyl, *d*-deprenyl, which would be metabolized in part to *d*-methamphetamine and *d*-amphetamine, generalized to *d*-amphetamine completely and dose-dependently at doses of 5.6 and 10.0 mg/kg under the stimulus-shock termination schedule and at a dose of 17.0 mg/kg under the food reinforcement schedule. *l*-Amphetamine also produced dose-dependent increases in *d*-amphetamine, appropriately responding and generalized completely to *d*-amphetamine at a dose of 2.0 mg/kg under the stimulus-shock termination schedule and at a dose of 3.0 mg/kg under the food reinforcement schedule. In general, the two procedures led to comparable results; however, there were some clear differences. For example, *l*-amphetamine and *d*-deprenyl appeared more potent under the shock-termination schedule then under the food-presentation schedule. When *l*-deprenyl (2.0 mg/kg, i.p.) was given as a pretreatment 60 min before *d*-amphetamine it did not shift the dose-response curve for *d*-amphetamine, which further indicates a lack of interaction of these compounds as discriminative stimuli.

It is well established that psychoactive drugs have the potential to serve as discriminative stimuli [27]. In particular, drugs with established human abuse liability have been found to serve as effective and robust discriminative stimuli in animal drug-discrimination studies, although the converse is not necessarily true (e.g., atropine can serve as a discriminative stimulus but has no abuse liability). Consequently, it was of interest to determine whether *l*-deprenyl, itself, could serve as an effective and robust discriminative stimulus. A series of experiments was conducted by Yasar et al. [30] in an attempt to establish *l*-deprenyl as a discriminative stimulus. Rats received over 180 days of training with initial doses of 5.6 or 10.0 mg/kg, i.p., *l*-deprenyl under both schedules, but none of the rats ever reached the training criterion. Further, manipulations such as lowering the *l*-deprenyl dose, changing pretreatment time, and altering dosing regimes were also unsuccessful in establishing *l*-deprenyl as a discriminative stimulus. Thus, in contrast to drugs with established human abuse liability, *l*-deprenyl did not appear to function as an effective and robust discriminative stimulus.

In summary, drug discrimination studies from different laboratories generally showed that *l*-deprenyl, even at doses 10 to 20 times higher than those relevant to clinical use, had only limited amphetamine-like, discriminative-stimulus properties in rats. In contrast, several studies have indicated that complete generalization can occur to cocaine but, again, this occurs at doses 10 to 20 times higher than the clinically-used therapeutic dose range within which *l*-deprenyl acts as a specific MAO-B inhibitor.

4.2. Pharmacological Modification of Intracranial Self-Stimulation Behavior

Operant responding can be maintained in rats at a high rate by electrical stimulation of the brain when electrodes are located in appropriate areas, and frequency and current intensity are maintained at appropriate levels (e.g., [39]). When drugs are administered before or during experimental sessions, decreases in the intensity or frequency of electrical stimulation needed to maintain levels of responding have been used as indicators of potential reinforcing effects of psychoactive drugs (e.g., [40]). O'Regan et al. [41] compared the effects of prolonged exposure via osmotic minipump to clorgyline or *l*-deprenyl (1.0 mg/kg/day) on hypothalamic self-stimulation behavior of rats. As in previous studies [42], clorgyline produced a shift to the left in the response rate/stimulation frequency function which would suggest enhanced sensitivity to the reinforcement effects of lateral hypothalamic self-stimulation. In marked contrast, *l*-deprenyl had no effect on any of the measures of hypothalamic self-stimulation behavior.

4.3. Intravenous Drug Self-Administration Behavior

Many of the factors which make interpretation of results of the previously described studies difficult can be eliminated by directly assessing the reinforcing effects of *l*-deprenyl using operant procedures in monkeys in which specified doses of *l*-deprenyl are made available for intravenous self-administration. Using an apparatus first described by Deneau et al. [43], and shown in Figure 4 [44], Winger (unpublished results) assessed the reinforcing effects of *l*-deprenyl in rhesus monkeys.

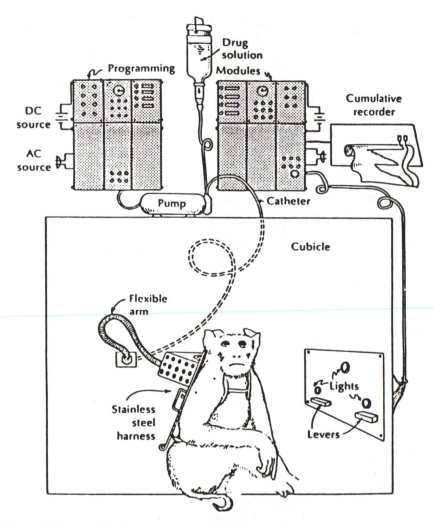

Figure 4. Diagram of an experimental chamber for the study of intravenous drug self-administration behavior in the rhesus monkey. The monkey is restrained by a metal harness and a flexible metal restraining arm which attaches to the rear wall of the chamber. A response key and a stimulus light are mounted on the rear wall of the chamber. The monkey's chronically implanted venous catheter passes through the arm and out the back of the chamber where it attaches to an automatic injection pump [44].

With these experimental procedures, monkeys are first surgically prepared with a chronic venous catheter and then individually housed 24 h a day in a stainless-steel cage containing a panel with response levers and stimulus lights. The monkey wears a harness which is connected to a hollow stainless-steel arm that is designed to allow the animal free movement within the cage and at the same time to protect the venous catheter. The catheter is led through the arm to an automatic-injection pump located behind the cage. Typically, the drug is made available such that depression of the response lever by the monkey activates the injection pump, resulting in delivery of an intravenous drug injection. When a drug is injected as a consequence of pressing the lever and the frequency of pressing the lever subsequently increases, then the drug is said to function as a reinforcer [45].

In 1989, Winger et al. [46] described a procedure for rapidly evaluating reinforcing effects of intravenously delivered drugs in rhesus monkeys using the apparatus described above. Catheters were implanted and monkeys were then returned to their home cages and given the opporunity to respond and receive injections of a drug such as cocaine. Experimental sessions when the drug was made available were limited to 130 min, and two sessions were scheduled each day, separated by at least 4 h. Each session was divided into four components; each component was signaled by illumination of a red stimulus light and was separated from the following component by a 10-min intercomponent interval. During the intercomponent interval, no lights were illuminated and responses on the lever had no consequences.

This rapid-evaluation procedure was used by Winger (unpublished results) to evaluate l-deprenyl for reinforcing effects in comparison with cocaine. A unique dose per injection of drug was available during each of four components. A component ended either after 20 injections of that particular dose were earned, or 25 min had passed, whichever occurred first. Thirty lever presses were required to produce each injection (a fixed-ratio 30 schedule of i.v. drug injection) and each injection was followed by a 45-s timeout period during which the red light was off and lever presses had no programmed consequences. Each injection was accompanied by illumination of a center green light. Drug concentration was kept constant throughout a session and, instead, doses were altered by adjusting duration of activation of the injection pump. Doses were evaluated in one-half logarithm unit steps. Monkeys were initially trained with l-cocaine. When saline was substituted, injection durations continued to be varied for each component, as they were with the drug. If rates of saline-maintained responding were higher than approximately 0.5 responses per second at any injection duration, saline was substituted again until rates were consistently below 0.5 responses per second. l-Deprenyl or l-cocaine were substituted during single sessions after rates of saline-maintained responding were low.

Figure 5 shows that, under these conditions, l-cocaine was a very effective reinforcer, maintaining rates of lever pressing of over two responses per second at the optimal injection dose of 0.01 mg/kg. In contrast, l-deprenyl failed to maintain self-administration responding above saline-control levels, although it was studied over a thousandfold dose range from 0.001 to 1.0 mg/kg/injection. It should be noted that at the 1.0 mg/kg injection dose a monkey could receive as much as

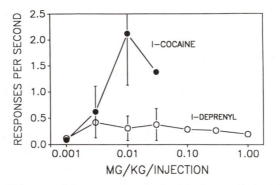

Figure 5. Rates of lever-pressing responses maintained by intravenously delivered *l*-cocaine (solid circles) or *l*-deprenyl (open circles) in rhesus monkeys. Ordinate is the rate of responding in responses per second; abscissa is dose of drug in mg/kg/injection. Data points represent the mean of observations in three monkeys where there are vertical, S.E.M. bars, and the mean of observations in two monkeys where there are no vertical bars.

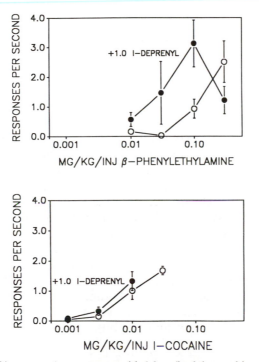

Figure 6. Effects of i.v. presession treatment with 1.0 mg/kg *l*-deprenyl i.v. (closed circles) on behavior maintained by i.v. injection of either β-phenylethylamine (top) or *l*-cocaine (bottom) (open circles). Ordinates are rates of responding in responses per second; abscissae are dose of drug in mg/kg/injection. Data points represent the average of observations in three or four monkeys. Vertical bars are the S.E.M. for the data points.

20 mg/kg i.v. *l*-deprenyl in about 25 min if responding occurred at a rapid rate, as it did when other drugs such as cocaine with known abuse liability were available.

A comparison was made of the effects of *l*-deprenyl on i.v. self-administration responding maintained by different doses of cocaine, with its effects on self-administration responding maintained by different doses of β-phenylethylamine, the preferred substrate for type B MAO enzyme (Winger, unpublished results). *l*-Deprenyl was given i.v. 30 min before the session. As shown in Figure 6, β-phenylethylamine functioned effectively as a reinforcer at injection doses of 0.1 to 0.3 mg/kg, with average response rates at the 0.3 mg/kg/injection dose of 2.5 responses per second.

Pretreatment with 1.0 mg/kg *l*-deprenyl produced no change in cocaine-maintained responding (bottom of Figure 6), but shifted the β-phenylethylamine dose-response curve to the left (top of Figure 6). A dose of 0.03 mg/kg/injection of β-phenylethylamine, which previously maintained a relatively low rate of 0.9 responses per second, maintained response rates of 3.1 responses per second after pretreatment with 1.0 mg/kg *l*-deprenyl. Similar interactions have been reported between *l*-deprenyl and β-phenylethylamine with other behavioral measures. For example, Timar and Knoll [47] found that s.c. treatment with 0.25 to 2.0 mg/kg doses of *l*-deprenyl greatly potentiated the intensity and duration of stereotyped behavior induced by a 40.0 mg/kg s.c. dose of β-phenylethylamine.

5. Conclusions

The series of physiological and behavioral studies reviewed in this chapter were performed in different laboratories, in different animal species, and with a wide variety of experimental procedures relevant to evaluation of abuse liability of drugs. In the clinically-relevant dose range within which *l*-deprenyl serves as a selective MAO-B inhibitor, it did not demonstrate signs of abuse liability. Even at very high parenteral doses (10.0 to 17.0 mg/kg, i.p.), at which *l*-deprenyl generalized to the discriminative stimulus effects of cocaine, it only partially generalized to *d*-amphetamine. Also, *l*-deprenyl could not be distinguished from saline placebo in self-administration studies with nonhuman primates, even at injection doses as high as 1.0 mg/kg, i.v. that would have allowed subjects to self-inject cumulative doses of *l*-deprenyl as high as 20.0 mg/kg within a 25-min period. Thus, the preclinical findings reviewed generally support the clinical experience that in over 20 years of therapeutic use there has been no established case of human abuse of *l*-deprenyl.

Summary

Since *l*-deprenyl is metabolized to *l*-methamphetamine and *l*-amphetamine and also inhibits dopamine reuptake, evaluation of *l*-

deprenyl for abuse liability is important. A series of preclinical studies in animals is reviewed which employed experimental procedures which are highly predictive of human abuse liability. Changes in EEG of rats induced by *l*-deprenyl and *l*-amphetamine were different from those produced by the *d*-enantiomers. After several weeks of chronic treatment in rats, withdrawal of *l*-deprenyl or *l*-amphetamine, in contrast to *d*-amphetamine or *d*-deprenyl, did not elicit any physiological or behavioral signs of physical dependence. In two-lever drug-discrimination studies in rats, *l*-amphetamine generalized completely to *d*-amphetamine, although it was less potent. *l*-Deprenyl showed only partial generalization to *d*-amphetamine and this occurred at a very high dose. *l*-Deprenyl did produce complete generalization to *l*-cocaine but, again, this only occurred at high doses above those with selective MAO-B activity. Finally, in intravenous self-administration studies with rhesus monkeys, *l*-deprenyl did not maintain self-administration responding above saline levels, while cocaine maintained high rates of responding. Also, pretreatment with *l*-deprenyl markedly increased self-administration behavior maintained by β-phenylethylamine, but had no effect on self-administration behavior maintained by cocaine. Thus, preclinical results confirm the clinical experience that therapeutically relevant doses of *l*-deprenyl are without abuse liability.

Acknowledgements

Portions of the cost of preparation of this manuscript and the cost of research relating to drug self-administration studies in rhesus monkeys conducted at the University of Michigan Medical School were provided by USPHS grants DA 04403 and DA 05951 from the National Institute on Drug Abuse.

The views expressed in this chapter are those of the authors, and do not necessarily reflect the views of the agencies or institutions with which the authors are affiliated.

References

[1] Reynolds GP, Elsworth JD, Blau K, Sandler M, Lees AJ, Stern GM. Deprenyl is metabolized to methamphetamine and amphetamine in man. Br J Clin Pharmacol 1978; 6: 542–544.
[2] Phillips SR. Amphetamine, p-hydroxyamphetamine and β-phenethylamine in mouse brain and urine after (−)- and (+)-deprenyl administration. J Pharmac Pharmacol 1981; 31: 739–741.
[3] Elsworth JD, Sandler M, Lees AJ, Ward C, Stern GM. The contribution of amphetamine metabolites of (−)-deprenyl to its antiparkinsonian properties. J Neural Trans 1982; 54: 105–110.
[4] Ritz MC, Lamb RJ, Goldberg SR, Kuhar MJ. Cocaine receptors on dopamine transporters are related to self-administration of cocaine. Science 1987; 237: 1219–1223.

[5] Knoll J. (−)-Deprenyl (selegiline, Movergan®) facilitates the activity of the nigrostriatal neuron. In: Riederer P, Przuntek J, editors. MAO-B inhibitor selegiline (R-(−)-deprenyl). J Neural Transm 1987; 25: [Supplement] 45−66.

[6] Knoll J. The pharmacology of selegiline ((−)-deprenyl). New aspects. In: Rinne UK, Pakkenberg H, Jensen NO, editors. New strategies in the treatment of Parkinson's disease. Acta Neurol Scand 1989; 80: [Supplement] 83−91.

[7] Winters WD. The continuum of CNS excitatory states and hallucinosis. In: Siegel RK, West W, editors. Hallucinations: behavior, experience and theory. New York: Wiley 1975: 53−75.

[8] Hermann WM. Development and critical evaluation of an objective procedure for the electroencephalographic classification of psychotropic drugs. In: Hermann WM, editor. Electroencephalography in drug research. Stuttgart: Gustav Fischer 1982: 249−351.

[9] Itil TM, editor. Psychotropic drugs and the human EEG. Vol. 8. Modern problems in pharmacopsychiatry. Basel: Karger 1974.

[10] Serafetinides EA, Willis BA. A method for quantifying EEG for psychopharmacological research. Int Pharmacopsychiatry 1973; 8: 245−247.

[11] Saphiro DM, Glasser M. Measurement and comparison of EEG drug effects. In: Itil TM, editor. Psychotropic drugs and human EEG. Vol. 8. Modern problems in pharmaco-psychiatry. Basel: Karger 1974: 327−349.

[12] Lukas SF. Brain electrical activity as a tool for studying drugs of abuse. In: Mello NK, editor. Advances in substance abuse. Behavioral and biological research. Vol. 4. London: Jessica Kingsley Publishers 1991: 1−88.

[13] Fink M. EEG and human psychopharmacology. Ann Rev Pharmacol 1969; 9: 241−258.

[14] Fink M, Saphiro DM, Itil TM. EEG profiles of fenfluramine, amobarbital and dextro-amphetamine in normal volunteers. Psychopharmacologia 1971; 22: 369−383.

[15] Nickel B, Schulze G, Szelenyi I. Effect of enantiomers of deprenyl (selegiline) and amphetamine on physical abuse liability and cortical electrical activity in rats. Neuro-pharmacology 1990; 29: 983−992.

[16] Dietsch G. Fourier-Analyse von Elektroencephalographologrammen des Menschen. Pflugers Arch Ges Physiol 1932; 230: 106−112.

[17] Nickel B, Zerrahn H. Pharmacoelectroencephalography in the rat as a method for characterization of different types of analgesics. Postgrad Med J 1987; 63: [Supplement] 3: 45−47.

[18] Nickel B, Szelenyi I. Comparison of changes in the EEG of freely moving rats induced by enciprazine, buspirone and diazepam. Neuropharmacology 1989; 28: 799−803.

[19] Hosoya E. Screening of dependence liability of drugs using rats. Pharmac Ther 1979; 5: 515−517.

[20] Blasig I, Herz H, Reinhold K, Zieglgansberger S. Development of physical dependence on morphine in respect to time and dosage and quantification of the precipitated withdrawal syndrome in rats. Psychopharmacologia 1973; 33: 19−38.

[21] Goldberg SR, Stolerman IP, editors. Behavioral analysis of drug dependence. London: Academic Press 1986.

[22] Skinner BF, editor. The behavior of organisms. New York: Appleton-Century-Crofts 1938.

[23] Ferster CB, Skinner BF, editors. Schedules of Reinforcement. New York: Appleton-Century-Crofts 1957.

[24] Skinner BF. Two types of conditioned reflex: a reply to Konorski and Miller. J Gen Psyehol 1937; 16: 272−279.

[25] Terrace HS. Stimulus control. In: Honig WK, editor. Operant behavior: areas of research and application. Englewood Cliffs, N.J.: Prentice-Hall 1966: 271−344.

[26] Young R, Glennon RA. Discriminative stimulus properties of amphetamine and struc-turally related phenylalkylamines. Med Res Rev 1986; 6: 99−130.

[27] Young AM. Discriminative stimulus profiles of psychoactive drugs. In: Mello NK, editor. Advances in substance abuse. Behavioral and biological research. Vol. 4. London: Jessica Kingsley Publishers 1991: 139−203.

[28] Schechter MD. Stimulus properties of d-amphetamine as compared to l-amphetamine. Eur J Pharmacol 1978; 47: 461−464.

[29] Glennon R, Young R. Further investigation of the discriminative stimulus properties of MDA. Pharmacol Biochem Behav 1984; 20: 501−505.

[30] Yasar S, Schindler CW, Cohen C, Thorndike EB, Goldberg SR, Szelenyi I. Drug discrimination analysis of *l*-deprenyl. 21st annual Meeting; 1991 November 10–15; New Orleans (LA), USA. Society for Neuroscience Abstracts 1991; 17: 1431.

[31] Yang HYT, Neff NH. Beta-phenylethylamine. A specific substrate for type B monoamine oxidase of brain. J Pharmacol Exp Ther 1973; 187: 365–371.

[32] Yang HYT, Neff NH. The monoamine oxidases of brain: Selective inhibition with drugs and the consequences for the metabolism of the biogenic amines. J Pharmacol Exp Ther 1974; 189: 733–740.

[33] Colpaert FC, Niemegeers CJE, Janssen PAJ. Evidence that preferred substrate for type B monoamine oxidase mediates stimulus properties of MAO inhibitors: a possible role for beta-phenylethylamine in the cocaine cue. Pharm Biochem Behav 1980; 13: 513–517.

[34] Johanson CE, Barrett JE. The discriminative stimulus effects of cocaine in pigeons. American College of Neuropsychopharmacology. 29th Annual Meeting; 1990 Dec. 10–14; San Juan, Puerto Rico.

[35] Heinionen EH, Myllyla V, Sotaniemi K, Lamintausta R, Salonem JS, Anttila M, et al. Pharmacokinetics and metabolism of selegiline. In: Rinne UK, Pakkenberg H, Jenssen NO, editors. New strategies in the treatment of Parkinson's disease. Acta Neurol Scand 1989; 80: [Supplement] 126: 83–91.

[36] Porsolt RD, Pawelec C, Jalfre M. Use of a drug discrimination procedure to detect amphetamine-like effects of antidepressants. In: Colpaert FC, Slangen JL, editors. Drug discrimination: applications in CNS pharmacology. Amsterdam: Elsevier, Biomedical 1982: 193–202.

[37] Porsolt RD, Pawelec C, Roux S, Jalfre M. Discrimination of the amphetamine cue. Effects of A, B and mixed type inhibitors of monoamine oxidase. Neuropharmacology 1984; 23: 569–573.

[38] Moser PC. Generalization of *l*-deprenyl, but not MDL-72974, to the amphetamine stimulus in rats. Psychopharmacol 1990; 101: S40.

[39] Kornetsky C, Bain G. Brain-stimulation reward: A model for drug-induced euphoria. In: Adler M, Cowan A, editors. Testing and evaluation of drugs of abuse. Vol. 6. Modern methods in pharmacology. New York: Wiley-Liss 1990: 211–231.

[40] Gallistel CR, Karaas D. Pimozide and amphetamine have opposite effects on the reward summation function. Pharmacol Biochem Behav 1984; 20: 73–77.

[41] O'Regan D, Kwok RPS, Yu PH, Bailey BA, Greenshaw AJ, Boulton AA. A behavioral and neurochemical analysis of chronic and selective monoamine oxidase inhibition. Psychopharmacologia 1987; 92: 42–47.

[42] Aulakh CS, Cohen RM, Pradhan SN, Murphy DL. Self-stimulation responses are altered following long-term but not short-term treatment with clorgyline. Brain Res 1983; 270: 383–386.

[43] Deneau GA, Yanagita T, Seevers MH. Self-administration of psychoactive substances by the monkey. A measure of psychological dependence. Psychopharmacologia 1969; 16: 30–48.

[44] Schuster CR, Johanson CE. The use of animal models for the study of drug abuse. In: Gibbins RJ, Israel Y, Kalant H, Popham R, Schmidt W, Smart R, editors. Research advances in alcohol and drug problems. Vol. 1. New York: Wiley and Sons 1974: 1–31.

[45] Schuster CR, Thompson T. Self-administration of and behavioral dependence on drugs. Ann Rev of Pharmacol 1969; 9: 483–502.

[46] Winger G, Palmer RK, Woods JH. Drug-reinforced responding: rapid determination of dose-response functions. Drug and Alcohol Dependence 1989; 24: 135–142.

[47] Timar J, Knoll B. The effect of repeated administration of (−)-deprenyl on the phenylethylamine-induced stereotypy in rats. Arch Int Pharmacodyn 1986; 279: 50–60.

Clinical Experience with Monoamine Oxidase B Inhibitors

Inhibitors of Monoamine Oxidase B
Pharmacology and Clinical Use in Neurodegenerative Disorders
ed. by I. Szelenyi
© 1993 Birkhäuser Verlag Basel/Switzerland

CHAPTER 12
The History of *l*-Deprenyl

M. J. Parnham

1   Introduction
2   The Synthesis of E-250
3   Biological and Clinical Characterization
4   MAO-A and MAO-B
5   The Link to Parkinson's Disease
6   The American Connection
6.1 Drugs for Jewels
6.2 MPTP and the Radical Dimension
7   FDA Approval: a Battle Against Bureaucracy
8   Postscript: a Child of Several Fathers
     Summary
     References

> "Research is to see what everyone has seen
> and to think what no-one has thought."
> A. Szent-Györgyi

1. Introduction

The above statement was quoted first to me many years ago by Iván Bonta during a successful four-year period I spent in his department in Rotterdam. It is particularly apt as the opening sentence to a history of *l*-deprenyl, since it was first said by a Hungarian Nobel Prizewinner, quoted to me by an ex-Hungarian emigré, and summarizes very succinctly the story of a Hungarian drug, published in a book by a Germano-Hungarian editor! But the history of *l*-deprenyl is much more than a parochial Hungarian affair; its see-saw fortunes have carried it on a roller-coaster developmental journey through many countries over 30 years. At each stage there have been a few clear thinkers who, while seeing the facts at their and others' disposal, still managed to think what others had not thought.

   Ideas, however, are very difficult to claim as personal property and are frequently incorporated into other people's thinking, their origin then becoming undetectable. Scientific obliteration may occur when an idea is so incorporated into scientific knowledge that its originator may be totally forgotten. Add to this process the desire of every researcher (admitted or not) to gain international recognition for his/her research ideas, and we have the potential for the misunderstandings, claims and counterclaims which arise when a scientific project gains public attention.

Another important factor in the impact of drugs and other biomedical discoveries is the Atlantic Ocean. The way things are seen in the New World is frequently at odds with the attitudes of the Europeans. There is a tendency to view discoveries and situations from a subjective geographical standpoint.

Since North America is the world's largest pharmaceutical market, it is often emphasized to the detriment of Europe. This is certainly the case in a recent book, "The Deprenyl Story" [1], which, while giving some interesting background facts, tends to give the impression that no drug is really a drug until it is sold in North America!

In an attempt to walk the razor's edge between fact and wishful thinking, I shall try to draw together a number of the strands of *l*-deprenyl's history in the hope that a balanced story will emerge.

2. The synthesis of E-250

It is common for a drug to be synthesized with a particular clinical indication in mind and, ultimately, to find therapeutic application in a totally different field. A number of examples spring to mind, including levamisol, an antihelminthic found to be useful as an immunomodulator. Iproniazid, the prototype monoamine oxidase (MAO) inhibitor, started life as a tuberculostatic agent before it was discovered to exert a marked antidepressant action in man. Shortly after it had been marketed by Hoffmann-La Roche to treat tuberculosis in 1952, Zeller demonstrated that iproniazid (which has a structure reminiscent of catecholamines) was a potent irreversible inhibitor of MAO [2]. Subsequent studies demonstrated that iproniazid potentiated the pharmacological actions of monoamines and of reserpine *in vivo*. In 1956, his curiosity aroused by the animal studies and attracted by the fact that tuberculosis patients treated with iproniazid "felt good", Kline submitted the drug to a thorough clinical trial and demonstrated its antidepressant or psychoenergizing properties [3]. This study provided the impetus for the search for other monoamine oxidase inhibitors as potential anti-depressants.

Iproniazid is a hydrazine derivative, and like other hydrazine derivatives, such as hydralazine, has antihypertensive activity. Chemists at Abbott seized upon this activity as an opening for a new selective antihypertensive agent and synthesized pargyline which, although developed from iproniazid, was marketed as an antihypertensive with a gradual onset of action [4]. The mechanism of action of pargyline appeared to be central via a depressant action on the cerebral vasomotor centre, in which it reduced noradrenaline turnover. Peripherally, though, pargyline increased the concentration of circulating catecholamines, an action which tended to antagonize its beneficial central antihypertensive activity.

The logical approach to improving the activity of pargyline would be to alter its structure so that its selectivity for the CNS would be increased.

At this point the Chinoin Pharmaceutical Company in Budapest enters the story. With a product palette of mostly generic products, Chinoin decided to develop a new antihypertensive to improve its image and turnover. The head of chemical research at Chinoin, Zoltan Ecseri had a particular interest in preparing me-too drugs and showed a penchant for drugs acting on the CNS. The young scientific advisor to Chinoin, Jozsef Knoll, now chairman, then a staff member of the Department of Pharmacology at the Semmelweiss University of Medicine in Budapest, was also actively interested in drug action on the CNS and had been studying the effects of amphetamines. According to Knoll's own account, he and his colleagues found in 1960 that low doses of amphetamine improved the performance of rats in a one-way avoidance test, and that they increased catecholaminergic tone in the brain [5]. High doses of amphetamine, on the other hand, selectively increased serotonergic tone and disturbed avoidance behaviour. Similar dose-dependency was seen with methamphetamine. The discovery initiated a series of investigations into the effects of derivatives of phenylalkylamine as possible drugs with selective effects on brain catecholamine release. During these investigations it was found that synthetic phenylalkylamine derivatives with substituents at the nitrogen moiety lost their ability to release biogenic amines from the cytoplasmic pools at the nerve endings [5]. A nitrogen-substituted pargyline derivative thus offered the potential of greater selectivity of action on CNS catecholamines and, possibly, less peripheral release of these biogenic amines. Consequently, Ecseri set his laboratory technician Mrs. Miklósné Müller to synthesizing derivatives of phenylalkylamine and pargyline, a task that took 2 years and resulted in the synthesis of 250 compounds.

At what point the strategic indication at Chinoin for this series of compounds changed from hypertension to mental depression is unclear. Knoll implies that, from the start, the compounds were synthesized in an attempt to derive a better MAO inhibitor as a "psychic energizer" [5]. Presumably, Knoll's interest and experience with animal behavioural tests inevitably biased the interest towards psycho-pharmacological effects. In his first publication on *l*-deprenyl in an English-language journal, Knoll implies that the compound was synthesized in a search for an acute psychostimulant like methamphetamine with the psychoenergetic effects characteristic of MAO inhibitors [6]. If this had been the primary reason for the project, then iproniazid would have been a better

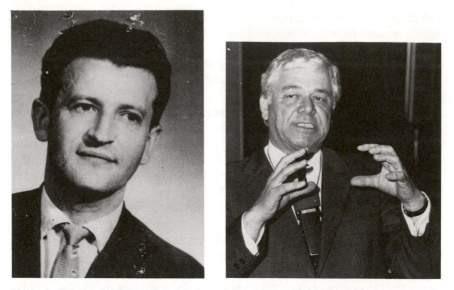

Figure 1. The chemist Zoltan Ecseri (left) and the pharmacologist Jozsef Knoll (right), who performed the first experiments on *l*-deprenyl (photographs reproduced with kind permission of the "Ärzte Zeitung").

starting candidate than pargyline in view of its more pronounced anti-depressant effects. Whatever the motive behind the synthetic approach, compound E-250 proved to be the most potent compound of the series, with both MAO inhibitory activity and acute psychostimulant activity. A patent was issued in Hungary on 13 December, 1962, and a report published in 1964 [7]. It should be noted that the patent does not mention Parkinson's disease as a possible indication.

3. Biological and Clinical Characterization

The first English-language publication on E-250 was received by Archives Internationales de Pharmacodynamie on 17 June, 1964 [6]. By this time the compound had been shown to inhibit brain MAO activity *in vivo* in rats, to antagonize reserpine-induced depression of jumping in rats, and to alter conditioned and unconditioned reflexes in rats and mice in the same manner as amphetamine. Motility in rats and mice was unaffected, but a clear hypertensive action in the cat was observed. The stimulation of the basal metabolic rate of rats was much less than that with amphetamine. The authors concluded that E-250 showed promise as a new type of central nervous excitant drug with acute psychostimulant and chronic psychic energizing actions. They also referred to preliminary investigatons in man which indicated that E-250 was efficacious in the treatment of depression. These clinical trials were performed by E. Varga in the Soviet Union.

In the mid-1960s reports of liver damage with MAO inhibitors began to appear and the "cheese effect" became a serious problem. The MAO inhibitors available at that time not only inhibited MAO in the brain, but also in the liver. Consequently, when the drugs were administered with foods such as aged cheese, broad beans, yeast, chocolate, and red wines, all of which contain large amounts of tyramine, this biogenic amine remained unmetabolized and precipitated severe hypertension and, on rare occasions, death by cardiac arrest. Varga never observed such adverse reactions, not even when he deliberately tried to provoke the "cheese effect" [8]. But the adverse effects were sufficiently serious with the marketed MAO inhibitors for several, including iproniazid and tranylcypromine, to be withdrawn, although tranylcypromine was subsequently reintroduced under stricter recommendations. In this hostile climate, it is no wonder that Chinoin lost interest in the development of E-250.

Knoll, however, was very persistent. E-250 itself was the racemic form of phenyl-isopropylmethylpropinylamine. Comparative investigation in Knoll's laboratory of the two optical isomers revealed that the (+)-enantiomer exhibited marked amphetamine-like activity in increasing motility and rectal temperature in rats, and in being a more potent psychostimulant than the (−)-enantiomer [9]. The latter, however, was 500 times more potent as a MAO inhibitor *in vitro*, and more effective on chronic administration as an inhibitor of reserpine-induced lowering of the threshold for convulsions in mice. These studies thus made it clear that the (−)-enantiomer showed the most promise as a psychic energizer.

4. MAO-A and MAO-B

Despite Knoll's persistence, the attractive biological activity of the (−)-enantiomer E-250 (*l*-deprenyl), and the lack of adverse effects in the Soviet clinical studies, it is highly unlikely that *l*-deprenyl would ever have been reconsidered as a suitable candidate for a drug had it not been for a discovery made in 1968 in England.

As early as 1961, it had been shown that at least two enzymes in rat liver were involved in the metabolism of tyramine, and that only one enzyme metabolized serotonin [10]. The actual existence of two forms of MAO was demonstrated by Johnston at May and Baker in Dagenham, who found that a new compound, MB 9302 (later named clorgyline), was a potent and selective inhibitor of the enzyme which preferentially deaminates serotonin [11]. This enzyme he termed MAO-A, and the enzyme with low sensitivity to clorgyline he named MAO-B. Subsequent investigations in the late 1970s revealed that MAO-A has selectivity for the substrates serotonin and noradrenaline, while MAO-B has selectivity for β-phenylethylamine and dopamine [12]. Clorgyline was extensively used as an experimental tool for the inhibition of MAO-A, but a selective inhibitor of MAO-B was apparently not available at the time.

In the same year that Johnston published his findings on clorgyline, Knoll and his colleagues published further investigations on $(-)$-E-250 in a German journal not widely read at the time by English-speaking pharmacologists [13]. In this paper they showed that $(-)$-E-250, in contrast to other MAO inhibitors, not only failed to potentiate the effects of tyramine, but actually antagonized the actions of this agonist *in vitro* and *in vivo* in the rat and cat (blood pressure and nictitating membrane). In other words, $(-)$-E-250 was a MAO inhibitor which did not produce the "cheese effect". These findings were communicated by Knoll in 1971 at a conference in Sardinia convened in honour of Hermann Blaschko, the discoverer of MAO [14]. This presentation familiarized the leading researchers on MAO with $(-)$-E-250, although there was some scepticism about an inhibitor without the "cheese effect", especially one coming from behind the Iron Curtain.

The year before, Moussa Youdim from Haifa, Israel, working at that time with Merton Sandler at the Queen Charlotte Hospital in London, had reported that MAO-B was particularly abundant in the brain [15], and that this now appeared to be the major site of action of $(-)$-E-250 [16].

But just as the penetrating smell of old camembert lingers in the nose long after the offending material has been removed, so the "cheese effect" was a label which no MAO inhibitor seemed to be able to shake off. $(-)$-E-250, now known as $(-)$- or *l*-deprenyl (or selegiline), was an interesting curiosity, but continued to suffer under the stigma of other antidepressant MAO inhibitors, despite its now acknowledged selectivity for MAO-B. It still did not appear to be destined for commercial use.

It is important to recognize that, in all experimental studies on selective MAO inhibitors, two major substrates were in general use at that time. These were serotonin for MAO-A and β-phenylethylamine for MAO-B. Endogenous catecholamines, such as noradrenaline and dopamine were considered to be specific substrates for MAO-A and not MAO-B on the basis of rodent data. This was clearly Knoll's understanding, even as late as 1975. He himself recognized that the Ciba Foundation Symposium on "Monoamine Oxidase and its Inhibition", held in London that year was a turning point in the recognition by clinicians of the importance of selective MAO inhibitors [5]. But throughout his paper presented at this symposium he continually referred to β-phenylethylamine as the target for *l*-deprenyl, and even cites experimental evidence for a physiological role of β-phenylethylamine in the brain, with regard to the etiology of depression [17].

The time was ripe for someone to see what others had seen and think what no-one had thought. A lecture by Moussa Youdim at the Neurological Institute of the University of Vienna in 1974 came at the crucial moment.

5. The Link to Parkinson's Disease

Vienna had been for several years one of the major centres of research on the mechanisms of Parkinson's disease. This reputation developed following the demonstration in the late 1950s by Carlsson in Stockholm of the presence of dopamine in the basal ganglia of the brains of rats, and that experimental depletion of this cerebral dopamine by reserpine was associated with extrapyramidal muscle dysfunction [18]. Obtaining human brain tissue from the Neurological Clinic of Walther Birkmayer, the Viennese pharmacologists H. Ehringer and O. Hornykiewicz demonstrated that brains of Parkinson's patients were deficient in dopamine [19]. The logical step of providing substitution therapy with a dopamine precursor able to pass the blood-brain barrier led to the introduction by Birkmayer and Hornykiewicz in 1961 of L-dopa for the treatment of Parkinson's disease [20].

They had also carried out some investigations at the same time with MAO inhibitors in an attempt to prevent the breakdown of any dopamine remaining in the basal ganglia of Parkinson's patients. But the side-effects of the drugs were too severe, because of the lack of selectivity of the products then available. During a visit to Queen Charlotte's Hospital in 1973, Peter Riederer, a co-worker of Birkmayer's in Vienna, told Youdim of these early studies on MAO inhibitors and Parkinson's disease and invited him to give a lecture in Vienna, which Youdim did in October 1974 [21]. Youdim's lecture on multiple forms of MAO also included a discussion of a MAO inhibitor which did not exhibit the cheese effect: *l*-deprenyl.

Over a well-lubricated dinner that evening Riederer suggested to Youdim that the on-off rhythm in Parkinson's patients appeared to be related to MAO activity, and that this might be treatable with *l*-deprenyl, since the drug is selective for MAO-B [21]. The next day, despite Youdim's scepticism about dopamine being a substrate for MAO-B, Birkmayer was informed of the proposal and agreed to perform the study in Parkinson's patients with *l*-deprenyl obtained from Youdim.

The trial was a success and demonstrated that *l*-deprenyl, given as an adjunct to L-dopa and peripheral decarboxylase inhibition therapy in 44 patients, was highly effective in sustaining motor function in the patients during their "off" periods, when they were normally most incapacitated [22]. Knoll, rather suprisingly, was not cited at all in this paper and

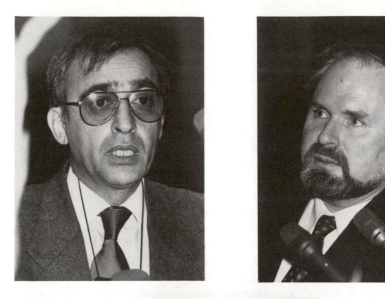

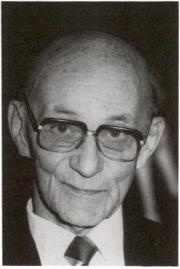

Figure 2. Moussa Youdim (top left), Peter Riederer (top right), and Walter Birkmayer (bottom), who first demonstrated the usefulness of *l*-deprenyl in Parkinson's disease (photographs reproduced with kind permission of the "Ärzte Zeitung").

apparently heard about the results of the clinical trial in a personal communication from Youdim, as stated during the Ciba meeting in London in 1975 [17]. He, like other participants at the conference, still thought that dopamine was a substrate for MAO-A and did not appear to recognize the importance of Youdim's news, suggesting that Birkmayer's findings may have indicated an involvement of β-phenylethylamine in Parkinson's disease. In fact, in the discussion to Knoll's paper, Fuller reported using the MAO inhibitor Lilly 51641 in Parkinson's patients with slight benefit, apparently independently of Birkmayer's work, but with the usual rise in blood pressure seen with MAO-A inhibitors. Sandler also mentioned having tried tranylcypromine in Parkinson's patients without benefit.

Clearly, the time had been ripe for testing a MAO-B inhibitor in Parkinson's disease, but it was Riederer who broke through the current dogma on dopamine as a substrate for MAO-A, Youdim who provided the information on *l*-deprenyl, and Birkmayer who performed the study. A more extensive long-term study (2 years) on 223 patients published by the same authors 2 years later in the Lancet confirmed the earlier findings and made the data on *l*-deprenyl available to a wider audience [23].

Youdim appears to have also interested his colleague Merton Sandler in *l*-deprenyl. Ater smuggling 1.5 kg of Chinoin's best *l*-deprenyl (courtesy of Knoll) through customs at London's Heathrow Airport, Sandler provided Gerald Stern, consultant neurologist at University College Hospital, with the contraband [1]. Their paper (also published in 1977 in the Lancet) corroborated Birkmayer's data in Parkinson's patients and provided sound data, acceptable to the British Commission on the Safety of Medicines, on the safety of *l*-deprenyl for human use [24].

l-Deprenyl was launched on the market in Hungary in 1977. Licensed by Chinoin through Farmos of Finland (in 1979) to Britannia Pharmaceuticals, *l*-deprenyl made rapid profit as an adjunct to L-dopa in the treatment of Parkinson's disease following its launching in the United Kingdom on 1 October, 1982 [1]. Europe-wide sales of *l*-deprenyl also increased as it became more widely used, first in combination with L-dopa/benserazide and, more recently, as monotherapy, depending on the stage of the disease.

6. The American Connection

6.1. Drugs for Jewels

In North America, though, *l*-deprenyl (or selegiline) was still practically unknown. Donald Buyske, the Research and Development Director of Warner-Lambert, after talking with Knoll, had actually tried to obtain the compound as an antidepressant under licence from Chinoin during a visit to Budapest in 1970, the year before Knoll gave his lecture in Sardinia [1]. However, MAO inhibitors were still under the stigma of the cheese effect which coloured Chinoin's attitude to their compound, and the Hungarian government at the time was not well-disposed to contacts with the west. Due to the intransigence of the Hungarian government lawyers the deal fell through, but Buyske's contacts with Chinoin were retained to good effect later. In 1978, when Hungary was already leaning westwards in foreign policy, at the request of Hungarian friends, he joined a group of Americans in persuading the U.S. government to return the Hungarian crown jewels to their rightful owners. These jewels included the 1000-year-old crown of St. Stephen and had been held at Fort Knox since World War II when US soldiers had taken them to keep them "safe" from the Red Army [25]. This act of philanthropy stood Buyske in good stead when, in 1981, acting on behalf of his new employer S.C. Johnson & Son (Johnson Wax), he successfully negotiated an agreement with Chinoin for the licensing in North America of the Hungarian company's drugs including *l*-deprenyl. This agreement did not last long. With litigation against pharmaceutical companies on the increase, Johnson Wax decided to pull out of the risky pharmaceutical branch, and Buyske took over the fledgling prescription drug business in his new company Somerset Pharmaceuticals.

A further incentive to launch the new company with *l*-deprenyl as its most promising research compound came from a discovery made in drug addicts in California in July 1982 (see next section).

6.2. MPTP and the Radical Dimension

1-Methyl-4-phenyl-1,2,3,6-tetrahydropyridine (MPTP) was first reported on in the early 1950s as one of a series of compounds synthesized in the search for a new analgesic [26]. MPTP not only failed to produce analgesia, but also produced toxic parkinsonian-like symptoms in monkeys. Because of its toxicity the compound was abandoned until it received the attention of scientists in 1977.

In the summer of 1976, Barry Kidston, a 23-year-old college student in Bethesda, Maryland, who was addicted to hard drugs, synthesized 1-methyl-4-propionoxy-4-phenyl-piperidine (MPPP), a compound structurally similar to the pain-killer meperidine which provides a high like heroin. The chemistry was performed in his parent's cellar but with inadequate facilities he failed to completely react the phenolic intermediate with propionic anhydride and generated MPTP as a by-product [1, 26]. This was confirmed by staff at the National Institute of Mental Health in Bethesda, after the young man had been admitted to a local hospital in a state of muteness, severe rigidity, weakness, tremor, and a flat facial expression; he had injected his own synthetic product intravenously. He responded well to L-dopa/carbidopa and bromocriptine, but later died after a self-inflicted overdose of cocaine and codeine [26]. The autopsy revealed degeneration of dopaminergic neurons in the substantia nigra, which provided clear evidence of parkinsonism in a 24-year-old. But this case report did not arouse much interest at the time.

Five years later, J. William Langston, a neurologist in San Jose, California, was called to treat a young prisoner in a local jail. Both the prisoner and his girlfriend showed the classical rigidity of Parkinson's disease, and both were heroin addicts. Langston found a total of four patients with parkinsonism, ages ranging from 26–42 years, all of whom had purchased illicit "synthetic heroin" and whose symptoms had appeared within 4 to 14 days. The Stanford University neurologists confirmed the presence of MPTP (by mass spectrometry) in the powders used [27].

Langston announced his findings to the press and soon an intensive study of MPTP toxicity was underway in many different laboratories. It soon became clear that MPTP is not particularly toxic itself. Being lipophilic, it is taken into glial cells where it is oxidized by MAO-B to MPDP$^+$ which further oxidizes non-enzymatically to MPP$^+$ [26]. The selectivity of the toxicity of MPP$^+$ is considered to lie in its redox-cycling with the neuromelanin within dopaminergic neurons in the substantia nigra. This results in the generation of the superoxide anion, a highly reactive oxygen radical (Figure 3). Such a mechanism not only offers an explanation for the action of MPTP, but also suggests a possible role of reactive oxygen species in the degeneration of dopaminergic neurons in Parkinson's disease. This may involve environmental toxins, but MAO-B also generates H_2O_2 during the metabolism of dopamine, and the generation may be exacerbated by the fact that radical scavenging enzymes in the brain lose their activity with increasing age [28].

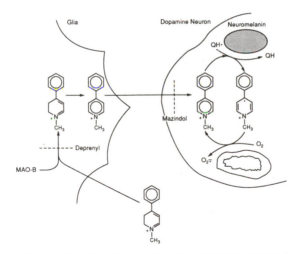

Figure 3. Proposed mechanism for the neurotoxicity of MPTP. MPTP is transported by diffusion due to its lipophilicity into glial cells, where it is oxidized by monoamine oxidase B (MAO-B) to MPDP$^+$ which oxidizes nonenzymatically to MPP$^+$. This is taken up by dopaminergic teminals where it can undergo redox cycling using neuromelanin as an electron source, and produce superoxide in mitochondria. Reproduced from [26] with permission (copyright John Wiley and Sons, New York).

By the mid-1980s a number of investigators had reported that *l*-deprenyl, as an inhibitor of MAO-B, was able to inhibit MPTP toxicity in experimental animals [26]. Then, in 1985, a clinical report by Birkmayer's group in Vienna provided the first clinical indication that *l*-deprenyl may indeed retard the degeneration of dopaminergic neurones in parkinsonism.

7. FDA Approval: a Battle Against Bureaucracy

In an open, uncontrolled study Birkmayer (together with the other main European actors in the *l*-deprenyl story: Knoll, Riederer, and Youdim) had investigated the effects of long-term (9 years) treatment of parkinsonian patients with Madopar (a combination of L-dopa and benserazide, a dopa decarboxylase inhibitor) alone (n = 377) and in combination with *l*-deprenyl (n = 564). They found that *l*-deprenyl not only produced remission in patients no longer responding to L-dopa, but also increased survival by an average of 15.3 months [29]. The study results were criticized because the study had been a retrospective analysis and the trial had not been originally started with the intention of measuring survival, although it did give an indication that *l*-deprenyl provided more benefit than just symptomatic relief.

Meanwhile, Buyske was still seeking approval for *l*-deprenyl from the FDA. The discovery of the action of MPTP had encouraged him to apply for an orphan drug approval in 1983, in order to extend patent coverage, but the FDA was still not satisfied with the documentation [1]. One of the problems lay in the fact that the FDA officially required 12-month toxicity tests in animals, whereas in Europe, where *l*-deprenyl had been developed, only 6-month tests were necessary. At the recent meeting to harmonize world drug-registration criteria the FDA agreed to accept 6-month studies [30], thus one wonders why they had held out so long for expensive, unnecessary tests and had jeopardized, not only *l*-deprenyl, but also other interesting new drugs. I suspect the "Atlantic Ocean Syndrome" was once again at work here, with the U.S. authorities wishing to be seen as a touch stricter than the Europeans. The FDA also demanded further clinical data from Somerset Pharmaceuticals despite the fact that the drug was doing well in Europe; fulfilling the demand nearly brought the company to financial ruin.

Further support came from Canadian physician, businessman, and TV personality Morton Shulmann. He suffered from Parkinson's Disease and had been greatly helped by *l*-deprenyl obtained through personal contacts in Europe. He then brought together sufficient investors to form Deprenyl Research Ltd., which received the rights to the drug in Canada and provided the necessary injection of capital to carry out the additional studies required [1]. The crucial, FDA-approved, controlled, double-blind U.S. study against placebo was carried out by Roger Duvoisin, Abraham Liebermann, Manfred Muenter, and their colleagues in 96 patients, and published in 1988 [31]. They concluded that *l*-deprenyl is of moderate benefit in a majority of patients with symptom fluctuations complicating Parkinson's disease, and that it is well tolerated.

The FDA finally approved *l*-deprenyl for addition to the standard therapy of L-dopa for Parkinson's disease in June 1989, thereby making the drug available to Parkinson's patients world-wide. The story does not end there. *l*-Deprenyl is now considered to be a potential drug for the retarding of the aging process and for Alzheimer's disease [1, 25]. The jury is still out regarding these indications, as the following chapters reveal, but *l*-deprenyl seems destined for a long and interesting life. It has also spawned a number of derivative compounds, including new aliphatic propargylamine compounds under development by Deprenyl Research Ltd. for parkinsonism.

8. Postscript: a Child of Several Fathers

In 1948, a Hungarian student of Szent-Györgyi, the biochemist I. Banga, discovered the enzyme elastase in the pancreas. For this, she was nominated to receive the highest Hungarian scientific award. Her husband and department head, J. Balo, a highly-esteemed pathologist, was extremely annoyed that his name had been omitted from the nomination. He protested to the jury that his wife could never have discovered the enzyme had he not shown her where to look! The jury acknowledged their oversight and honoured both husband and wife with the prize.

Not all scientific prize juries have been so perspicacious, and some have inadvertently stirred up a hornet's nest of conflicting individual claims to recognition. Like the elastase discovery, the worldwide introduction of selegiline or *l*-deprenyl as an anti-parkinsonian drug has been made possible by several crucial, although individually incomplete contributions. Knoll proposed and selected the compound, but failed to recognize the Parkinson connection. Youdim recognized the importance of the selectivity of *l*-deprenyl and the lack of the cheese effect, but was sceptical about the relevance of dopamine as a target. Riederer, on the other hand, had expertise in Parkinson's disease and was able to put Youdim's information into context. Birkmayer also lacked Youdim's specialist knowledge, but as the clinical doyen of parkinsonism, he carried sufficient weight to approve and substantiate the ideas of the younger scientists. Finally, the initiative of Sandler and the business acumen of Buyske helped to overcome regulatory barriers. In this sense, selegiline is a child of several fathers.

Summary

l-Deprenyl was originally synthesized in the early 1960s by the Chinoin company in Budapest as a "me-too" monoamine oxidase (MAO) inhibitor with anti-depressant activity. The drug received international attention following a lecture by Knoll in 1971, when he reported that *l*-deprenyl did not potentiate the hypertensive effect of exogenous catecholamines, i.e., it did not elicit the cheese effect. This was due to a selective action on brain MAO-B. Riederer and Youdim subsequently recognized the relevance of the finding for Parkinson's disease, and in 1975, Birkmayer et al. reported the first use of *l*-deprenyl for this indication. The drug made little impact in North America until the parkinsonian-like toxicity of MPTP was reported by Langston and shown to be inhibited by *l*-deprenyl. An arduous struggle with the U.S. Food and Drug Administration finally led to its approval of *l*-deprenyl for use in the treatment of Parkinson's disease in 1989, which gave the drug world-wide accessibility.

References

[1] Dow A. The Deprenyl Story. Toronto: Stoddart, 1990.
[2] Zeller EA. Monoamine oxidase and its inhibitors in relation to antidepressive activity. In: Parnham MJ, Bruinvels J, editors. Psycho- and Neuro-pharmacology. Discoveries in Pharmacology. Vol. 1. Amsterdam: Elsevier, 1983: 223–232.
[3] Lehmann HE, Kline NS. Clinical discoveries with anti-depressant drugs: In: Parnham MJ, Bruinvels J, editors. Psycho- and Neuro-pharmacology. Discoveries in Pharmacology. Vol. 1. Amsterdam: Elsevier, 1983: 209–222.
[4] Schier O, Marxer A. Antihypertensive agents 1962–1968: Progr Drug Res 1969; 13: 101–135.
[5] Knoll J. Deprenyl (selegiline): the history of its development and phamacological action. Acta Neurol Scand, 1983; [Supplement] 95: 57–80.
[6] Knoll J, Ecseri Z, Kelemen K, Nievel J, Knoll B. Phenyl-isopropylmethylpropinylamine (E-250), a new spectrum psychic energizer. Arch Int Pharmacodyn 1965; 155: 154–164.
[7] Ecseri Z, Müller M, Knoll J, Somfai E. Hungarian Patent Nr. 151090, 1964.
[8] Varga A, Tringer L. Clinical trial of a new type of promptly acting psychoenergetic agent (phenyl-isopropyl-methyl-propinylamine·HCl) (E-250). Acta Med Acad Sci Hung 1967; 23: 289–295.
[9] Magyar K, Vizi ES, Ecseri Z, Knoll J. Comparative pharmacological analysis of the optical isomers of phenyl-isopropyl-methyl-propinylamine (E-250). Acta Physiol Acad Sci Hung 1967; 32: 377–387.
[10] Hardegg W, Heilbron E. Oxidation of tyramine and serotonin by liver mitochondrial monoamine oxidase. Biochim Biophys Acta 1961; 51: 533–559.
[11] Johnston JP. Some observations upon a new inhibitor of monoamine oxidase in brain tissue. Biochem Pharmacol 1968; 17: 1285–1297.
[12] Youdim MBH, Finberg JPM. Monoamine oxidase B inhibition and the "cheese effect". J Neural Transm 1987; [Supplement] 25: 27–33.
[13] Knoll J, Vizi ES, Somogyi G. Phenylisopropyl-methyl-propinylamine (E-250), a monoamine oxidase inhibitor antagonizing effects of tyramine. Arzn-Forsch 1968; 18: 109–112.
[14] Knoll J, Magyar K. Some puzzling effects of monoamine oxidase inhibitors. Adv Biochem Psychopharmacol 1972; 5: 393–408.

[15] Collins GGS, Sandler M, Williams ED, Youdim MBH. Multiple forms of human brain mitochondrial monoamine oxidase. Nature 1970; 225: 817–820.

[16] Squires R. Multiple forms of monoamine oxidase in intact mitochondria as characterized by selective inhibitors and thermal stability. A comparison of eight mammalian species. Adv Biochem Psychopharmacol 1972; 5: 355–370.

[17] Knoll J. Analysis of the pharmacological effects of selective monoamine oxidase inhibitors. In: Wolstenholme GEW, Knight J, editors: Monoamine oxidase and its inhibition. Amsterdam: Elsevier 1976: 135–161.

[18] Carlsson A. Antipsychotic agents: elucidation of their mode of action. In: Parnham MJ, Bruinvels J, editors. Psycho- and Neuro-pharmacology. Discoveries in Pharmacology. Vol. 1. Amsterdam: Elsevier 1983: 197–206.

[19] Birkmayer W. 10 Jahre L-DOPA-Therapie des Parkinson-Syndroms. Wien Klin Wschr 1971; 83: 221–227.

[20] Birkmayer W, Hornykiewicz O. Der L-Dioxyphenylalanin (L-DOPA)-Effekt bei der Parkinson-Akinesie. Wien Klin Wschr 1961; 73: 787–794.

[21] Riederer P. Besuch beim "Heurigen" brachte den entscheidenden Entschluß. In: Morbus Parkinson. Eine Dokumentation der Ärzte Zeitung 1991: 20–22.

[22] Birkmayer W, Riederer P, Youdim MBH, Linauer W. Potentiation of anti-akinetic effect after L-dopa treatment by an inhibitor of MAO-B, *l*-deprenyl. J Neural Transm 1975; 36: 303–323.

[23] Birkmayer W, Riederer P, Ambrozi L, Youdim MBH. Implications of combined treatment with Madopar and *l*-deprenyl in Parkinson's disease. Lancet 1977; ii: 439–443.

[24] Lees AJ, Shaw KM, Kohout LJ, Stern GM, Elsworth JD, Sandler M, Youdim MBH. Deprenyl in Parkinson's disease. Lancet 1977; ii: 791–796.

[25] Waldholz M. Medical odyssey. The Wall Street Journal 1990 Nov 28; p. 1 (col. 1).

[26] Markey SP, Schmuff NR. The pharmacology of the parkinsonian syndrome producing neurotoxin MPTP (1-methyl-4-phenyl-1,2,3,6-tetrahydropyridine) and structurally related compounds. Med Res Rev 1986; 6: 389–429.

[27] Langston JW, Ballard P, Tetrud JW, Irwin I. Chronic parkinsonism in human due to a product of meperidine-analog synthesis. Science 1983; 219: 979–980.

[28] Ceballos I, Javoy-Agid F, Delacourte A, Defossez A, Nicole A, Sinet P-M. Parkinson's disease and Alzheimer's disease: neurodegenerative disorders due to brain antioxidant deficiency? Adv Exp Med Biol 1990; 264: 493–498.

[29] Birkmayer W, Knoll J, Riederer P, Youdim MBH, Hars V, Marton J. Increased life expectancy resulting from addition of *l*-deprenyl to Madopar treatment in Parkinson's disease: a longterm study. J Neural Transm 1985; 64: 113–127.

[30] Press release. International Conference on Harmonisation of Technical Requirements for Registration of Pharmaceuticals for Human Use; 1991 Nov 5–7; Brussels.

[31] Golbe LI, Liebermann AN, Muenter MD, Ahlskog J, Gopinathan G, Neophytides AN, Foo SH, Duvoisin RC. Deprenyl in the treatment of symptom fluctuations in advanced Parkinson's disease. Clin Neuropharmacol 1988; 11: 45–55.

Inhibitors of Monoamine Oxidase B
Pharmacology and Clinical Use in Neurodegenerative Disorders
ed. by I. Szelenyi
© 1993 Birkhäuser Verlag Basel/Switzerland

CHAPTER 13
MAO-B Inhibitors in Neurological Disorders with Special Reference to Selegiline

K. Wessel

1   The Physiological Role of MAO-B
2   Potential Therapeutic Use of MAO-B Inhibitors
3   Selegiline in the Treatment of Parkinson's Disease
4   Side-Effects of MAO Inhibitors in Parkinson's Disease with Special Reference to
         Selegiline
4.1   Comparison with Non-Selective MAOI
4.2   Side-Effects During Combination Therapy
4.3   Side-Effects During Monotherapy
5   How Do MAO-B Inhibitors Work in Parkinson's Disease?
         Summary

1. The Physiological Role of Monoamine Oxidase B (MAO-B)

It has been shown that monoamines like serotonin and noradrenaline are preferentially metabolized in man by MAO-A, while benzylamine, phenylethylamine, and phenylethanolamine are specific substrates for MAO-B. Other monoamines are metabolized by both forms, but regional differences exist [1]. In the intestine, MAO-A is the dominant form, while MAO-B is preferentially found in platelets and in the brain, especially in the glial cells [2] (see Chapters 2, 6, 9).

In the central nervous system, MAO is also responsible for protection against exogenous monoamines, and it is involved in maintaining a constant, physiological, monoamine tonus [3]. This seems also to be true for the regulation of the intraneuronal monoamine level [4]. In this context, it is interesting that MAO-B is preferentially expressed in serotonergic neurons and in the glia, while MAO-A occurs in noradrenergic and dopaminergic neurons [3, 5]. It is important to mention, however, that in human striatal synaptosomes the MAO-activity outside the neuron (MAO-B) is up to five times higher than intraneuronally [6]; this is indicative of the importance of MAO-B inhibition. By histochemical techniques it has been shown that dopaminergic neurons in the substantia nigra do not have MAO-B activity, but serotonergic neurons in the raphe nuclei and noradrenergic neurons in the locus coeruleus do, as do glial cells [7] (see Chapter 2). Experi-

ments with cAMP-induced dopamine flux support physiological relevance of extraneuronal metabolism of dopamine by MAO-B [8] (see
Chapters 6, 7).

Despite the role in regulating the monoamine level, it should be noted
that the regulation of the concentration of trace amines is also of
physiological importance. Especially phenylethylamine, an endogenous
enhancer of dopaminergic function, is selectively metabolized by MAO-
B [9]. In addition to the importance of MAO-B in the metabolism of
several monoamines, it becomes evident that N-actylated polyamines
like N-acetylputrescine are substrates for MAO-B [10]. In this way,
MAO-B may indirectly interplay with the NMDA-receptor [11, 12].
Antagonism of polyamines like spermine can be used to modulate the
NMDA receptor [13] (see Chapters 2, 9).

It has also been shown that there is a relationship between the
mitochondrial respiratory state and the MAO-activity [14]. It has been
suggested that an oxidase or oxygenase is involved in the regulation of
oxygen-supply in the brain [15]. Studies investigating the relation between the local cerebrocortical microflow and local cerebrocortical
oxygen tension during normoxia and hypoxemia suggest that local
regulatory mechanisms are responsible for an increase in microflow if
cortical pO_2 falls below a critical level [16]. This increase can be
inhibited by selegiline (l-deprenyl), a selective MAO-B-inhibitor, and
suggests a possible role of MAO-B in regulating local cerebrocortical
capillary blood flow [17].

The dopaminergic system plays a role in ischemic neuronal death
[18]. An activation of dopamine metabolism and, thereby, the induction
of oxidative stress has been reported [19, 20]. Deamination of
monoamines by MAO-B inhibits, in sarcoplasmic reticulum vesicles, the
activity of Ca^{2+}-Mg^{2+}-dependent ATPase and the active Ca^{2+} transport [21]. This is probably due to the toxic effects of the aldehydes
produced.

The level of monoamine oxidase in the human brain increases with
age [22–24] and in neurodegenerative diseases like Alzheimer's disease
(AD) [25]. This is probably linked to the increase of glial cells in the
brain with age [26]. The deamination of biogenic amines by MAO-B
causes lipid peroxidation due to the H_2O_2 produced, even in the
presence of free iron, leading to an increase of radical formation and
oxidative stress [27–29] in brains of parkinsonian patients (see Chapters
7, 8, 9).

Another function of MAO is the metabolism of exogenous substances, working as neurotoxins like 1-methyl-4-phenyl-1,2,3,6-tetrahy-
dropyridine (MPTP) and its toxic metabolite MPP^+. MPTP is a
possible model substance for environmental agents. This matter has
been reviewed in detail [30, 31] (see Chapter 8).

2. Potential Therapeutic Use of MAO-B Inhibitors

It is generally accepted that the actual history of MAO-inhibitors (MAOI) began the 1950s with the introduction of iproniazid in the treatment of depression [32]. Interestingly, as early as 1929, the first MAOI, banisterine, was used in the management of Parkinson's disease (PD) (based on experience in natural medicine) [33]. Following the introduction of iproniazid, a phase of development of new MAOI started. This class of substances, however, had to be used with care because of side-effects. The most serious side-effect, the so-called "cheese effect", led to a temporary discontinuation of MAOI development. A rebirth of MAO inhibitors took place after the finding that two forms of monomaine oxidase with different substrate specificities exist [34]. Specific inhibitors have been described for type A (clorgyline) and type B (selegiline) [35].

When selegiline was first developed [36, 37] the potential first clincial application was not clear. And even today, after selegiline has been established as a standard therapeutic compound in PD, several other applications may still be possible.

In the beginning of its clinical development, selegiline was also tested in several clinical trials to investigate the "classical" indication of MAO inhibitors, the treatment of depression [38–42] (see Chapter 17).

Neuroleptic drugs induce extrapyramidal side-effects such as tardive dyskinesias. These may be due to decreased dopaminergic release after chronic neuroleptic treatment [43]. Another alternative is the oxidative stress hypothesis of tardive dyskinesias [44]. Therefore it might be possible to use antioxidants or MAOI to prevent tardive dyskinesias.

There are some reports about the action of dopaminergic agents in the treatment of brain injury. An improvement of behavior was observed with amantadine therapy [45]. A cognitive and behavioral improvement was observed with L-dopa after traumatic brain injury [46]. A possible beneficial effect of MAO-B inhibition, however, remains to be investigated.

Alzheimer's disease (AD) is characterized by several pathological and physiological changes. The neurofibrillary tangles and amyloid deposition as well as the cholinergic deficit possibly accompanied by cognitive dysfunction are well described [47]. But other transmitter systems are also affected. Dopamine deficits have been reported as well as an increase in MAO-B activity. This can be explained by an increase in glial cells. Based on these observations and the preclinical profile of selegiline, several clinical trials have been performed with this drug [48–56]. The studies suggest that selegiline has an effect on certain cognitive functions and perhaps a positive influence on social interaction (see Chapter 16). As an antioxidant the drug may even have an impact on the progression rate of the disease. Increased lipid peroxidation has been shown in the cortex of Alzheimer's patients after autopsy [49]. Further long-term studies based on the results of preclinical studies are needed to clarify the beneficial role of selegiline in the (symptomatic and/or neuroprotective) treatment of AD.

There are several reports about an extension of life-span by selegiline in rodents [57, 58]. The interpretation of these results in respect to healthy humans is unclear and could only be clarified in long-term prospective studies. It is likely that selegiline may prolong the life of parkinsonian patients [59].

3. Selegiline in the Treatment of Parkinson's Disease

In the early 1960s, nonspecific MAO inhibitors were tested for the treatment of PD, but they were undesirable because of the risk of hypertensive crisis. Selegiline was developed in 1964 by Knoll and coworkers. As a selective MAO-B inhibitor it was free of the risk of hypertensive crisis. But it was not until 1975 that the first clinical trial with selegiline was conducted in the treatment of PD by Birkmayer and coworkers [60]. This group, and others, have shown that by inhibiting the breakdown of dopamine [61] selegiline improves the efficacy of L-dopa. It reduces fluctuations of disability, especially "wearing-off", prolongs "on"-time, and reduces "off"-periods. Long-term treatment of parkinsonian patients with selegiline in combination with L-dopa resulted in a prolongation of life-span of 15 months, as has been shown by a retrospective analysis of more than 900 patients [59]. A reduction of the L-dopa dose by about 20–50% is also possible because selegiline potentiates the antiakinetic effect of L-dopa [62–85, 88]. A greater improvement in the degree of disability (27% vs. 37%) was found for the combination of L-dopa with selegiline [68]. The dose of 10 mg/day seems to be optimal; higher doses do not improve efficacy of selegiline [74]. The L-dopa dose can be dramatically reduced by combination of selegiline with L-dopa in long-term treatment over a period of 4 years. L-Dopa-treated patients needed 668 mg L-dopa after 4 years' therapy, while with combination therapy, patients needed only 403 mg. The addition of a dopamine agonist to the combined treatment allows the reduction of L-dopa by another 100 mg daily. Consequently, combination therapy has a positive impact on the occurrence of fluctuations of disability [69]. There is evidence that early combination of L-dopa with selegiline results in a better improvement than a late onset of combination therapy [86]. The degree of improvement over a period of up to 4 years was better in a group of 65 patients of disease stages 2–3 (55%) than in a group of fluctuating patients (44%). In a group of 17 advanced stage-4 patients only a slight improvement (14%), if any, was observed.

Table 1. Results from open controlled clinical trials with selegiline in the combination therapy of Parkinson's disease with L-dopa

Reference	No. of patients	Duration of the disease	Study duration and design	Dose (mg/day)	Clinical score	Fluctuations	L-dopa dose
Fornadi & Ulm [70]	133 113 33	8.5 y 10.3 y 11.7 y	max 3 y, o, p	control 10 Sel Ergots	WRS + + WRS + +	—	414 mg 367 mg 447 mg
Ulm & Fornadi [71]	15 15	9.3	3 w, o, p	10 Sel Bromocriptin	CURS − 11.3% CURS − 10.6%	—	—
Liebermann et al. [72]	40	8.1 y	25 d 22 mo, o, p	10 Sel	NYUDS + + +	+ + +	− 6.5%
Birkmayer et al. [56]	564 377	—	5 y, o, p	5–10 Sel	extension of survival	—	—
Rinne [69]	25 30 26 27	— — —	4 y, o, p	— 10 Sel 1.1 Lisurid 0.8 Lisurid + 10 Sel	CURS +/−	— + + + + + + +	668 mg 403 mg 484 mg 302 mg

Abbreviations: y: year; m: month; w: weeks; d: day; db: double-blind; sb: single-blind; o: open; co: cross-over; p: parallel; Pl: placebo; Sel: selegiline; HY: Hoehn & Yahr stage; CURS: Columbia University Rating Scale; WRS: Webster Rating Scale; UPDRS: Unified Parkinson's Disease Rating Scale; NUDS: North-Western University Disability Scale; RNE: Rated Neurological Examination; +/−: no difference; +: slight improvement; ++: moderate improvement; +++: strong improvement

Table 2. Results from double-blind controlled clinical trials comparing selegiline with placebo in the combination with L-dopa/peripheral decarboxylase inhibitor in parkinsonian patients

Reference	No. of patients	PD stage/duration	Study duration and design	Dose (mg/day)	Clinical score	Fluctuations	L-dopa dose
Broderson et al. [64]	19	11 y	8 w, db, co	5 Sel / Pl	WRS +/-	+ + +	- 20%
Eisler et al. [73]	11	1–6 y	4 w, db, co	10 Sel / Pl	CURS +/-	—	- 42% (50% patients)
Frankel et al. [74]	12	13.3 y	5 * 3 w, db, co	10 Sel / 20 Sel / 30 Sel / 40 Sel / Pl	UPDRS + + / UPDRS + + / UPDRS + + / UPDRS + +	—	—
Goldstein [75]	5	12 y	12 d, db, co	10 Sel / Pl	RNE + +	+/-	—
Golbe et al. [76]	50	HY 2–4	6 w, db, p	10 Sel / Pl	—	+ +	- 17%
Duvoisin et al. [77]	49 / 46	9.5 y / 8.5 y	8 w, db, p	10 Sel / Pl	CURS +/-	+ + +	- 33%
Heinonen et al. [78]	19	13.3 y	12 w, db, co	10 Sel / Pl	CUDS +	+ +	- 100 mg

Study	n	Stage/Duration	Design	Dose	Scale		
Lander et al. [79]	60	10 y / 11 y	4 w, db, p	10 Sel / Pl	—	++	− 100 mg
Lees et al. [80]	41	9 y	4 w, db, co	10 Sel / Pl	CURS & NUDS +/−	+++	− 35%
Presthus & Hajba [67]	20 / 18	max 3 y	8 w, db, p	10 Sel / Pl	WRS ++	++	− 32% / − 20%
Przuntek et al. [31]	25	de novo	18 w, db, co	10 Sel / Pl	CURS ++	—	—
Rascol et al. [82]	15	HY 2–4	2 w, db, co	10 Sel / Pl	+/−	—	—
Schacter et al. [33]	19	2–5 y	2 w, db, co	10 Sel / Pl	+++	+++	+/−
Sivertson et al. [34]	39	HY 1–3	8 w, db, co	10 Sel / Pl	CURS ++	+/−	− 24%
Stern et al. [62]	85	1–4 y	1 m, db, co	10 Sel / Pl	++	++	− 200 mg
Teychenne & Parker [85]	10	max 5 y	16 w, db, co	10 Sel / Pl	UPDRS ++	++	—

Abbreviations.: y: year; m: month; w: weeks; d: day; db: double-blind; sb: single-blind; o: open; co: cross-over; p: parallel; Pl: Placebo; Sel: Selegiline; HY: Hoehn & Yahr stage; CURS: Columbia University Rating Scale; WRS: Webster Rating Scale; UPDRS: Unified Parkinson's Disease Rating Scale; NUDS: North-Western University Disability Scale; RNE: Rated Neurological Examination; +/−: no difference; +: slight improvement; ++: moderate improvement; +++: strong improvement

Table 3. Results from studies with selegiline in the monotherapy of previously untreated "de-novo" patients

Reference	No. of patients	PD stage/duration	Study duration and design	Dose (mg/day)	Clinical score	Patients requiring L-dopa	Time L-dopa is required
Allain et al. [92]	48 45	HY 1.8 HY 1.7	3 m, db, p	10 Sel Pl	UPDRS 21.4 UPDRS 24.7	4.5% 18.4%	26–79 d 25–71 d
Csanda & Tarczy [140]	30	HY 1.3	6 m, uc	10 Sel	10% improvement	67%	—
Elizan et al. [141]	22	2.3 y	7–84 m, uc	10 Sel	17 responders	27%	—
Myllylä et al. [90]	27 25	HY 1.5 HY 1.5	3–52 w, db, p	10 Sel Pl	CURS 32–45 CURS 38–45	44% 56%	18 m 12 m
Parkinson Study Group (DATATOP) [91]	375 377	HY 1.6 HY 1.7	12 m, db, p	10 Sel +/− Toc Pl +/− Toc	UPDRS 22 UPDRS 52	26% 47%	26 m 15 m
Terävainen [142]	20	HY 2.7	3 m, db, co	5–30 Sel	+/−	—	—
Tetrud & Langston [89]	22 22	HY 1.6 HY 1.5	3 y, db, p	10 Sel PL	UPDRS 6–35 UPDRS 35–63	—	18 m 10 m

Abbreviations.: y: year; m: month; w: weeks; d: day; db: double-blind; sb: single-blind; o: open; co: cross-over; p: parallel; uc: uncontrolled; Pl: placebo; Sel: Selegiline; HY: Hoehn & Yahr stage; CURS: Columbia University Rating Scale; WRS: Webster Rating Scale; UPDRS: Unified Parkinson's Disease Rating Scale; NUDS: North-Western University Disability Scale; RNE: Rated Neurological Examination; TOC: Tocopherol

In addition to combination therapy with L-dopa (Tables 1 and 2), which is based on the enhancing effect of selegiline on dopaminergic neurotransmission, clinical trials have been performed with selegiline in the monotherapy of PD. The rationale for these studies is based on the neuroprotective properties of the substance. Selegiline protects against MPTP-induced dopaminergic cell destruction [34, 35] and protects against oxidative stress induced by increased dopamine turnover [87] (see Chapters 6, 7, 9). A weak dopaminergic effect of selegiline in monotherapy has been reported from an uncontrolled study [88]. Therefore, long-term trials have been performed with newly diagnosed, untreated patients who did not yet need dopaminergic therapy; the trials have attempted to prove the clinical efficacy of selegiline in monotherapy and to elucidate the influence of selegiline treatment on the progressin of the disease [89–91].

As summarized in Table 3, three double-blind, randomized, parallel, placebo-controlled prospective studies have been performed. The main endpoint was the need for additional L-dopa treatment. Selegiline was superior to placebo by 237 days [89] or 173 days [90] in studies involving 54 and 52 patients, respectively. A study with 800 patients showed in an average follow-up period of 12 months that only 97 selegiline-treated patients needed L-dopa vs. 176 in the placebo group [91]. These data show efficacy of selegiline monotherapy in the treatment of early parkinsonism. Selegiline-treated patients were able to remain employed for a longer time period. Disability, as measured by clinical scores, progressed more slowly in the selegiline group (see Chapter 15). The efficacy of selegiline in the monotherapy of early diagnosed parkinsonian patients has recently been confirmed by a 3-month, double-blind, placebo-controlled study with 93 patients [92]. After 3 months, selegiline was superior in the UPDRS total score. L-Dopa had to be started more frequently in the placebo group.

The long-term efficacy of selegiline has clearly been proved. Four-week wash-in and 4-week wash-out periods during the above-mentioned clinical trial [91] showed a weak initial effect and no rapid deterioration 4 weeks after withdrawal of medication. Therefore, one pharmacological explanation for the clinical efficacy is based on the neuroprotective properties of this drug. As discussed in detail in [93] (see also Chapter 8), an otherwise dopaminergic effect should have occurred first, at more than 4 weeks after initiation of therapy, and would have lost efficacy shortly before reaching the end-point. This is very unlikely as patients in the selegiline group needed twice the time to reach the end-point and their level of disability after wash-out should have been much worse than in the placebo group when reaching the end-point, if the mode of action of selegiline were only symptomatic. The initial responders (patients who had an initial symptomatic benefit) in the selegiline group and in the placebo group showed similar group differences in respect to reaching the end-point compared with the non-responders (see Chapters 15).

In summary, selegiline monotherapy is superior to placebo in long-term treatment, but it has only weak acute effects on symptoms. The explanation may be found in its neuroprotective profile. In addition, first data from a post-mortem study [99] seem to prove the hypothesis that selegiline slows degeneration of dopaminergic neurons in the substantia nigra, but the number of cases involved in that study should be extended.

Preliminary data [95] shows that the start of selegiline monotherapy treatment in *de novo* patients led to a clear reduction of the L-dopa dose, when this compound was introduced into therapy later on. It seems unlikely that this reduction in L-dopa can be explained only by the dopaminergic-like effect. Therefore, it may be advisable to start selegiline treatment as early as possible. The L-dopa-free interval can be prolonged by selegiline. Later in the time-course of the disease, when additional symptomatic therapy is necessary, L-dopa can be added to the selegiline basic therapy and it may be kept at a very low level for a long time. If the patient needs L-dopa from the beginning, it is recommended to start with combined therapy [89]. Possible oxidative damage from the metabolism of L-dopa can be prevented by this strategy [59, 87, 94]. If necessary, dopamine agonists can be added to the regime (see Chapter 14).

4. Side-Effects of MAOI in Parkinson's Disease with Special Reference to Selegiline

4.1. Comparison with Nonselective MAOI

One principal problem with regard to the use of MAO inhibitors is related to the inhibition of metabolism of dietary amines. The most frequent dietary amine, tyramine, is metabolized by MAO-A. Noradrenaline released by tyramine from nerve endings in turn increases blood pressure. The blockade of MAO-A by nonspecific MAOI or by MAO-A inhibitors potentiates the indirect pressor effect of these amines, sometimes inducing a hypertensive crisis [96]. Selective MAO-B inhibition (selegiline, 10 mg/day) leaves the intestinal MAO-A active and tyramine can be metabolized [97]. Unlike other MAO-B inhibitors, selegiline blocks tyramine-induced hypertensive effects by inhibiting the uptake of tyramine into the nerve endings [98] (see Chapter 6). No clinically relevant increase of tyramine sensitivity has been described [99–102], even after a treatment period of 2 months. No significant increase of tyramine sensitivity was seen, even after 30 mg/day of selegiline, or after long-term use [103]. Other typical MAOI side-effects are not known in the case of the selective MAO-B inhibitor selegiline. Only a minimal occurrence of orthostatic hypotension has been occasionally reported in depressed patients [104].

4.2. Side-Effects During Combination Therapy

Concerning the combination therapy with selegiline and L-dopa much experience has been reported in respect to side-effects. Orthostatic hypotension in a few patients has been reported [59, 67, 105]. Two cases of syncope have been observed [76, 80]. Dyskinesias have been mentioned after combined therapy in an average of 28% of patients [63, 64, 76, 80, 84]. These problems occurred shortly after addition of selegiline to L-dopa, and are related to peak-concentrations of L-dopa; they can be prevented by reducing the L-dopa dose [76]. Edema is a MAOI side-effect currently under discussion. It has been reported that edema after treatment with nonselective MAOI reversed after switching to selegiline [104]. This suggests that altered vascular tone resulting from nonspecific MAOI treatment might be responsible for this side-effect. Several other side-effects have been reported when selegiline has been used together with L-dopa, including headache, nausea, vomiting, confusion, dizziness, sleep disturbances, hallucinations, anxiety, akathisia, dry mouth, and psychosis. An increase in some liver enzymes has also been mentioned [105]. These effects are well known from L-dopa therapy and may be related to the indirect dopaminergic activity of selegiline when combined with L-dopa. Therefore, it seems advisable to reduce L-dopa after selegiline has been added to the therapy.

4.3. Side-Effects During Monotherapy

To get a definite insight into the intrinsic potential of side-effects of selegiline, it might be useful to compare the groups of placebo-controlled selegiline monotherapy trials. Table 4 shows reported adverse effects with group differences as observed during the trials. The adverse effects of selegiline are very mild. Most of the common side-effects known from combination therapy with L-dopa do not occur. It seems that only the events "dry mouth" and "transient elevation of liver enzymes" may be more common in the selegiline-treated patients. No evidence exists of withdrawal symptoms after discontinuation of selegiline therapy or of increased sexual activity during selegiline treatment. In summary, it can be concluded that selegiline is safe and well tolerated.

Table 4. Side-effects from placebo-controlled studies with selegiline in the monotherapy of previously untreated "*de-novo*" patients

Reference	No. of patients	PD stage/duration	Study duration and design	Dose (mg/day)	Item	Placebo	Selegiline
Allain et al. [92]	48	HY 1.8	3 m, db, p	10 Sel	Vertigo	2	5
	45	HY 1.7		Pl	Nausea/Vomiting	5	3
					Headache	—	2
					Unpleasant taste	—	2
					Insomnia	2	—
					Anxiety	2	—
Myllylä et al. [92]	27	HY 1.5	3–52 w, db, p	10 Sel	Depression	1	1
	25	HY 1.5		Pl	Headache	1	1
					Fatigue	2	3
					Memory disturbance	—	1
					Insomnia	4	—
					Dizziness	1	2
					Dry mouth	—	3
					Nausea	—	3
					Gastrointest. pain	1	—
					Invol. mouth movement	1	—
					Heart trouble	1	—
Parkinson Study Group (DATATOP) [91]	375	HY 1.6	12 m, db, p	10 Sel +/− Toc	Trans. ALAT elevation	2	15
	377	HY 1.7		Pl	Dry mouth	5	14
					Depression	1	2

Reference	n	HY	Design	Treatment	Adverse event	Sel	Pl
Teräväinen [142]	20	HY 2.7	3 m, db, co	5–30 Sel / Pl	Urinary hesitancy	1	—
					Urinary frequency	1	—
					Hematuria	1	—
					Arrhythmia	1	—
					Orth. hypotension	1	1
					Chest pain	—	1
					Diarrhea	—	1
					Myopathy	—	1
					Vertigo	1	—
					Insomnia	1	—
					Back pain	—	1
					Headache	1	—
					Influence on blood pressure (30 mg/die)	1	—
Tetrud & Langston [89]	22 / 22	HY 1.6 / HY 1.5	3 y, db, p	10 Sel / Pl	Insomnia	14	4
					Headache	7	10
					Dizziness	8	6
					Vertigo	5	5
					Euphoria	1	1
					Trans. elevation liver enzymes	—	1
					Elevation kreatin-phos. kinase	—	—

Abbreviations.: y: year; m: month; w: weeks; d: day; db: double-blind; sb: single-blind; o: open; co: cross-over; p: parallel; uc: uncontrolled; Pl: placebo; Sel: Selegiline; HY: Hoehn & Yahr stage

5. How Do MAO-B Inhibitors Work in Parkinson's Disease?

To explain the mode of action of MAO-B inhibitors in PD, it is necessary to differentiate between monotherapy and combination with L-dopa. Even in the latter case, where huge amounts of external L-dopa reach the brain, the indirect dopaminergic effect due to the inhibition of dopamine metabolism may be dominant for its therapeutic effect. Post-mortem studies on human brain demonstrated virtually complete inhibition of MAO-B activity in L-dopa-treated patients compared with patients who had received L-dopa and selegiline in combination. Enhanced levels of dopamine were found in the substantia nigra of selegiline-treated patients in post-mortem studies [9].

In addition to MAO-B inhibition, selegiline offers some other mechanisms that probably contribute to the indirect dopaminergic mode of action. It inhibits the uptake of dopamine into striatal slices from rats after treatment with selegiline, as has been shown in animal ex-vivo studies [107, 108]. This effects seems to be reversible because the uptake inhibition is not reduced after 24 h. This may explain the necessity of daily selegiline dosing.

Another mechanism possibly responsible for the therapeutic effect of selegiline is the enhancement of turnover of dopamine synthesis [109, 110]. This can probably be mediated by a blockade of the presynaptic dopamine receptor, leading to an increased dopamine release [108]. The last possible mode of action may involve the enhanced level of phenylethylamine after selegiline treatment [9]. Phenylethylamine releases catecholamines [111] and has a direct stimulating effect on postsynaptic dopamine receptors [112].

The enhancement of L-dopa efficacy has been demonstrated in 6-hydroxydopamine (6-OHDA) lesioned rats, where selegiline alone induces an ipsilateral rotation, but enhances the L-dopa-induced contralateral rotation [113]. The latter effect is induced by MAO-B inhibition, but the ipsilateral rotation is possibly related to dopamine-uptake inhibition. The central action of selegiline in combination therapy has been confirmed in a clinical trial, where an effect on peripheral pharmacokinetics of L-dopa has been excluded [114] (see Chapters 10, 14).

Selegiline offers several modes of action that could possibly be responsible for the known effects in combination therapy (reduction in L-dopa dose, prolongation of L-dopa efficacy, reduction in fluctuations of disability) and, thereby, it is more than a simple MAO-B inhibitor. To explain the efficacy of selegiline its neuroprotective pharmacological profile should also be taken into consideration. It has been demonstrated during the last few years that oxidative damage may contribute to the pathophysiology of PD [115–118]. Metabolism of catecholamines by monoamine oxidase leads to the production of H_2O_2, aldehydes, and ammonia, leading to the production of toxic free radicals. Antioxidative detoxification mechanisms are reduced in PD [115, 119–122]. Finally, the enhanced oxidative stress may cause cell death via Ca^{2+}-overload. Selegiline can counteract this damaging effect [21] (see Chapter 9).

As it is known that dopamine turnover is enhanced in the remaining dopaminergic neurons in PD and, in addition, elevated by exogenous L-dopa, it is of importance that selegiline can decrease the concentration of oxidized glutathione while keeping the concentration of the reduced form constant. Oxidized glutathione has been elevated by increased dopamine turnover provoked by haloperidol in rats [87]. Selegiline inhibits *in vitro* lipid peroxidation induced by ascorbate and NADPH [123]. It also induces activity of superoxide dismutase and of catalase in rat striatum [124]. Inhibition of MAO-B and MAO-A by selegiline and pargyline reduces neuromelanine synthesis in tissue from rat and human substantia nigra [125]. Neuromelanine is probably involved in oxidative cell damage [116] (see Chapter 7).

As summarized in Table 5, there is a second neuroprotective pharmacological rationale for selegiline in PD. The neurotoxin MPTP causes a Parkinson-like symptomatology in humans, primates and, to a lesser extent, in rodents [126–128]. Selegiline treatment is able to prevent the neuronal degeneration in the substantia nigra induced by MPTP exposure in primates and rodents [129, 130]. MPTP is not toxic by itself, but is converted to the potent toxin MPP^+ [131]. MPP^+ preferentially enters dopaminergic neurons via the dopamine-uptake carrier system [132] and then interferes inside the mitochondria with complex I of the respiratory chain, which induces ATP depletion [133]. In addition to the protective effect mediated by MAO-B inhibition, selegiline seems to prevent neuronal damage by inhibiting the uptake of MPP^+ [134] (see Chapter 8).

This mechanism has also been postulated to explain the prevention of toxicity of DSP-4 (N-(2-chloroethyl)-N-ethyl-2-bromobenzylamine hydrochloride)-induced neurotoxicity by selegiline. DSP-4 acts preferentially on noradrenergic nerve terminals. It is unlikely that MAO-B inhibition *per se* is involved in this effect, because other MAO-B inhibitors (Ro 16-6491, Ro 19-6327, MDL 72974) fail to prevent cell death [135, 136]. This neuroprotective effect seems to be reversible, because selegiline (10 mg/kg, i.p.) is protective when DSP-4 is administered 1 h after selegiline, but only about 50% protection was observed when the toxin was given 24 h after selegiline [136]. There is evidence that selegiline, by uptake inhibition, also prevents neurotoxicity of 6-OHDA, a neurotoxin that may be generated endogenously during dopamine autoxidation. Pretreatment with selegiline prevents the ouabain-induced release of acetylcholine from striatal slices obtained from rats exposed to 6-OHDA [137]. This effect might be of particular interest with regard to a possible neuroprotective effect in combination therapy with L-dopa. Indeed, it has been shown that selegiline patially prevents L-dopa-induced neurotoxicity *in vitro* [138].

Table 5. Pharmacological activities of selegiline that may be related to the therapeutic efficacy in Parkinson's disease

MAO-B dependent	MAO-B independent	
– Inhibition of dopamine degradation [9] – Inhibition of phenylethylamine degradation [9, 111, 112]	– Inhibition of dopamine reuptake [107, 108] – Enhancement of dopamine turnover [109–110]	*Enhancement of monoamine transmission*
– Reduction of H_2O_2 generation and subsequent toxic radical production [2–6, 87, 123] – Reduction of NH_3 generation [2–6] – Reduction of aldehyde generation [2–6] – Reduction of neurotoxin generation (MPTP-metabolism) [129, 130]	– Increase of SOD activity [124] – Increase of catalase activity [124] – Reduction of neuromelanin synthesis [125] – Inhibition of neurotoxin uptake (6-OH-DA, DSPA, MPP^+) [134–138]	*Neuroprotective effects*

Abbreviations: DSP-4: N-(2-chloroethyl)-N-ethyl-2-bromobenzylamine hydrochloride; MPP^+: 1-methyl-4-phenylpyridinium ion; MPTP: 1-methyl-4-phenyl-1,2,3,6-tetrahydropyridine; 6-OHDA: 6-hydroxydopamine; SOD: superoxide dismutase

Another, so far unknown, action has recently been reported. MPTP-pretreated mice were treated with selegiline for 20 days (0.25 mg/kg and 10 mg/kg) after a 5-day exposure to MPTP (30 mg/kg) and an additional wash-out period of 3 days. Even in this model selegiline increased survival of neurons, as measured by histochemical and immunohistological methods. This neuroprotective effect is independent of the MAO-B-mediated protection against acute MPTP intoxication. The mechanism is unknown and probably MAO-B independent [139].

Other properties of selegiline may contribute to the observed neuroprotective effects. Selegiline is able to prevent catecholamine-induced inhibition of Ca^{2+}/Mg^{2+} dependent ATPase *in vitro* [21]. The substance has a positive effect on cerebrocortical microflow [17] and may reduce cerebral ischemic damage [18]. A possible modulating effect on the NMDA receptor complex via the polyamine binding site may be possible by interfering with the metabolism of N-acetylated polyamines due to MAO-B inhibition [10–14].

In summary, selegiline can be characterized both as an indirect dopaminergic and as a neuroprotective agent. The substance shows effects that could be related to MAO-B inhibition and also to MAO-B-inhibition-independent mechanisms. Therefore, selegiline is more than a simple MAO-B inhibitor. It is still uncertain whether pure MAO-B inhibitors will show similar clinical efficacy in the treatment of PD in monotherapy in the early phase, and in combination with L-dopa.

Summary

Selegiline can be characterized both as an indirect dopaminergic and as a neuroprotective agent. The substance shows effects that could be related to both monomaine oxidase type B (MAO-B) inhibition and MAO-B-inhibition-independent mechanisms. Therefore, selegiline seems to be more than a MAO-B inhibitor, but it has not yet been tested if pure MAO-B inhibitors show similar clinical efficacy in the monotherapy of Parkinson's disease (PD) (in the early phase) and in combination with L-dopa.

References

[1] Kabins D, Gershon S. Potential applications for monoamine oxidase inhibitors. Dementia 1990; 1: 323–348.
[2] Riederer P, Youdim MBH, Rausch WD. On the mode of action of l-deprenyl in the human nervous system. J Neural Transm 1978; 43: 217–226.
[3] Finberg JPM. Effects of selective inhibition of MAO types A and B on peripheral symphatetic function. In: Kamijo K, Usdin E, Nagatsu, editors. Monoamine oxidase: Basic and clinical frontiers. Princeton: Excerpta Medica 1982, 174–182.
[4] Green AR, Mitchell BD, Tordoff A, Youdim MBH. Evidence for dopamine deamination by both type A and B monoamine oxidase in rat brain in vivo and for the degree of inhibition of enzyme necessary for increased functional activity of dopamine and 5-hydroxytryptamine. Br J Pharmac 1977; 60: 343.
[5] Demarest KT, Smith DJ, Azzaro AJ. The presence of type A form of monoamine oxidase within nigrostriatal dopamine containing neurons. J Pharmac Exp Ther 1980; 215: 461–468.
[6] Oreland, L, Arai Y, Stenström A. The effect of deprenyl (selegiline) on intra- and extraneuronal dopamine oxidation. Acta Neurol Scand 1983; 95 (Supplement): 81–95.
[7] Konradi C, Kornhuber J, Froelich L, Fritze J, Heinsen H, Beckmann H, Schulz E, Riederer P. Demonstration of monoamine oxidase-A and -B in the human brainstem by a histochemical technique. Neuroscience 1989; 33: 383–400.
[8] Liccione J, Azzaro AJ. Different roles for type A and type B monoamine oxidase in regulating synaptic dopamine at D-1 and D-2 receptors associated with adenosine-3′,5′-cyclic monophosphate (cyclic AMP) formation. Naunyn-Schmiedeberg's Arch Pharmacol 1988; 337: 151–158.
[9] Riederer P, Youdim MBH. Monomaine oxidase activity and monoamine metabolism in brains of Parkinsonian patients treated with l-deprenyl. J Neurochem 1986; 46: 1359–1365.
[10] Youdim MBH, Finberg JPM. New directions in monomaine oxidase A and B selective inhibitors and substrates. Biochem Pharmacol 1990; 41: 155–162.
[11] Ransom RW, Deschenes NL. Polyamines regulate glycine interaction with the N-methyl-D-aspartate receptor. Synapse 1990; 5: 294.
[12] Sacaan AI, Johnson KM. Spermine enhances binding to the glycine site associated with the NMDA receptor complex. Mol Pharmacol 1989; 36: 758.
[13] Ransom RW. Polyamine and ifenprodil interactions with the NMDA receptor's glycine site. Eur J Pharmacol 1991; 208: 67–71.
[14] Smith GS, Reid RA. The influence of the respiratory state on monoamine oxidase activity in the rate liver mitchondria. Biochem J 1978; 176: 1011–1014.
[15] Traystman RJ, Gurtner GH, Koehler RC, Jones MD, Rogers MC. Central chemoreceptor and oxygenase regulation of cerebral blood flow. J Cerebral Blood Flow Metab 1983; 3: 180–181.
[16] Kozniewska E, Weller L, Höper J, Harrison DK, Kessler M. Cerebrocortical microcirculation in different stages of hypoxic hypoxia. J Cerebral Blood Flow Metab 1987; 7: 464–470.

[17] Höper J, Kozniewska E. Attentuation of hypoxic response in cerebral microcirculation following deprenyl. Int J Microcirc. 1992.

[18] Globus MYT, Ginsberg MD, Dietrich WE, Busto R, Scheinberg P. Substantia nigra lesions protects against ischemic damage in the striatum. Neurosci Lett 1987; 80: 251–256.

[19] Kumagae Y, Matsui Y, Iwata N. Participation of type A monoamine oxidase in the activated deamination of brain monoamines shortly after perfusion in rats. Jpn J Pharmacol 1990; 54: 407–413.

[20] Damsa G, Boisvert DP, Mudrick LA, Wenkstein D, Fibiger HC. Effects of transient forebrain ischemia and pargyline on extracellular concentrations of dopamine, serotonin, and their metabolites in the rat striatum as determined by in vivo microdialysis. J Neurochem 1990; 54: 801–808.

[21] Tatýanenko LV, Raikhman LM, Gorkin VZ. Type B monoamine oxidase and function of Ca^{2+}, Mg^{2+}-dependent adenosine tri-phosphate in preparations from sarcoplastic reticulum vesicles. Byulleten Eksperimental noi Biologii Meditsiny 1977; 83: 283–284.

[22] Robinson DS, Nies A, Davis JN, Bunney WE, Devies JM, Colbuin RW. Ageing, monoamines, and monoamine levels. Lancet 1972; i: 290–291.

[23] Sparks DL, Woeltz van M, Markesberry WR. Alterations of brain monoamine oxidase activity in ageing, Alzheimer's disease and Pick's disease. Arch Neurol 1991; 48: 718–721.

[24] Fowler CJ, Wiberg A, Oreland L, Marcusson J, Winblad B. The effect of age on the activity and molecular properties of human brain monoamine oxidase. J Neural Transm 1990; 49: 1–20.

[25] Jossan SS, Gilberg PG, Karlsson I, Gottfries CG, Oreland L. Visualisation of brain monoamine oxidase B (MAO-B) in dementia of the Alzheimer's type of means of large cryosection autoradiography; a pilot study. J Neural Transm 1990; (Supplement 32): 61–65.

[26] Oreland L, Fowler CJ, Carlsson A, Magnusson T. Monoamine oxidase A- and -B activity in the rat brain after hemitransection. Life Sci 1990; 26: 139–146.

[27] Cohen G. Oxygen radicals and Parkinson's disease. Upjohns Symposium/Oxygen Radicals April 1987; 130–135.

[28] Perry TL, Godin DV, Hansen S. Parkinson's disease: A disorder due to nigral glutathione deficiency? Neurosci Lett 1982; 33: 305–310.

[29] Riederer P, Sofic E, Rausch W-D, Schmidt B, Reynolds GP, Jellinger K. Transition metals, ferritin, glutathione, and ascorbic acid in parkinsonian brains. J Neurochem 1989; 52: 515–520.

[30] Burns RS. Subclinical damage of the nigrostriatal dopamine system by MPTP as a model of preclinical Parkinson's disease: a review. Acta Neurol Scand 1991; 136 (Supplement 84): 29–36.

[31] Heikkila RE, Terleckyj I, Sieber BA. Monoamine oxidase and the bioactivation of MPTP and related neurotoxins: relevance to DATATOP. J Neural Transm 1990; 32: 217–227.

[32] West ED, Dally PJ. Effect of iproniazid in depressive syndromes. Br Med J 1959; 1: 1491–1494.

[33] Sanchez-Ramos, JR. Banisterine and Parkinson's disease. Clin Neuropharmacol 1991; 14: 391–402.

[34] Squires R. Multiple forms of monoamine oxidase in intact mitochondria as characterized by selective inhibitors and thermal stability. Adv Biochem Psychopharmacol 1972; 5: 335–370.

[35] Johnston JP. Some observations upon a new inhibitor of monoamine oxidase in brain tissue. Biochem Pharmacol 1968; 17: 335–370.

[36] Knoll J, Magyar K. Some puzzling pharmacological effects of monoamine oxidase inhibitors. Adv Biochem Psychopharmacol 1972; 5: 393–408.

[37] Knoll J, Ecseri Z, Kelemen K, Nievel J, Knoll B. Phenylisopropylmethylpropinylamine (E-250), a new spectrum psychic energizer. Arch Int Pharmacodyn 1965; 155: 154–164.

[38] Mann J, Gershon S. l-Deprenyl: A selective monoamine oxidase-B inhibitor in endogenous depression. Life Sci 1980; 26: 877–882.

[39] Mann J, Frances A, Kaplan RD, Kocsic J, Peselow ED, Gershon S. The relative efficacy of l-deprenyl, a selective monoamine oxidase type B inhibitor, in endogenous and nonendogenous depression. J Clin Psychopharmacol 1982; 2: 54–57.

[40] Quitkin FM, Leibowitz MR, Stewart W, McGrath PJ, Harrison W, Rabkin JG. *l*-Deprenyl in atypical depressives. Arch Gen Psychiarty 1983; 142: 508–511.

[41] Wender PH. Minimal brain dysfunction: An overview. In: Lipton MA, DiMascio A, Killam KF, editors. Psychopharmacol: A generation of progress. New York: Raven Press, 1978: 1429–1435.

[42] Mann J, Aarons SF, Wilner PJ. A controlled study of the antidepressant efficacy and side effects of deprenyl: A selective monoamine oxidase inhibitor. Arch Gen Psychiatry 1989; 46: 45–50.

[43] Ichikawa J, Meltzer H. The effect of clozapine and haloperidol on the basal dopamine release and metabolism in the rat striatum and nucleus accumbens studied by *in vivo* microdialysis. Eur J Pharmacol 1990; 176: 371–374.

[44] Cadet JL, Lohr JB. Possible involvement of free radicals in neuroleptic-induced movement disorders. In: Vitamin E: Biochemistry and health implications. Ann NY Acad Sci 1989; 570: 176–185.

[45] Lal S, Merbtiz LP, Grip JG. Modification of function in headinjured patients with sinemet. Brain Inj 1988; 2: 225–233.

[46] Gaultieri T, Chandler M, Coons T, Brown LT. Amantadine: A new clinical profile for traumatic brain injury. Clin Neuropharmacol 1989; 12: 258–270.

[47] Hardy J, Allsop D. Amyloid deposition as the central event in the etiology of Alzhemier's disease. TiPS 1991; 12: 383–388.

[48] Tariot PN, Sunderland T, Cohen RM, Newhouse PA, Mueller EA, Murphy DL. Tranylcypromine compared with *l*-deprenyl in Alzheimer's disease. J Clin Psychopharmacol 1988; 8: 23–27.

[49] Tariot PH, Cohen RM, Sunderland T, Newhouse PA, Yount D, Mellow A. *l*-Deprenyl in Alzheimer's disease. Arch Gen Psychiat 1987; 44: 427–433.

[50] Sunderland T, Tariot PH, Cohen RM, Newhouse PA, Mellow A, Mueller EA. Dose-dependent effects of deprenyl on CSF monoamine metabolites in patients with Alzheimer's disease. Psychopharmacol 1987; 91: 293–296.

[51] Agnoli A, Martucci N, Fabbrini G, Buckley AE, Fioravanti M. Monomaine oxidase and dementia: Treatment with an inhibitor of MAO-B activity. Dementia 1990; 1: 109–114.

[52] Campi N, Todeschini GP, Scarella L. Seleginine versus *l*-acetylcarnitine in the treatment of Alzheimer-type dementia. Clin Therap 1990; 12 (4): 306–314.

[53] Martignoni E, Bono G, Blandini F, Sinforiani E, Merlo P, Nappi G. Monoamines and related metabolite levels in the cerebrospinal fluid of patients with dementia of Alzheimer-type. Influence of treatment with *l*-deprenyl. J Neural Transm (PDSect) 1991; 3: 15–25.

[54] Monteverde A, Gnemmi P, Rossi F, Monteverde A, Finali GC. Seleginine in the treatment of mild or moderate Alzheimer-type dementia. Clin Therap 1990; 12: 315–322.

[55] Piccinin GL, Finali G, Piccirilli M. Neuropsychological effects of *l*-deprenyl in Alzheimer's type dementia. Clin Neuropharmacol 1990; 12 (2): 147–163.

[56] Schneider LS, Pollock VE, Zemansky MF, Gleason RP, Palmer R, Sloane RB. A pilot study of low-dose *l*-deprenyl in Alzheimer's disease. J Geriatric Psych Neurol 1991; 4: 143–148.

[57] Knoll J. The striatal dopamine dependency of life span in male rats. Longevity study with (−)-deprenyl. Mech Ageing Dev 1988; 46: 237–262.

[58] Milgram NW, Racine RJ, Nellis P, Mendonca A, Ivy GO. Effect of selective monoamine oxidase inhibitors on the morphine-induced hypothermia in retrained rats. Gen Pharmac 1987; 18: 185–188.

[59] Birkmayer W, Knoll J, Riederer P, Youdin MBH, Hars V. Increased life expectancy resulting from addition of *l*-deprenyl to Madopar treatment in Parkinson's disease: a long term study. J Neural Transm 1985; 64: 113–127.

[60] Birkmayer W, Riederer P, Youdim MBH, Linauer W. The potentiation of the anti-akinetic effect of L-dopa treatment by the inhibitor of MAO-B, deprenyl. J Neural Transm 1975; 36: 303–326.

[61] Riederer P, Youdim MBH, Rausch WD, Birkmayer W, Sellinger K. On the mode of action of *l*-deprenyl in human central nervous system. J Neural Transm 1978; 43: 217–226.

[62] Stern GM, Elsworth JD, Sandler M, Lees AS, Kohout LS, Shaw KM. Deprenyl in Parkinson's disease. Lancet 1977; i: 791–796.

[63] Birkmayer W, Riederer P, Ambrozi L. Implications of combined treatment with Madopar and *l*-deprenyl in Parkinson's disease. Lancet 1977; : 439–444.

[64] Broderson P, Philbert A, Gulliksen G, Stigard A. The effect of *l*-deprenyl on the on-off phenomena in Parkinson's disease. Acta Neurol Scand 1985; 71: 494.

[65] Csanda E, Antal J, Antony M, Csanady A. Experience with *l*-deprenyl in parkinsonism. J Neural Transm 1978; 43: 263–269.

[66] Rinne UK, Siirtola T, Sonninen V. *l*-Deprenyl treatment of on-off-phenomena in Parkinson's disease. J Neural Transm 1978; 43: 253–262.

[67] Presthus J, Hajba A. Deprenyl combined with levodopa and a decarboxylase inhibitor in the treatment of Parkinson's disease. Acta Neurol Scand 1983; 95 (Supplement 68): 127–133.

[68] Birkmayer W, Knoll J, Riederer P, Youdim MBH. Deprenyl leads to prolongation of L-dopa efficacy in Parkinson's disease. Mod Probl Pharmacopsych 1983; 19: 170–176.

[69] Rinne UK. New Strategies in the treatment of early Parkinson's disease. Acta Neurol Scand 1991; 136 (Supplement 84): 95–98.

[70] Fornadi F, Ulm G. Early combination with deprenyl: a retrospective study. Adv Neurol 1990; 53: 437–440.

[71] Ulm G, Fornadi F. R-(–)-deprenyl in the treatment of end-of-dose akinesia. J Neural Transm 1987; 25 (Supplement): 163–172.

[72] Liebermann AN, Gopinathan G, Neophytides A, Foo SH. Deprenyl in the treatment of Parkinson's disease. NY State J Med 1984; 84: 13–16.

[73] Eisler T, Teräväinen H, Nelson R, Krebs H, Weise V. Deprenyl in Parkinson's disease. Neurology 1981; 31: 19–23.

[74] Frankel JP, Kempster PA, Stibe CM, Eatough VMH, Nathanson M, Lees AJ. A double-blind, controlled study of high-dose *l*-deprenyl in the treatment of Parkinson's disease. Clin Neuropharmacol 1989; 12: 448–451.

[75] Goldstein L. The "on-off" pheomena in Parkinson's disease – treatment and theoretical considerations. The Mount Sinai J Med 1980; 47: 80–84.

[76] Golbe LI, Liebermann AN, Muenter MD. Ahlskog JE, Gopinathan E. Deprenyl in the treatment of symptom fluctuations in advanced Parkinson's disease. Clin Neuropharmacol 1988; 11: 45–55.

[77] Duvoisin RC, Golbe LI, Liebermann AN. Double-blind, randomized parallel placebo-controlled clinical trial of 10 mg *l*-deprenyl per day for 6 weeks as adjunctive therapy with Sinemet in Parkinson patients who are achieving less optimal response to Sinemet therapy. Study report. Data on file.

[78] Heinonen E, Rinne UK, Tuominen J. Selegiline in the treatment of daily fluctuations in disability of parkinsonian patients with long-term levodopa treatment. Acta Neurol Scand 1989; 126 (Supplement 90): 113–118.

[79] Lander CM, Lees A, Stern G. Oscillations in performance in levodopa-treated parkinsonians: Treatment with bromocrip-tine and *l*-deprenyl. Clin Exp Neurol 1979; 16: 197–203.

[80] Lees AJ, Kohout LJ, Shaw KM, Stern GM, Elsworth JD. Deprenyl in Parkinson's disease. Lancet 1977; ii: 791–795.

[81] Przuntek H, Kuhn W. The effect of R-(–)-deprenyl in *de novo* Parkinson patients on combination therapy with levodopa and decarboxylase inhibitor. J Neural Transm 1987; 25 (Supplement): 97–104.

[82] Rascol O, Montastruc JL, Senard JM. Two weeks of treatment with deprenyl (selegiline) does not prolong L-dopa effect in parkinsonian patients: a double-blind cross-over placebo-controlled trial. Neurology 1988; 38: 1387–1391.

[83] Schachter M, Marsden CD, Parkes JD, Jenner P, Testa B. Deprenyl in the management of response fluctuations in patients with Parkinson's disease on levodopa. J Neurol Neurosurg Psychiatry 1980; 40: 1016–1021.

[84] Sivertson B, Dupont E, Mikkeslson B, Mogensen P, Rasmussen C. Selegiline and levodopa in early or moderately advanced Parkinson's disease: a double-blind controlled short- and long-term study. Acta Neurol Scand 1989; 126: 147–152.

[85] Teychenne PF, Parker S. Double-blind, cross-over placebo controlled trial of selegiline in Parkinson's disease – an interim analysis. Acta Neurol Scand 1989; 126: 119–125.

[86] Liebermann A, Fazzini E. Experience with selegiline and levodopa in advanced Parkin-
      son's disease. Acta Neurol Scand 1991; 136 (Supplement 84): 66–69.
[87] Cohen G, Spina MB. Deprenyl suppresses the oxidant stress associated with increased
      dopamine turnover. Ann Neurol 1989; 26: 689–690.
[88] Csanda E, Tarczy M, Takats A, Mogyoros I, Köves A. (−)-Deprenyl in the treatment
      of Parkinson's disease. J Neural Transm 1983; 19: 283–290.
[89] Tetrud JW, Langston JW. The effect of deprenyl (selegiline) on the natural history of
      Parkinson's disease. Science 1989; 245: 519–522.
[90] Myllylä VV, Sotaniemi KA, Vuorinen JA, Heinonen E. Selegiline as a primary treatment
      of Parkinson's disease. Acta Neurol Scand 1991; 136 (Supplement 84): 70–72.
[91] The Parkinson Study Group. Effect of deprenyl on the progression of disability in early
      Parkinson's disease. N Engl J Med 1989a; 321: 1364–1371.
[92] Allain H, Coungnard J, Neukirch HC, the FSMT members. Selegiline in *de novo*
      parkinsonian patients: the French selegiline multicenter trial (FSMT). Acta Neurol
      Scand 1991; 136 (Supplement 84): 73–84.
[93] Langston JW. Selegiline as neuroprotective therapy in Parkinson's disease: concepts and
      controversies. Neurology 1990; 40: 61–69.
[94] Rinne JO. Nigral degeneration in Parkinson's disease in relation to clinical features.
      Acta Neurol Scand 1991; 136 (Supplement 84): 87–90.
[95] Tetrud JW, Langston JW. Comparison of patients with Parkinson's disease treated with
      selegiline (deprenyl) and levodopa compared to treatment with levodopa alone: a
      prospective, double-blind study. 5th Int Con Movement Disorders 1990; Washington
      D.C.; Abstract 179.
[96] Marley E, Blackwell B. Interactions of monoamine oxidase inhibitors, amines and
      foodstuffs. Adv Pharmacol Chemother 1970; 8: 186–239.
[97] Elsworth JD, Glover V, Reynolds GP. Deprenyl administration in man: A selective
      monoamine oxidase inhibitor without the cheese effect. Psychopharmacol 1978; 57:
      33–38.
[98] Heinonen EH, Lammintausta R. A review of the pharmacology of selegiline. Acta
      Neurol Scand 1991; 84 (Supplement 136): 44–59.
[99] Pickar D, Cohen RM, Jimerson DC, Murphy LD, Tyramine infusions and selective
      monoamine oxidase inhibitor treatment. Psychopharmacol 1981; 74: 4–7.
[100] Prasad A, Glover V, Goodwin BL. Enhanced pressor sensitivity to oral tyramine
      challenge following high doses of selegiline treatment. Psychopharmacol 1988; 95:
      540–543.
[101] Sunderland T, Mueller EA, Cohen RM, Jimerson DC, Picker D, Murphy DL.
      Tyramine pressor sensitivity changes during deprenyl treatment. Psychopharmacol 1985;
      86: 432–437.
[102] Schulz R, Antonin K-H, Hoffman E, Jedrychowsky M, Nillson E, Schick C. Tyramine
      kinetics and pressor sensitivity during monoamine oxidase inhibition by selegiline. Clin
      Pharmacol Therap 1989; 46: 528–536.
[103] Stern GM, Lees AJ, Sandler M. Recent observations on the clinical pharmacology of
      deprenyl. J Neural Transm 1978; 43: 245–251.
[104] Mann J, Aarons SF, Frances AJ, Browns RD. Studies of selective and reversible
      monoamine oxidase inhibitors. J Clin Psychiatry 1984; 45: 62–66.
[105] Waters CH. Side effects of selegiline (Elderpryl). Abstract 938p. Neurology 1990; 40
      (Supplement): 370.
[106] Golbe LI. Long term efficacy and safety of deprenyl (selegiline) in advanced Parkinson's
      disease. Neurology 1989; 39: 1109–1111.
[107] Zsilla G, Földi P, Held G, Szekely Am, Knoll J. The effect of repeated doses of
      (−)-deprenyl on the dynamics of monoaminergic transmission. Comparison with
      clorgyline. Pol J Pharmacol Pharm 1986; 38: 57–67.
[108] Knoll J. R-(−)-deprenyl facilitates the activity of the nigrostriatal dopaminergic
      neuron. J Neural Transm 1987; 25 (Supplement): 45–66.
[109] Knoll J. Deprenyl (selegiline): The history of its development and pharmacological
      action. Acta Neurol Scand 1983; 95: 57–80.
[110] Zsilla G, Knoll J. The action of (−)-deprenyl on monoamine oxidase turnover rate in
      rat brain. In: Costa E, Racagni G, editors. Typical and atypical antidepressants:
      molecular mechanisms. New York: Raven Press, 1982; 211–217.

[111] Fuxe K, Grobecker H, Jonsson J. Effect of beta-phenylethylamine on central and peripheral monoamine containing neurons. Eur J Pharmacol 1967; 2: 203–207.

[112] Antelmann SM, Edwards DJ, Lin M. Phenylethylamine: evidence for a direct, post-synatpic dopamine-receptor stimulating action. Brain Res 1977; 127: 317–322.

[113] Heikkila RE, Cabbat FS, Manzoni L, Duvoisin RC. Potentiation by deprenil of L-dopa induced circling in nigral lesioned rats. Pharmacol Biochem Behav 1981; 15: 75–79.

[114] Cedarbaum JM, Silvestri M, Clark M, Hart A, Kutt H. l-Deprenyl, levodopa pharmacokinetics, and response fluctuations in Parkinson's disease. Clin Neuropharmacol 1990; 13: 29–35.

[115] Halliwell B. Oxidants and central nervous system: some fundamental questions. Is oxidant damage relevant to Parkinson's disease, Alzheimer's disease, traumatic injury or stroke? Acta Neurol Scand 1989; 80 (Supplement 126): 23–34.

[116] Youdim MBH, Ben-Shachar D, Riederer P. Iron in brain function and dysfunction with emphasis on Parkinson's disease. Eur Neurol 1991; 31 (Supplement 1): 34–40.

[117] Olanow CW. Oxidation reactions in Parkinson's disease. Neurology 1990; 40 (Supplement 3): 32–37.

[118] Spina MB, Cohen G. Dopamine turnover and glutathione oxidation: implications for Parkinson's disease. Proc Natl Acad Sci USA 1989; 86: 1398–1400.

[119] Kish SJ, Morito C, Hornykiewicz O. Glutathione peroxidation activity in Parkinson's disease brain. Neurosci Lett 1985; 58: 343–346.

[120] Ambani LM, van de Woert MH, Murphy S. Brain peroxidase and catalase in Parkinson's disease. Arch Neurol 1975; 32: 114–118.

[121] Sofic E, Paulus W, Jellinger K, Riederer P, Youdim MBH. Selective increase of iron in substantia nigra zona compacta of parkinsonian brains. J Neurochem 1991; 56: 978–982.

[122] Dexter DT, Carter CJ, Wells FR, Javoy-Agid F, Agid Y, Lees A. Basal Lipid peroxidation in the substantia nigra in increased in Parkinson's disease. J Neurochem 1989; 52: 381–389.

[123] Szökö E, Bathory G, Tekes K, Magyar K. Effect of l-deprenyl on lipid peroxidation in rat brain homogenate. Eur J Pharmacol 1990; 183: 1549.

[124] Carillo M-C, Kanai S, Nokubo M, Kitani K. (−)-Deprenyl induced activities of both superoxide dismutase and catalase but not of glutathione peroxidase in the striatum of young male rats. Life Sci 1991; 48: 517–521.

[125] Rabey JM, Hefti F. Neuromelanin synthesis in rat and human substantia nigra. J Neural Transm (PDSec) 1990; 2: 1–14.

[126] Davies GC, Williams AC, Markey SP, Ebert MH, Caine ED, Reichert CM. Chronic parkinsonism secondary to intravenous injection of meperidine-analogues. Psychiatry Res 1979; 1: 249–254.

[127] Langston JW, Ballard P, Tetrud JW. Irwin I. Chronic parkinsonism in humans due to a product of meperidine-analog synthesis. Science 1983; 219: 249–254.

[128] Mallard PA, Tetrud JW, Langston JW, Permanent human parkinsonism due to MPTP. Neurology 1985; 35: 949–980.

[129] Langston JW, Forno LS, Rebert CS, Irwin I. Selective nigral toxicity after systemic administration of MPTP in the squirrel monkey. Brain Res 1984; 292: 390–394.

[130] Fuller RW, Hemrick-Luecke SK, Perry KW. Deprenyl antagonises acute lethality of MPTP in mice. J Pharmacol Exp Therap 1988; 247: 531–535.

[131] Markey SP, Johannson JN, Chiueh CC, Burns RS, Herkenham MA. Intraneuronal generation of a pyridinium metabolite may cause drug-induced parkinsonism. Nature 1984; 311: 464–467.

[132] Javitch JA, D'Amato RJ, Strittmatter SM, Snyder SH. Parkinsonism-inducing neurotoxin, N-methyl-4-phenyl-1,2,3,6-tetrahydropyridine: Uptake of the metabolite N-methyl-4-phenylpyridine by dopamine neurons explains selective toxicity. Proc Natl Acad Sci USA 1985; 82: 2173–2177.

[133] Mizuno Y, Saitoh T, Sone N. Inhibition of mitochondrial NADH-ubiquinone oxidoreductase activity by 1-methyl-4-phenyl-pyridinium ion. Biochem Biophys Res Commun 1989; 163: 1450–1455.

[134] Mytiliuneou C, Cohen G. Deprenyl protects dopamine neurons from neurotoxic effect of 1-methyl-4-phenylpyridinium ion. J Neurochem 1985; 45: 1951–1953.

[135] Bertocci B, Gill G, Da Prada M. Prevention of the DSP-4-induced noradrenergic neurotoxicity by irreversible, not by reversible MAO-B inhibitors. Pharmacol Res Commun 1988; 20 (Supplement 4): 131–132.
[136] Finnegan KT, Skrati JJ, Irwin I, DeLanney LE, Langston JW. Protection against DSP-4 induced neurotoxicity by deprenyl is not related to its inhibition of MAO-B. Eur J Pharmacol 1990; 184: 119–126.
[137] Knoll J. The possible mechanism of action of (−)-deprenyl in Parkinson's disease. J Neural Transm 1978: 43: 177–198.
[138] Mena MA, Pardo B, Casarejos MJ, Fahn S, Garcia de Yebenes J. Neurotoxicity of levodopa on catecholamine-rich neurons. Movement Disorders 1992; 7: 23–31.
[139] Tatton WG, Greenwood CE. Rescue of dying neurons: a new action for deprenyl in MPTP parkinsonism. J Neurosci Res 1991; 30: 666–672.
[140] Csanda E, Tarczy M. Selegiline in the early and late phase of Parkinson's disease. J Neural Transm 1987; 25 (Supplement): 105–113.
[141] Elizan TS, Yahr MD, Moros DA, Mendoza MR, Pang S, Bodian CA. Selegiline use to prevent progression of Parkinson's disease. Arch Neurol 1989; 46: 1275–1279.
[142] Teräväinen H. Selegiline in Parkinson's disease. Acta Neurol Scand 1990; 81: 333–336.

Inhibitors of Monoamine Oxidase B
Pharmacology and Clinical Use in Neurodegenerative Disorders
ed. by I. Szelenyi
© 1993 Birkhäuser Verlag Basel/Switzerland

CHAPTER 14
(−)-Deprenyl Combined with L-Dopa in the Treatment of Parkinson's Disease

T. S. Elizan

1   Introduction
2   Historical Background
2.1 L-Dopa
2.2 Monoamine Oxidase Inhibitors
2.3 *l*-Deprenyl (Selegiline)
    Summary
    References

Introduction

The fundamental cause of idiopathic Parkinson's disease (PD) has remained unknown since its original description in the 19th century. Despite this fact, a rational therapeutic approach (exogenous replacement of the missing neurotransmitter, dopamine) was successfully introduced by Cotzias in 1967 [1], following the conceptual framework of Carlsson in 1959 [2], who suggested that dopamine may be a transmitter in the central nervous system involved in the control of motor function and may be involved in the parkinsonian syndrome; and the impressive neurochemical data of Hornykiewicz in 1963 [3] which definitively demonstrated a significant reduction in nigrostriatal dopamine concentration in both idiopathic and postencephalitic Parkinson's disease. Since then, the major therapeutic efforts have been primarily focused on modifications of the "delivery" of L-dopa [4–8], the use of dopamine agonists [9–12], and, more recently, the use of monoamine oxidase inhibitors, either alone or as adjuvants to levodopa therapy [13–18]. The latter therapeutic approach (specifically the use of a selective MAO-B inhibitor, selegiline (*l*-deprenyl) in combination with levodopa) is the focus of this review.

2. Historical Background

2.1. L-Dopa

After more than 20 years since its introduction into the clinical practice of neurology, L-dopa (L-3-4-dihydroxyphenylalanine) has remained the single most effective agent in the symptomatic treatment of PD [19, 20]. This aromatic amino acid precursor of dopamine, given in combination with a selective extracerebral decarboxylase (DC) inhibitor, has continued to produce the most remarkable therapeutic results in the control of parkinsonism, including improvement in the quality and duration of life [21, 22]. About 75–80% of parkinsonian patients are responsive to conventional levodopa (in combination with an inhibitor of DC, e.g. Madopar®, Sinemet®) therapy, with varying degrees of clinically significant (average of 70%) improvement. These therapeutic results are optimal during the initial 3 to 4 years of levodopa use. After this time, there is usually a slow, gradual, but definite decline in therapeutic efficacy (even with increased drug dosages) to about 40% or less over the succeeding years. Moreover, there is an increasing occurrence of distressing side-effects with long-term use of levodopa, in the form of abnormal involuntary movements, fluctuating diurnal motor responses, and occasionally, acute confusional states and hallucinations [23, 24]. Short of reducing the levodopa dose, even at the almost certain risk of markedly limiting the drug's optimal anti-parkinsonian therapeutic effect, there has been no effective means of controlling these side-effects. It is against this background of therapeutic benefits and limitations of long-term L-dopa therapy that the role of other anti-parkinsonian agents, including the MAO-B inhibitor, selegiline (l-deprenyl), has to be considered.

2.2. Monoamine Oxidase Inhibitors

A paper by Zeller and Barsky in 1952 [25] on the central role of the enzyme monoamine oxidase (MAO) in the catabolism of dopamine and the development of agents for its inhibition was of particular interest. Shortly after Hornykiewicz's group in Vienna showed the association of PD with nigrostriatal dopamine deficiency [26, 3], they made attempts to elevate the levels of brain dopamine with MAO inhibitors [27], as did Barbeau and Duchastel [28] in 1962, but with poor results. Moreover, dietary restrictions were required to avoid the risk of hypertensive crises [29, 30]. With the advent of L-dopa therapy in 1968 [19, 20], further clinical use of MAO inhibitors ceased since they could not be given concomitantly without the risk and consequence of excessive noradrenergic activity.

The discovery by Johnston in 1968 [31] that MAO exists in at least two types, A and B, each with substrate specificity and sensitivity to inhibition by selected agents, caused renewed interest in the use of MAO inhibitors. Clorgyline was found to inhibit the A-type enzyme selectively, with substrate preference for norepinephrine and serotonin. l-Deprenyl (selegiline), developed by the Hungarian scientists Knoll and colleagues [32] in the early 1960s (see Chapters 6, 7) was found to inhibit selectively the B-type enzyme [33, 34] whose substrate preference was for β-phenylethylamine and benzylamine. Dopamine, tyramine, and tryptamine were equally good substrates for both forms of the enzyme. This finding was particularly fortuitous and offered consider- able potential in the treatment of PD. Firstly, the striata of humans and nonhuman primates primarily utilize MAO-B for the catabolism of dopamine [35]. Secondly, l-deprenyl could be given together with L- dopa without risk of inducing a hypertensive crisis [13, 36]. And thirdly, dietary restrictions were not necessary since MAO in the gut is the A variety, and would not be inhibited, thus allowing tyramine to undergo oxidative deamination and avoiding the "cheese effect" [36, 37]. l- Deprenyl had the potential of safely allowing a more modulated and prolonged effect of striatal dopamine derived from exogenously admisis- tered levodopa.

2.3. l-Deprenyl (Selegiline)

l-deprenyl, a phenylalkylamine derivative, and a potent, irreversible inhibitor of monoamine oxidase type B (MAO-B), has been under clinical investigation as a new therapeutic agent in PD since the mid- 1970s [13]. Although originally designed as an anti-depressant, the drug's pharmacologic features, ably reviewed by its discoverer over the years [33, 38, 39], have led to its use as an adjuvant to levodopa therapy. Briefly, l-deprenyl has been shown in animal studies to retard the degradation of dopamine, and to promote its release and prevent reuptake into presynaptic storage sites, as well as to facilitate L-dopa transport across the blood-brain barrier when striatal dopamine is reduced [38].

In 1975, Birkmayer et al. [13] first reported on the potentiation of the L-dopa anti-kinetic effect by deprenyl, based on their first 44 PD patients treated with l-deprenyl for 7 months. These patients had had PD for an average of 9 years and had been on Madopar (benserazide/L- dopa) therapy for an average of 4.6 years at the time l-deprenyl was added. l-Deprenyl was given orally at 10 mg daily or every second or third day. The authors reported an improvement of 56% in motor disability scores with the addition of l-deprenyl, and noted this potenti- ating effect only when l-deprenyl was combined with a peripheral decarboxylase inhibitor (benserazide) and L-dopa (as Madopar), and not with L-dopa alone. The improvement was apparently still demon- strable at the seventh month of follow-up. The authors hypothesized that "deprenyl causes potentiation of dopamine storage in the damaged neurons of the substantia nigra, leading to an increase of dopamine concentration available for neurotransmission".

Several other short-term and longer-term open uncontrolled and double-blind studies [23, 40–43] have reported on the potential and limitations of *l*-deprenyl. The motor fluctuations that were most responsive to the addition of *l*-deprenyl were those occurring at the end of a dosing interval, whereas the more random "off" periods were less so. Most authors failed to find a beneficial effect on akinetic phenomena *per se*, beyond that which could be obtained from an optimal dose of L-dopa alone. Patient selection and the small numbers of these studies may have unduly biased the generally negative results.

In 1983, Birkmayer et al. [44] initially proposed the idea that adding *l*-deprenyl leads to "prolongation of L-dopa efficacy in Parkinson's disease". They compared 323 patients on Madopar (L-dopa/benserazide) or Sinemet (carbidopa/L-dopa) alone and 285 patients on Madopar or Sinemet combined with *l*-deprenyl. The average motor improvement (anti-akinetic efficacy) in the patients on conventional therapy was 27%, versus 37% in the patients on additional *l*-deprenyl. There were 141 deaths in the group on conventional therapy and 96 deaths in the group with *l*-deprenyl. Their average motor improvement during life was almost the same as that in their respective group. The authors concluded that *l*-deprenyl addition to conventional L-dopa therapy leads to a "significant prolongation of the evolution of the disease in both the living and deceased patients". The average daily dose of L-dopa required for these results in the two treatment groups was not included as a variable in this analysis.

In 1985, Birkmayer et al. [45] updated their previous clinical data of 1983 [44], and presented data that led them to conclude that *l*-deprenyl "may favorably increase life expectancy" in Parkinson's disease. This important paper was based on an open, uncontrolled, retrospective study comparing the effects of treatment with Madopar alone or in combination with *l*-deprenyl in 941 PD patients who were followed for 9 years. The patients who had lost their response to conventional Madopar therapy reportedly improved when *l*-deprenyl was added. Survival analysis apparently showed a significant increase in life expectancy in the group on combined Madopar + *l*-deprenyl, compared to the group on Madopar alone. The authors suggested that the selective MAO inhibition may have the ability "to prevent or retard the degeneration of striatal dopaminergic neurons", and compared this hypothesis with the selective protective effect of *l*-deprenyl in experimental animals that had been given MPTP [45–47]. This is the first time that a drug has been considered potentially effective against the basic neuronal degeneration of a human disease. In this key paper by Birkmayer et al. [45], 377 patients were treated with Madopar and compared with 564 patients treated with Madopar and *l*-deprenyl. In the latter group, *l*-deprenyl was started at the same time as Madopar in 81 patients, while it was added at varying intervals after the start of Madopar treatment in the remaining 483 patients; in this latter subgroup, *l*-deprenyl was added at the time of worsening motor disabilities despite increasing doses of Madopar. How soon this motor improvement occured, and how long it was maintained after additional *l*-deprenyl, is not clear from the data. The average duration of *l*-deprenyl treatment in this group of 564 patients was 3.92 ± 0.09 years. In 88 of these patients the duration of *l*-deprenyl treatment was 2 years or less; in 38 of this group, *l*-deprenyl was given for more than 8 years. The mean age at the start L-dopa therapy was 69.5 ± 0.42 years in the Madopar group, and 66.8 ± 0.36 years in the Madopar + *l*-deprenyl group. The time from onset of PD to start of L-dopa therapy was longer (3.9 ± 0.14 years) in the group on combined Madopar/*l*-deprenyl than in the group treated with Madopar alone (2.7 ± 0.14 years). Other differences were noted between the groups with regard to sex ratios and baseline disability scores. A most interesting difference between the two therapeutic groups was the observation that the average daily L-dopa dose for the whole period of therapy was lower (524.0 ± 15 mg) in the Madopar group than in the group on combined Madopar + *l*-deprenyl (627.6 ± 11.1 mg) The estimated survival times calculated from distribution curves was 129.2 ± 5.7 months in the Madopar group, compard to 144.5 ± 4.1 months for the Madopar + *l*-deprenyl group. These figures were based on the time interval between the start of L-dopa therapy and death, and did not include survival time from onset of PD or from time of initial PD diagnosis. The patients who died while on Madopar + *l*-deprenyl apparently lived an average of 15.3 months longer ($144.5 - 129.2$) than those on Madopar alone. On the basis of these data, the authors were able to conclude that the effect of *l*-deprenyl was positively significant regarding life expectancy. Whether it was the presence of *l*-deprenyl, or the higher, more "optimally adequate" dose of L-dopa (627 ± 11.1 mg vs. the lower dose of 524.0 ± 15 mg in the group on Madopar alone) that allowed this observed longer life expectancy remains an unproven explanation for these interesting results. This provocative paper by Birkmayer et al. [45] has remained the most extensive study on *l*-deprenyl/L-dopa combination covering a period of 9 years.

Sometime in 1976, our group at the Mount Sinai Medical Center started a prospective, open trial of *l*-deprenyl in carbidopa/L-dopa (Sinemet)-treated PD patients who were having increasingly limited or poor global motor response to conventional L-dopa therapy, or who were experiencing daily episodic motor deterioration that was either dose-related or unpredictably random. We initially reported our 10-year experience on 200 such patients at the 9th International Symposium on Parkinson's Disease held in Jerusalem in June, 1988 [48], and gave a more detailed account in a subsequent paper [17]. These 200 patients with typical idiopathic PD were of a median age of 63 years, had been on conventional L-dopa therapy for 8 years, and had had the disease for

10 years at the start of the *l*-deprenyl trial. *l*-Deprenyl was given at 10 mg daily for varying periods from less than 6 months to more than 24 months (28% of patients had the drug for longer than 2 years). *l*-Deprenyl did improve parkinsonian disability (by at least 25% compared with before-*l*-deprenyl motor disability scores) during the first 6, 12, and 24 months of combined therapy in one-third to almost one-half patients with an end-of-dose type of response to long-term L-dopa therapy. However, even this particular class of patients was unable to maintain such an improvement by 36 months, much less so by 48 months from start of the *l*-deprenyl trial. About one-fourth of poor responders to L-dopa and those with random deterioration also showed some mild improvement in their parkinsonian status in the first 6 months of the *l*-deprenyl trial, but their condition quickly deteriorated by 1 year. The two variables that were predictive of risk of failure with *l*-deprenyl were the predominant pattern of response to previous L-dopa therapy, and the severity of the total disability score at the initiation of the *l*-deprenyl trial. There were more patients "failing" with *l*-deprenyl than even the data on number of patients stopping the drug treatment would suggest. No significant reduction of the L-dopa dose was possible in most of these advanced PD cases and, indeed, the dose had to be increased in many instances after *l*-deprenyl had become ineffective and treatment with it was discontinued. There were no major side-effects that were primarily attributable to *l*-deprenyl. The drug did not significantly decrease the expected mortality rate beyond that already known for patients receiving L-dopa alone. We were thus unable to confirm the dramatic therapeutic role of *l*-deprenyl in the long-term management of PD as reported by Birkmayer et al. [13, 44, 45]. Our results with *l*-depenyl added to long-term L-dopa therapy were more in agreement with the later studies of Fischer and Baas [49], who studied 30 patients for 1 year, and by Poewe et al. [50], who studied 28 patients for a mean duration of 18.8 months. Both groups reported some improvement in end-of-dose akinesia, with loss of initial therapeutic benefit within an average of 12 months. Fischer and Baas [49] noted no marked positive influence on motor fluctuations, and only end-of-dose akinesia improved slightly. They concluded that *l*-deprenyl as an adjuvant therapy in advanced parkinsonism had "about the same effect as the addition of an anti-cholinergic". In the patients of Poewe et al. [50], peak-dose dyskinesias tended to increase with *l*-deprenyl, while biphasic and off-period involuntary movements improved in some cases. But patients already on maximally tolerated doses of L-dopa and those with severe on/off swings did not gain significant benefit. One-third of their initial responders to *l*-deprenyl lost beneficial effects within the first 15 months of combined treatment. They concluded that *l*-deprenyl's relatively short-lived effect "temporarily compensated for declining L-dopa efficacy in advanced PD".

Our results on *l*-deprenyl as an adjunctive agent to long-term conventional L-dopa therapy [17] were not unduly impressive as the Birkmayer results [13, 44, 45], with regard to preventing progression of the parkinsonian syndrome. Our concurrent data on *l*-deprenyl monotherapy [16] tended to reinforce our conclusion that *l*-deprenyl had only a modest effect as primary symptomatic therapy in PD. Twenty-two *de novo* cases of PD (mean age 58 years; mean PD duration 2.3 years; stages I–II) were given *l*-deprenyl (10 mg daily) for periods ranging from 7 to 84 months. At the time of their latest neurologic examination, 17 (77%) of the 22 patients had demonstrably worsened with *l*-deprenyl monotherapy at an average of 10.8 months from the start of the drug trial. Six of these 17 patients with worsening parkinsonism (or 27% of the original 22) eventually required the addition of L-dopa with carbidopa (Sinemet) at an average of 13 months from the start of *l*-deprenyl trial. An updated analysis of the above data 10 months later had shown that 20 (91%) of the original 22 patients had significant worsening of their parkinsonian state while receiving *l*-deprenyl alone. Fifteen (68%) of these patients were already receiving additional L-dopa, and another 5 would shortly require such addition. One patient had an unchanged stage and mildly improving motor disability scores at 18 months while receiving *l*-deprenyl alone. One other patient who had modest motor improvement at 12.5 months on *l*-deprenyl alone had been unavailable for follow-up.

We had elected to define disease progression in these *de novo* cases of PD [16] as the appearance of new (objective) signs and/or a definite, persistent worsening (greater than 25%) of those previously present, after the initiation of *l*-deprenyl trial. Clinical progression invariably occurred in 77% of our patients within less than 1 year (mean 10.8 months), with 27% requiring L-dopa therapy at 13 months. Unlike the DATATOP study [15] (which compared *l*-deprenyl-treated *de novo* PD cases with a totally untreated control group), we did not deliberately use the "need for L-dopa" as an end-point or outcome measure for disease progression. It is of interest, though, that the DATATOP study and ours [16] found remarkably similar figures for percentage of *l*-deprenyl-treated patients requiring L-dopa therapy at 1-year follow-up (24% vs. 27%, respectively).

We concluded from our results [16] that the use of *l*-deprenyl alone, even in the early phase of PD, did not prevent the progression of parkinsonism. The possibility that *l*-deprenyl may slow down the speed of clinical progression, as suggested by the DATATOP study [15] (by as yet unproven hypothesized mechanisms [51–53]) remains an open one.

In following the course of our *de novo* patients taking *l*-deprenyl alone [16], we were impressed with the observation that almost immediately (within weeks) after the addition of a starting minimal dose of

L-dopa, the worsening parkinsonism dramatically improved, with such improvement being maintained. Additionally, we know from our extensive experience with L-dopa since 1968, that an optimal L-dopa dose is generally reached within the first year of treatment and, when combined with a peripheral decarboxylase inhibitor in the form of Sinemet, within weeks to months after initiation of treatment. In 1991 [18], we reported our experience in 26 patients newly diagnosed as having PD (mean age 57.3 years; mean PD duration 2.7 years; mean Hoehn/Yahr stage 2; mean motor disability scores 11.4), who received an early combination of *l*-deprenyl and low-dose L-dopa (Sinemet) for an average of 26 (8.5 to 99) months. These patients were given a daily dose of 10 mg *l*-deprenyl and started on low-dose Sinemet, $25/100 \times 3-4$ doses per day. Twenty-four (92%) of these 26 patients taking the combined therapy for 26 months showed a dramatic improvement in their parkinsonism shortly after the addition of L-dopa, with significant decreases in their rated motor scores, such improvement being maintained at their latest neurologic evaluation. Eighteen (75%) of these 24 patients responded to the combination therapy with degrees of improvement equal to or greater than 50%, compared with their motor status at the start of combined therapy just before the addition of L-dopa. This degree of "reversal" of parkinsonism on addition of L-dopa (mean carbidopa/L-dopa dose, $98 + 398$ mg) was not observed in any of these same patients receiving *l*-deprenyl alone for an average of 13.8 months. Four patients taking combined therapy developed mild, transient, abnormal involuntary movements, and an end-of-dose pattern of response after more than 2 years of combined therapy (24.75 and 33.5 months, respectively).

Our results on combined *l*-deprenyl + L-dopa therapy [18] re-emphasized the continuing dominant role of L-dopa as the primary drug for the symptomatic treatment of Parkinson's disease. Additionally, the results again showed the paucity of anti-parkinsonian effect ("symptomatic" or "protective") of *l*-deprenyl alone. The possible synergistic role of *l*-deprenyl with L-dopa in these early PD cases is, however, suggested by the sustained therapeutic effectiveness of even low doses of L-dopa for a period of 26 months, with a delay in the appearance of relatively minor side-effects developing only after more than 2 years of combined therapy. A smoother induction period seems easier to accomplish with this early combination of *l*-deprenyl and L-dopa. A concurrently studied control group of patients treated optimally with low-dose L-dopa alone, or one treated with a combination of low-dose L-dopa and a dopamine agonist like bromocriptine, pergolide, or lisuride, may have further clarified the additional role of *l*-deprenyl in this combination trial, but such control subjects were not available to us at that time. We now have data on a population of PD patients on L-dopa alone (carbidopa/L-dopa, Dopicar®) followed regularly by the same neurologist for at least 4 years of initial therapy (Sroka, Elizan, unpublished data, 1992), which will be analyzed and compared with various combination therapies, with L-dopa as a common denominator. Whether one would still be able to demonstrate in such studies the singular role of the monoamine oxidase inhibitor, or the dopamine agonist, in various combination trials with the original amino acid precursor of dopamine, remains uncertain at this time.

The old question of whether L-dopa has a potential role in the pathogenesis of PD itself, especially if oxidative reactions and free radical formation were indeed involved in nigral cell death in PD [51−53], has been raised recently in connection with our early combined trial with *l*-deprenyl [54]. We can only reiterate that there are no conclusive data supporting the idea that L-dopa, particularly that derived from an exogenous source, induces cell death in experimental systems [55−57]. There is also no convicing evidence in the literature that L-dopa induces neuronal degeneration or accelerates the progression of human PD, even after long-term administration of the drug. The development of erratic pharmacological effects with long-term L-dopa therapy may be delayed or minimized with deliberate maintenance of low optimal dosage levels for as long as feasible. *l*-Deprenyl added to L-dopa from the start of combined therapy may allow this slow, careful titration of the latter, with a resultant smoother, easier induction period than would otherwise be possible.

Summary

The development of combined selegiline/L-dopa therapy in Parkinson's disease (PD) is reviewed. The historical origins and rational basis for this combination and the results of selected key studies in the literature are critically surveyed.

l-Deprenyl (selegiline) as a selective MAO-B inhibitor plays a modest role in improving the course of parkinsonism, both as monotherapy and when used concomitantly with L-dopa in *de novo* PD, or as a late adjunct to long-term conventional L-dopa therapy. *l*-Deprenyl's antiparkinsonian efficacy, by whatever hypothesized mechanisms, is not as dramatic as that of the dopamine precursor itself, L-dopa. But its addition to L-dopa early in PD allows for a smoother titration of the L-dopa dose and an easier maintenance of the latter drug to low optimal levels for as long as possible, and longer than would otherwise be the case. *l*-Deprenyl, by itself, is a relatively safe drug, but can accentuate the well-known L-dopa side-effects.

The hypothesis that *l*-deprenyl as a MAO-B inhibitor will provide a "protective" effect on nigral degeneration and slow the progression of PD remains unproven, to date.

A "triple" combination of *l*-deprenyl or another MAO-B inhibitor, a dopamine agonist (bromocriptine, pergolide or lisuride), and low-dose L-dopa may be tried as initial therapy in *de novo* cases of PD. A prospective, adequately controlled, long-term comparison of such combinations with L-dopa alone remains to be done.

References

[1] Cotzias GC, Van Woert MH, Schiffer LM. Aromatic amino acids and modification of Parkinsonism. N Engl J Med 1967; 276: 374–379.

[2] Carlsson A. The occurrence, distribution and physiological role of catecholamines in the nervous system. Pharmacol Rev 1959; 11: 490–493.

[3] Hornykiewicz O. Die topische Lokalisation und das Verhalten von Noradrenalin und Dopamin (3-hydroxytryptamin) in der substantia nigra des normalen und parkinsonkranken Menschen. Wien Klin Wschr 1963; 75: 309–312.

[4] Yahr MD, Duvoisin RC, Mendoza MR, Schear MJ, Barrett RE. Modification of L-dopa therapy of parkinsonism by alpha-methyl-dopa hydrazine (MK-486). Trans Am Neurol Asso 1971; 96: 55–58.

[5] Eckstein B, Shaw K, Stern G. Sustained release levodopa in parkinsonism. Lancet 1973; i: 431–432.

[6] Hardie RJ. Lees AJ, Stern GM. On-off fluctuations in Parkinson's disease. A clinical and neuropharmacological study. Brain 1984; 107: 487–506.

[7] Mouradian MM, Juncos JL, Fabbrini G, Chase TN. Motor fluctuations in Parkinson's disease: pathogenetic and therapeutic studies. Ann Neurol 1987; 22: 475–479.

[8] Cederbaum JM, Breck L, Kutt H, McDowell FH. Controlled-release levodopa/carbidopa. I. Sinemet CR3 treatment of response fluctuations in Parkinson's disease. Neurology 1987; 37: 233–241.

[9] Olanow CW, Alberts MJ. Double-blind controlled study of pergolide mesylate in the treatment of Parkinson's disease. Clin Pharmacol 1987; 10: 178–185.

[10] Libman I, Gawd MJ, Riopelle RJ, Bouchard S. A comparison of bromocriptine (Parlodel) and levodopa-carbidopa (Sinemet) for treatment of "de novo" Parkinson's disease patients. Can J Neurol Sci 1987; 14: 576–580.

[11] Rinne UK. Early combination of bromocriptine and levodopa in the treatment of Parkinson's disease: A 5-year follow-up. Neurology 1987; 37: 826–828.

[12] Rinne UK. Lisuride, a dopamine agonist in the treatment of early Parkinson's disease. Neurology 1989; 39: 336–339.

[13] Birkmayer W, Riederer P, Youdim MBH, Linauer W. The potentiation of the anti-akinetic effect after L-dopa treatment by an inhibitor of MAO-B, deprenyl. J Neural Transm 1975; 36: 303–326.

[14] Riederer P, Przuntek H. MAO-B inhibitor selegiline (R-(−)-deprenyl): a new therapeutic concept in the treatment of Parkinson's disease. J Neural Transm 1987; [Supplement] 25: 1–197.

[15] The Parkinson Study Group. Effect of deprenyl on the progression of disability in early Parkinson's disease. N Engl J Med 1989; 321: 1364–1371.

[16] Elizan TS, Yahr MD, Moros DA, Mendoza MR, Pang S, Bodian CA, Selegiline use to prevent progression of Parkinson's disease. Experience in 22 *de novo* patients. Arch Neurol 1989; 46: 1275–1279.

[17] Elizan TS, Yahr MD, Moros DA, Mendoza MR, Pang S, Bodian CA. Selegiline as an adjunct to conventional levodopa therapy in Parkinson's disease. Experience with this type B monoamine oxidase inhibitor in 200 patients. Arch Neurol 1989; 46: 1280–1283.

[18] Elizan TS, Moros DA, Yahr MD. Early combination of selegiline and low-dose levodopa as initial symptomatic therapy in Parkinson's disease: Experience in 26 patients receiving combined therapy for 26 months. Arch Neurol 1991; 48: 31–34.

[19] Cotzias GC, Papavasilou PS, Gellene R. Modifications of parkinsonism—chronic treatment with L-dopa. New Engl J Med 1969; 280: 337–345.

[20] Yahr MD, Duvoisin RC, Schear MJ, Barrett RE, Hoehn MM. Treatment of parkinsonism with levodopa. Arch Neurol 1969; 21: 343–354.

[21] Marsden CD, Parkes JD. Success and problems of chronic levodopa therapy in Parkinson's disease. Lancet 1977; i: 345–349.

[22] Yahr MD. Evaluation of long-term therapy in Parkinson's disease: mortality and therapeutic efficacy. In: Birkmayer W, Hornykiewicz O, editors. Advances in Parkinsonism. Basel: Roche, 1976; pp. 435–444.

[23] Yahr MD. Overview of present day treatment of Parkinson's disease. J Neural Transm 1978; 43: 227–238.

[24] Yahr MD. Limitations of long-term use of anto-parkinson drugs. Can J Neurol Sci 1984; 2: 191–194.

[25] Zeller AA, Barsky V. In vivo inhibition of liver and brain monoamine oxidase by 1-isonicotinyl-2-isopropylhydrazine. Proc Soc Exp Biol Med 1952; 81: 459.

[26] Ehringer H, Hornykiewicz O. Verteilung von Noradrenalin und Dopamin im Gehirn des Menschen und ihr Verhalten Bei Erkrankungen des extrapyramidalen Systems. Wien Klin Wschr 1960; 72: 1236.

[27] Bernheimer V, Birkmayer W, Hornykiewicz O. Verhalten der Monoaminooxydase im Gehirn des Menschen Nach Therapie mit Monoaminooxydase-Hemmern. Wien Klin Wschr 1962; 74: 558–559.

[28] Barbeau A, Duchastel Y. Tranylcypromine and the extrapyramidal syndrome. Can J Psychiat 1962; 7: 91–95.

[29] Blackwell B. Hypertensive crisis due to monoamine-oxidase inhibitors. Lancet 1963; ii: 849–851.

[30] Horwitz D, Lorenberg W, Engelman K, Sjoerdsma A. Monoamine oxidase inhibitors, tyramine and cheese. JAMA 1964; 188: 1108–1110.

[31] Johnston JP. Some observations upon a new inhibitor of monoamine oxidase in brain tissue. Biochem Pharmacol 1968; 17: 1285–1297.

[32] Knoll J, Ecsery Z, Kelemen, K, Nievel J, Knoll B. Phenylisopropyl-methylpropinylamine (E-250), a new spectrum psychic energizer. Arch Int Pharmacodyn Ther 1965; 155: 154.

[33] Knoll J. Magyar K. Some puzzling effects of monoamine oxidase inhibitors. Adv Biochem Psychopharmacol 1972; 5: 393–408.

[34] Youdim MBH, Collins GGS, Sandler M, Pare CMB, Bervan Jones AB, Nicolson WJ. Human brain monoamine oxidase: multiple forms and selective inhibition. Nature 1972; 236: 225–228.

[35] Glover V, Sandler M, Owen R, Riley GV. Dopamine is a monoamine oxidase-B substrate in Man. Nature 1977; 265: 80–81.

[36] Sandler M, Glover V, Ashford A, Stern GM. Absence of "cheese effect" during deprenyl therapy: some recent studies. J Neural Transm 1978; 43: 209–215.

[37] Elsworth JD, Glover V, Reynolds GP, Sandler M, Lees AJ, Phuapradit P, Shaw KM, Stern GM, Kumar P. Deprenyl administration in man: a selective monoamine oxidase B inhibitor without the "cheese effect". Psychopharmacology 1978; 57: 33–38.

[38] Knoll J. The possible mechanisms of action of (−)-deprenyl in Parkinson's disease. J Neural Transm 1978; 43: 177–198.

[39] Knoll J. Extension of life span of rats by long-term (−)-deprenyl treatment. Mt Sinai J Med 1988; 55: 67–74.

[40] Lees A, Shaw KM, Kohent LJ, Stern GM, Elsworth JD, Sandler M, Youdim MBH. Deprenyl in Parkinson's disease. Lancet 1977; ii: 791–796.

[41] Rinne UK, Siirtola T, Sonninen V. l-Deprenyl treatment of on-off phenomena in Parkinson's disease. J Neural Transm 1978; 43: 253–262.

[42] Stern GM, Lees AJ, Sandler M, Recent observations on the clinical pharmacology of deprenyl. J Neural Transm 1978; 43: 245–251.

[43] Schacter M, Marsden CD, Parkes JD, Jenner P, Testa B. Deprenyl in the management of response fluctuations in patients with Parkinson's disease on levodopa. J Neurol Neurosurg Psychiat 1980; 43: 1016–1021.

[44] Birkmayer W, Knoll J, Riederer P, Youdim MBH. (−)-Deprenyl leads to prolongation of L-dopa efficiency in Parkinson's disease. Med Probl Pharmacopsychiat 1983; 19: 170–176.

[45] Birkmayer W, Knoll J, Riederer P, Youdim MBH, Hars V, Morton J. Increased life expectancy resulting from addition of l-deprenyl to Madopar treatment in Parkinson's disease: a long-term study. J Neural Transm 1985; 64: 113–127.

[46] Heikkila RE, Manzino L, Duvoisin RC, Cabbat FS. Protection against the dopaminergic neurotoxicity of 1-methyl-4-phenyl-1,2,3,6-tetrahydropyridine (MPTP) by monoamine oxidase inhibitors. Nature 1984; 311: 467–469.

[47] Cohen G, Pasik P, Cohen B, Leist A, Mytilineou C, Yahr MD. Pargyline and deprenyl prevent the neurotoxicity of 1-methyl-4-phenyl-1,2,3,6-tetrahydropyridine (MPTP) in monkeys. Eur J Pharmacol 1984; 106: 209–210.

[48] Elizan TS, Yahr MD, Moros DA, Mendoza MR, Pang S, Bodian CA. *l*-Deprenyl, a MAO-B inhibitor, as an adjunct to conventional L-dopa therapy in Parkinson's disease: experience in 200 patients. Adv Neurol 1990; 53: 431–435.

[49] Fischer PA, Baas H. Therapeutic efficacy of R-(−)-deprenyl as adjuvant therapy in advanced parkinsonism. J Neural Transm 1987; [Supplement] 25: 137–147.

[50] Poewe W, Gerstenbrand F, Ransomayr G. Experience with selegiline in the treatment of Parkinson's disease. J Neural Transm 1987; [Supplement] 25: 131–135.

[51] Cohen G. Monoamine oxidase, hydrogen peroxide, and Parkinson's disease. Adv Neurol 1986; 45: 119–125.

[52] Spina MB, Cohen G. Dopamine turnover and glutathione oxidation: implications for Parkinson's disease. Proc Natl Acad Sci USA 1989; 86: 1398–1400.

[53] Cohen G, Spina MB. Deprenyl suppresses the oxidant stress associated with increased dopamine turnover. Ann Neurol 1989; 28: 689–690.

[54] Hauser AR, Olanow CW. Early therapy for Parkinson's disease (letter to the editor). Arch Neurol 1991; 48: 1009.

[55] Hefti F, Melamed E, Bhawan J, Wurtman RI. Long-term administration of L-dopa does not damage dopaminergic neurons in the mouse. Neurology 1981; 31: 1194–1195.

[56] Melamed E. Role of the nigrostriatal dopaminergic neurons in mediating the effect of exogenous L-dopa in Parkinson's disease. Mt Sinai J Med 1988; 55: 35–42.

[57] Brannan T, Martinez-Tica J, Yahr M. Effect of long-term L-dopa administration on striatal extracellular dopamine release. Neurology 1991; 45: 596–598.

Inhibitors of Monoamine Oxidase B
Pharmacology and Clinical Use in Neurodegenerative Disorders
ed. by I. Szelenyi

CHAPTER 15
Neuroprotective Effects of MAO-B Inhibition: Clinical Studies in Parkinson's Disease

P. A. LeWitt

1 Introduction
2 Clinical Trials
3 Discussion
  Summary
  References

1. Introduction

Parkinson's Disease (PD), characterized by a marked loss of nigro-striatal neurons [1], is generally a disorder of progressive disability. While additional neuronal systems of the PD brain are altered [2], the change most closely linked to the clinical symptomatology of Parkinsonism is the impaired generation of striatal dopamine. Dopamine production may also figure in the special vulnerability of substantia nigra pars compacta neurons in PD. Several hypotheses for the decline in dopaminergic neurons have been advanced. One speculation has been that one or more exogenous toxins might produce a metabolic effect damaging these neurons. Several neurotoxins with highly specific actions against nigrostriatal dopaminergic neurons are known. These produce parkinsonian symptomatology both in animal models and, in the case of manganese and 1-methyl-4-phenyl-1,2,3,6-tetrahydropyridine (MPTP), in man. MPTP has been the most intriguing of these because of its need for conversion in the brain prior to exerting toxicity to nigrostriatal dopamine neurons via their mitochondrial metabolism. The unique properties of MPTP have provided grist for speculation that PD could conceivably be the outcome of intermittent or continuous neurotoxicity from exposure to similar types of compounds [3–5].

The analogy of MPTP has prompted the consideration of ways in which putative toxins might produce neuronal damage. Because MPTP is a pro-toxin needing oxidative deamination to produce the toxic species, this compound has served to focus attention on the possible involvement of monoamine oxidase-B (MAO-B) in the pathogenesis of PD. Inhibition of MAO-B effectively prevents toxicity of MPTP to dopaminergic neurons. While other neurotoxins against dopaminergic neurons such as 6-hydroxydopamine and manganese do not require enzymatic activation for their neurotoxicity, there is another compound which serves as a substrate for generating oxidative stress. That compound is dopamine itself. Increasing attention has been given to roles that dopamine might play in the downfall of those neurons which produce it [6].

Dopamine contributes to oxidative stress of neurons in at least 2 ways: through its catabolism by oxidative deamination, and by auto-oxidation. The metabolic degradation of dopamine, which leads primarily to homovanillic acid, yields hydrogen peroxide as a byproduct. Hydrogen peroxide can react, in turn, via the Fenton and Haber-Weiss reactions to form superoxide and hydroxyl radicals. These highly reactive substances, if not promptly quenched by protective mechanisms, can be damaging to the intracellular environment. The extent of oxidative stress produced by the metabolism of dopamine appears to rise with an increase in the neurotransmitter's turnover [7]. In order to survive, the dopaminergic neuron needs to be equipped with adequate capacity to protect against the initiation of the cascade of oxidant reactions, and the damaging effects of oxidative free radicals [8, 9]. The relative importance of the various protective factors is not fully understood in the dopaminergic neuron and its surrounding environment. Among these are enzymatic defense mechanisms (e.g., superoxide dismutase, catalase, glutathione synthesis and reductase), small molecule antioxidants (e.g., ascorbate, tocopherol, urate), and other chain-breaking protective factors (e.g., transferrin, ceruloplasmin) [10]. Dopamine is also capable of reacting spontaneously to form cysteinyl adducts and other oxidation products within the neuron [6]. This process of auto-oxidation has been shown to be increased in the PD substantia nigra, in correlation to the extent of parkinsonian severity.

If the initiation or advance of PD involves the inadequate detoxification of oxygen radicals derived from dopamine catabolism, this etiological mechanism would predict that intraneuronal oxidative stresses might worsen if dopamine synthesis increases. In fact, there is evidence that, in PD, the remaining nigral neurons have increased their per-neuron production of dopamine synthesis [11, 12]. A consequence of this process would be the further imposition of demands on the cell's antioxidative mechanisms.

This model for self-injury of dopaminergic neurons has fostered several concepts of neuroprotection. The cascade of free radical damage ultimately leads to lipid peroxidation as a major means for cellular damage [8–10]. Efforts to quench these oxy-radicals by means of consumable antioxidants such as tocopherol have been advocated. Because much of the oxidative stress of a dopaminergic neuron is derived from the metabolism of the neurotransmitter, another strategy has been proposed which would accomplish neuroprotection through blockade of monoamine oxidase (MAO) [13]. With selective inhibition of this enzyme, oxidative deamination of dopamine is halted, along with the generation of hydrogen peroxide and the cytotoxic reactions ultimately derived from it [13]. Though MAO blockade appears to slow the rate of dopamine breakdown, its metabolism proceeds by diversion to alternative pathways such as sulfation and catechol-O-methylation. These routes, while inactivating dopamine, do not lead to reactive metabolites. The majority of striatal dopamine was once thought to be metabolized exclusively via MAO-B. However, intraneuronal MAO is now known to be predominantly the A-isoform (MAO-A), and so its metabolism of dopamine may also be of importance [14].

As mentioned above, with the loss of projections from substantia nigra in PD, there is increased dopamine turnover as the remaining neurons compensate for inadequate neurotransmission [11, 12]. Other factors enhancing the vulnerability of substantia nigra dopaminergic neurons to oxidant-mediated cytotoxicity have been identified. For example, increased nigral concentrations of iron [15] (a catalyst in the Haber-Weiss reaction when in the ferrous form) and a diminution of striatal glutathione synthesis [16] have been described in the PD brain.

Animal experiments in which dopamine turnover was correlated to effects on glutathione as a function of oxidative stress have shown that, with use of the MAO-B inhibitor l-deprenyl (selegiline), the consumption of reduced glutathione was decreased [7, 13]. Results such as these gave impetus to the notion that pharmacological interventions such as MAO inhibition might be able to limit ongoing oxidative stresses in PD. The hypothesis for this application would be that the continuing turnover of dopamine creates an ongoing oxidative stress which exceeds the capacity of detoxifying mechanisms. If so, then continuing inhibition of MAO-B might prevent the progressive damage to dopaminergic nigrostriatal neurons. Other effects from use of the MAO-B inhibitor deprenyl such as increased striatal superoxide dismutase activity [17] might further improve anti-oxidant defenses. Additionally, if there was endogeneous or exogenous neurotoxic substances that, like MPTP, happened to require activation by MAO-B [3–5], there might be another rationale for MAO inhibition as a protective agent against the advance of PD.

2. Clinical Trials

Because of the suspicion that free radicals or similar mechanisms may be involved in the pathogenesis of PD, there has been a strong interest for investigating various antioxidant strategies to determine whether the disease can be halted. While there is a long legacy of clinical trials for symptomatic treatments against parkinsonism, there was little prior experience at studying treatments for protecting against the development of the disease. Several studies have focused upon the mortality of PD after the introduction of L-dopa or other therapies, but the relationship between premature death and PD is obviously a complex matter. The first study devoted to deprenyl's long-term effects in fact claimed that mortality was improved and equated this outcome with benefits against the underlying PD [18]. Though uncontrolled and lacking other objective clinical indicators, this study emphasized the potential that MAO-B inhibition might offer for influencing the progressive disorder and not just its signs and symptoms.

Several studies have been conducted to determine if the progression of parkinsonian signs or disabilities might be lessened with use of *l*-deprenyl as a monotherapy. The largest has been a project entitled "Deprenyl and Tocopherol Antioxidative Therapy of Parkinsonism" (DATATOP) [19, 20]. This study was carried out in 28 North American centers with a group of 800 patients. DATATOP was a randomized entry, placebo-controlled trial providing the opportunity to test whether the 2 different but potentially complementary antioxidative strategies might be effective in altering the course of worsening in parkinsonian disability. The study evaluated outcomes from treatments with *l*-deprenyl (selegiline), 10 mg/day, and alpha-tocopherol (vitamin E), 2000 I.U./day, in mild forms of PD. The choice of these compounds came from an interest in the 2 ways that oxidative stresses to dopaminergic nigral neurons might be lessened: by limiting the production of hydrogen peroxide-derived free radicals (via MAO-B inhibition), and by enhancing CNS concentrations of a compound which might protect against peroxidation in lipid membranes (alpha-tocopherol). The format of the study permitted each of these regimes to be assessed versus placebo, either alone or in combination. Each treatment arm involved 200 subjects. The reasons behind the inclusion of so many patients came from power analysis estimates of the natural rate at which parkinsonian disability progresses over the course of 2 years following diagnosis. While the possible magnitude of detectable drug effect was not known, the study was designed for sensitivity to even partial protective actions.

Analysis of the treatment groups was directed at the differences that might emerge in the number of individuals progressing in their parkinsonism after 2 years, using a uniform study end-point (defined as sufficient disability to require symptomatic therapy). Survival analysis using the methods of Kaplan and Meier was chosen to be the means for comparing placebo treatment to the 2 drug interventions. The DATATOP trial was planned to follow patients whose initially mild symptomatology would be expected to progress over the trial period so that the majority would have reached the stage of requiring symptomatic therapy (e.g., L-dopa). Other measures of the parkinsonian state were also carried out during the study, using standardized ratings of clinical signs and disability assessments from the Unified PD Rating Scale. However, the survival analysis to the drug-treatment endpoint constituted the primary study end-point because of a belief that this outcome constituted the most practical and global measure of worsening. Although such an endpoint is necessarily subjective, each investigator enrolled a large enough group of patients to ensure a statistically valid sample in each treatment arm for comparisons.

No interaction between tocopherol and *l*-deprenyl was anticipated, as based upon their independent actions at exerting anti-oxidant effects. With the daily dose of *l*-deprenyl used, a selective inhibition of MAO-B was expected. Post-mortem studies have indicated that this dose results in nearly complete inhibition of brain MAO-B, with little effect with respect with MAO-A [21]. Although *l*-deprenyl slows the breakdown of dopamine and can augment the symptomatic effects of L-dopa [22], the use of this MAO inhibitor in otherwise untreated subjects was not anticipated to produce any symptomatic effects against parkinsonism. The study design incorporated ratings that permitted evaluation of "wash-in" effects (symptomatic actions of the therapies at 1 and 3 months after their start, for comparison to baseline) and "wash-out" effects (for assessment of the parkinsonian state 4 weeks after discontinuation of medications).

Subjects chosen for the study were stage I or II by the Hoehn and Yahr scale, and had highly typical parkinsonism of no more than 5 years' duration. Symptomatic medications had been discontinued for several weeks before subjects entered into the study (if such drugs had been used before). Patients were followed at regular intervals to assess for end-point criteria and to conduct clinical ratings. In addition to these evaluations, subjects performed a battery of neuropsychological tests and some quantitative ratings, including the step-second walking test and the Purdue pegboard task of manual dexterity and speed. Cerebrospinal fluid (CSF) studies of homovanillic acid (the major metabolite of dopamine) were also carried out in a drug-free state before entering the study, and after "wash-out" of study medications.

In September, 1987, enrollment began. Although the study was planned to continue with follow-up of each patient on original treatment assignments for 2 years, an interim analysis by an independent monitoring committee led to a premature termination of the initial study. The findings prompting the discontinuation of the placebo phase (with respect to deprenyl treatment) was the markedly slower rate of endpoints occurring in the deprenyl-treated group [20, 23]. At a mean ($\pm$S.D.) of 12 ± 5 months, only 97 of 399 *l*-deprenyl-treated subjects had reached end-point, as compared to 176 of 401 placebo-treated individuals. This difference was assessed by a survival analysis, which indicated that the divergence between the 2 groups (analyzed by Fisher's exact test for the differences between proportions of subjects who reached end-point in each group) was highly significant $(p < 10^{-8})$. The increased avoidance of end-point in the l-deprenyl group was not found to be associated with any differences in baseline characteristics, such as clinical or demographic features, or the results of neuropsychological testing [23]. Further support for the study's hypothesis came from the non-parallel divergence of end-point occurrences over time, as indicated by Kaplan-Meier cumulative survival plots. These analyses projected that, at 2 years, l-deprenyl reduced the risk for progression to end-point criteria from a probability of 0.66 to 0.46. In further support of global benefits for preserving a milder parkinsonian state with the MAO-B inhibitor regimen were the diversity of improved clinical and disability ratings in the l-deprenyl-treated group. Plotting of the hazard ratios (the probability of reaching end-point over time) suggested that the risk of end-pointing started to diverge in l-deprenyl- and placebo-treated subjects from the first few months of the study.

Additional analyses in the DATATOP study will assess the possibility of symptomatic rather than protective effects from the use of l-deprenyl treatment. While the interim analysis has stressed that the magnitude of apparent protective action could not be accounted for by l-deprenyl's mild symptomatic actions against parkinsonism, a more complete scrutiny of "wash-in" and "wash-out" effects will be provided in subsequent publications. The results of the alpha-tocopherol arm will also be revealed in reports that are planned to be published in late 1992.

Other l-deprenyl studies have yielded similar results. A study by Tetrud and Langston began prior to DATATOP and reached similar conclusions which were published shortly before the DATATOP interim results [24]. These investigators (who are also participants in the DATATOP trial) found a dramatic difference between l-deprenyl and placebo treatment with respect to the progression of PD disability. Their prospective study involved 54 patients, randomized in double-blind fashion to l-deprenyl 10 mg/day or placebo. These investigations found that monotherapy with l-deprenyl resulted in a highly significant delay in reaching the need for symptomatic therapy with L-dopa, almost doubling the "survival" time. Delay of the need for symptomatic treatment with L-dopa was similar to the results from the DATATOP study, with the placebo group having a mean $(\pm S.D.)$ of 372 ± 28 versus 545 ± 90 days. This study concluded that symptomatic improvements could not account for the enhanced "survival" against the study end-point of L-dopa need. In fact, the Tetrud and Langston data provided no evidence for "wash-in" or "wash-out" effects from l-deprenyl treatment, in contrast to the DATATOP study results. The issue of whether effects reported by these 2 studies are truly protective or symptomatic in nature has not been resolved. One concern is that such effects might be combined, possibly changing their relative actions over time.

Several other *l*-deprenyl monotherapy studies have been carried out [e.g., 25, 26]. In the French Selegiline Multicenter Trial [27], the symptomatic effects of *l*-deprenyl were assessed in otherwise unmedicated subjects. Motor improvements at 4 weeks continued through the 3-month assessment. These symptomatic effects (recognized from blinded ratings) were not associated with the subjective appreciation of improvement in most instances. A smaller group of patients (18.4% versus 45%) advanced in the course of this 3-month evaluation to parkinsonian symptomatology requiring the use of L-dopa. Unlike the DATA-TOP study, "wash-out" from *l*-deprenyl was not conducted.

Myllylä and colleagues in Finland have been carrying out a trial since 1985 in which *l*-deprenyl has been used as a monotherapy in a placebo-controlled double-blind prospective trial with 54 PD subjects. A recent interim report [28] indicated benefits with *l*-deprenyl monotherapy: there was greater "survival" against need for L-dopa in the *l*-deprenyl-treated group. Of interest were data showing that the highly significant improvements on several measures of parkinsonism (including the Northwestern University Disability Scale, the Columbia University Rating Scale, and the Webster Rating Scale) lasted only through the first 8 months; the ratings conducted at 12 months showed that the placebo group did not differ from the *l*-deprenyl treatment group. The symptomatic effect on these 3 rating scales appeared to be greater at 8 months as compared to 4 months after start of treatment. Despite the differences in study designs among clinical trials, the long-term follow-up of patients on *l*-deprenyl and placebo therapies may help to elucidate the nature of the apparent protective action. Whether other outcomes related to parkinsonism are changed (such as mortality, development of cognitive decline, or motor fluctuations and dyskinesias when L-dopa is used) remains to be learned. The DATATOP study is continuing to follow all subjects who have reached the study end-point and have gone to receive L-dopa.

3. Discussion

While the cause for PD is unknown, research has contributed to an increasing appreciation for the possible involvement of oxidative stress mechanisms in the neurodegenerative process. This perspective has fostered the first generation of experimental strategies directed at halting progression of the underlying disease. The outcome of the tocopherol trial in the DATATOP study has not yet been reported, nor the results past the interim analysis published in November, 1989. Despite the promising results of *l*-deprenyl trials, there is no conclusive proof at present that this drug or other antioxidative strategies block the pathogenesis of PD. Even in the most optimistic portrayals of the DATATOP

and similar studies, the continuing progression of parkinsonism in
l-deprenyl-treated subjects is evident.

The relative short-term follow-up of patients in the DATATOP
study [23] poses one problem to determining the interaction of *l*-
deprenyl with the natural history of PD progression. Another chal-
lenge to understanding these results might be some of the underlying
assumptions made in these and other studies. For example, while the
research subjects have been regarded as manifesting *early* or *mild* PD,
in actuality the extent of neuronal dropout is likely to be quite extensive despite mild symptomatology [1, 2]. Whether the worsening of the
clinical state results solely from the additional loss of nigrostriatal
neurons remains to be studied.

There may be alternative explanations for the progression of parkinsonian disability. One possibility is a decline of dopamine production within the remaining neurons, irrespective of further loss in their
population. Studies of the dopaminergic terminal fields in striatum
of PD brains have found depletion of 80% or more of the previous
neuronal population [12]. Dopaminergic neurons are capable of increasing their production of dopamine in response to feedback from
effector sites, and there is evidence in the striatal regions of PD brain
for an increased turnover of dopamine. The decline in this compensatory response may be indistinguishable from the clinical outcome
of further loss in nigrostriatal dopamine neurons. Methods proven
to differentiate these possibilities have not been developed. There
are some indications of neurochemical clues found in CSF which
might correlate to the compensatory response of increased dopamine
synthesis [29].

Clinical trials do not necessarily announce the mechanisms by which
treatment acts. In the case of the DATATOP trial, the interpretation of
results is confounded by the occurrence of anti-parkinsonian effects
after the start of the drug. While the data at 1 and 3 months found these
to be mild and unable to account for the magnitude of apparent
protective action, other explanations are certainly tenable. *l*-Deprenyl
probably exerts some of its effects against parkinsonism by augmenting
central concentrations of dopamine. In patients already receiving L-
dopa, the addition of *l*-deprenyl permits reduction of the dopamine
precursor by 30–50% in order to maintain the same clinical effects [22].
Inhibition of MAO-B may not be the only way in which sustained
l-deprenyl therapy might influence parkinsonian features. MAO-B
blockade can markedly increase central concentrations of 2-phenylethyl-
amine, an endogenous monoamine which acts as a modulator of dopamine effects [30]. 2-Phenylethylamine produces behavioral actions
resembling those of dopamine and activates dopamine receptors [31].
Sustained use of *l*-deprenyl may have actions with respect to other
neurotransmitter systems as well. Although the drug is predominantly

an MAO-B inhibitor at the daily intake of 10 mg/day, it is conceivable that a cumulative action of MAO-A inhibition might have evolved over time (as will occur with administration of higher daily *l*-deprenyl doses). If so, serotonergic and noradrenergic facilitation may have direct or indirect effects on the features of parkinsonism. Another means for *l*-deprenyl to alter functions of the nigrostriatal dopaminergic system might be through actions of its *l*-amphetamine and *l*-methamphetamine metabolites. While only small amounts of these are produced (and they are less active than their corresponding dextro-rotatory forms), chronically administered amphetamine compounds can directly alter the sensitivity of dopaminergic receptors [32] and thereby might influence the parkinsonian state.

If the clinical outcomes of the *l*-deprenyl neuroprotection trials are in fact due to increased survival of dopamine neurons, then inhibition of MAO-B need not be the only explanation. Other actions of the drug may also be tenable, including the as yet unexplained means by which it enhances survival of substantia nigra neurons several days after MPTP exposure [33]. One of the ways for clarifying the observed effects of *l*-deprenyl is through the outcome of a trial underway with another MAO-B inhibitor, lazabemide (Ro 19-6327). This compound, which differs from *l*-deprenyl in its competitive action at the enzyme and freedom from any MAO-A inhibition at high dose, is not metabolized to amphetamine compounds [34]. If lazabemide fails to exert the same protective or symptomatic actions shown by *l*-deprenyl, then it would be reasonable to conclude that *l*-deprenyl may be acting through mechanisms beyond MAO-B inhibition.

The outcomes of studies assessing neuroprotective actions will require further tools to explore changes in the parkinsonian state. While the clinical end-point used in the DATATOP and other studies appears to have been useful, more objective biological markers of PD are needed for improving the sensitivity and the monitoring of disease progression [35]. Another largely unexplored direction of neuroprotective actions is the role which neurotrophic factors for dopaminergic neurons might play in retarding their attrition. Since these substances have been described to counteract even potent neurotoxins like MPP$^+$ [36], the current fancy for antioxidative mechanisms as the likely cause for PD may have to be reconsidered in light of many alternatives for the etiology of PD.

Summary

The interim results from a study of 800 mildly-affected parkinsonians allows the conclusion that the progression of disability can be attenuated with *l*-deprenyl, 10 mg/day. This prospective controlled clinical trial ("Deprenyl and Tocopherol Antioxidative Therapy of Parkinson-ism", or DATATOP) investigated subjects for a mean of 12 ± 5 months. During this time, l-deprenyl treatment produced a steady decrease in the risk for parkinsonism advancing to the point at which L-dopa becomes a necessary therapeutic option. Other clinical ratings also support the improved outcome from regular use of l-deprenyl. Another investigation still underway is assessing whether protective effects might come from an additional anti-oxidative strategy with alpha-tocopherol (2000 I.U./day).

Acknowledgment

This work was supported by grants from the National Institute of Neurological Diseases and Stroke, U.S. Public Health Service (NS-24778 and NS-27892).

References

[1] Forno LS. Pathology of Parkinson's disease: the importance of the substantia nigra and Lewy bodies. In: Stern GM, editor. Parkinson's Disease. Baltimore: Johns Hopkins Press 1990; 185–238.

[2] Agid Y, Javoy-Agid F, Ruberg M. Biochemistry of neurotransmitters in Parkinson's disease. In: Marsden CD, Fahn S, editors. Movement Disorders 2. London: Butterworths 1987; 166–230.

[3] Cohen G. Monoamine oxidase, hydrogen peroxide, and Parkinson's Disease. Adv Neurol 1986; 45: 119–125.

[4] Kopin IJ, Markey SP. MPTP toxicity: implications for research in Parkinson's disease. Ann Rev Neurosci 1988; 11: 81–96.

[5] Ballard PA, Tetrud JW, Langston JW. Permanent human parkinsonism due to 1-methyl-4-phenyl-1,2,3,6-tetrahydropyridine (MPTP): seven cases. Neurology 1985; 35: 949–956.

[6] Fornstedt B, Brun A, Rosengren E, Carlsson A. The apparent autoxidation rate of catechols in dopamine-rich regions of human brains increases with the degree of depigmentation of substantia nigra. J Neural Transm [P-D Sect] 1989; 1: 279–295.

[7] Spina MB, Cohen G. Exposure of striatal synaptosomes to L-dopa increases levels of oxidized gluthathione. J Pharmacol Exptl Therap 1988; 247: 502–507.

[8] Halliwell B. Oxidants and the central nervous system: some fundamental questions. Acta Neurol Scand 1989; 126: 23–33.

[9] Adams JD, Odunze IN. Oxygen free radicals and Parkinson's Disease. Free Radical Biol Med 1991; 10: 161–169.

[10] Halliwell B, Gutteridge JMC. Free Radicals in Biology and Medicine. Oxford: 1989; Oxford Press.

[11] Mogi M, Harada M, Kiuchi K, Kojima K, Kondo T, Narabayashi H, Rausch D, Riederer P, Jellinger K, Nagatsu T. Homospecific activity (activity per enzyme protein) of tyrosine hydroxylase increases in Parkinson's Disease. J Neural Transm 1988; 72: 77–81.

[12] Hornykiewicz O, Kish SJ. Biochemical pathophysiology of Parkinson's Disease. Adv Neurol 1986; 45: 19–34.

[13] Cohen G, Spina BM. Deprenyl suppresses the oxidant stress associated with increased dopamine turnover. Ann Neurol 1989; 26: 689–690.

[14] Kato T, Dong E, Iskii K, Kinemuchi H. Brain dialysis. *In vivo* metabolism of dopamine and serotonin by monoamine oxidase A but not B in the striatum of unrestrained rats. J Neurochem 1986; 48: 1277–1282.

[15] Dexter DT, Wells FR, Lees AJ, Agid Y, Jenner P, Marsden CD. Increased nigral iron content and alterations in other metals occurring in brain in Parkinson's disease. J Neurochem 1989; 52: 1830–1836.

[16] Riederer P, Sofic E, Rausch WD et al. Transition metals, ferritin, glutathione, and ascorbic acid in parkinsonian brains. J Neurochem 1989; 52: 515–520.

[17] Knoll J. The striatal dopamine dependency of life span in male rats. Longevity study with (−)deprenyl. Mech Ageing Devel 1988; 46: 237–262.

[18] Birkmayer W, Knoll J, Riederer P, Youdim MBH, Hars V, Marton J. Increased life-expectancy resulting from the addition of l-deprenyl to Madopar treatment in Parkinson's disease: a longterm study. J Neural Transm 1985; 65: 113–127.

[19] The Parkinson Study Group: DATATOP: a multicenter controlled clinical trial in early Parkinson's disease. Arch Neurol 1989; 46: 1052–1060.

[20] LeWitt PA, The Parkinson Study Group. Deprenyl's protective effect against the progression of Parkinson's Disease: the DATATOP study. Acta Neurol Scand 1991; 84 (Supplement 136): 79–86.

[21] Riederer P, Youdim MB. Monoamine oxidase activity and monoamine metabolism in brains of parkinsonian patients treated with l-deprenyl. J Neurochem 1986; 46: 1359–1365.

[22] Golbe LI. Deprenyl as symptomatic therapy in Parkinson's disease. Clin Neuropharmacol 1988; 11: 387–400.

[23] The Parkinson Study Group. Effect of deprenyl on the progression of disability in early Parkinson's disease. N Engl J Med 1989; 321: 1364–1371.

[24] Tetrud JW, Langston JW. The effect of deprenyl (selegiline) on the natural history of Parkinson's disease. Science 1989; 145: 519–522.

[25] Elizan TS, Yahr MD, Moros DA, Mendoza MR, Pang S, Bodian CA. Selegiline use to prevent progression of Parkinson's disease. Experience in 22 de novo patients. Arch Neurol 1989; 46: 1275–1279.

[26] Terävainen H. Selegiline in Parkinson's disease. Acta Neurologica Scand 1990; 81: 333–336.

[27] Allain H, Cougnard J, Neukirch H-C, French Selegiline Multicenter Trial Members. Selegiline in de novo parkinsonian patients: The French Selegiline multicenter trial. Acta Neurol Scand 1991; 84 (Supplement 136): 73–78.

[28] Myllylä VV, Sotaniemi KA, Vuorinen JA, Heinonen EH. Selegiline as a primary treatment of Parkinson's disease. Acta Neurol Scand 1991; 84 (Supplement 136): 70–72.

[29] LeWitt PA, Galloway MP, Matson W, Milbury P, McDermott M, Oakes D, The Parkinson Study Group. Markers of endogenous dopamine synthesis in Parkinson's Disease. Neurology 1992; 42 (Supplement 3): 420.

[30] Antelman SM, Edwards DJ, Lin M. Phenylethylamine: evidence for a direct, post-synaptic dopamine-receptor stimulatory action. Brain Res 1977; 127: 317–322.

[31] Jackson DM. 2-phenylethylamine, dopamine, and behaviour. In: Sandler M, Dahlstrom A, Belmaker RH, editors. Progress in catecholamine research. Part B: Central aspects. New York: Alan R Liss 1988; 429–432.

[32] Robinson TE, Becker JB. Enduring changes in brain and behavior produced by chronic amphetamine administration: a review and evaluation of animal models of amphetamine psychosis. Brain Res Rev 1986; 11: 157–198.

[33] Tatton WG, Greenwood CE. Rescue of dying neurons: a new action for deprenyl in MPTP parkinsonism. J Neurosci Res 1991; 30: 666–672.

[34] Da Prada M, Kettler R, Keller HH et al. From moclobemide to Ro 19-6327 and Ro 41-1049: the development of a new class of reversible, selective MAO-A and MAO-B inhibitors. J Neural Transm 1990; 29 (Supplement): 279–292.

[35] LeWitt PA, Galloway MP. Neurochemical markers of Parkinson's Disease. In: Koller WC, Paulson G, editors. Therapy of Parkinson's Disease. New York: Marcel Dekker 1990; 63–93.

[36] Hyman C, Hofer M, Barde Y-A et al. BDNF is a neurotrophic factor for dopaminergic neurons of the substantia nigra. Nature 1990; 350: 230–232.

Inhibitors of Monoamine Oxidase B
Pharmacology and Clinical Use in Neurodegenerative Disorders
ed. by I. Szelenyi
© 1993 Birkhäuser Verlag Basel/Switzerland

CHAPTER 16
Alzheimer's Disease and *l*-Deprenyl: Rationales and Findings

P. N. Tariot, L. S. Schneider, S. V. Patel and B. Goldstein

1   Introduction
2   Rationale for Short-Term Administration
2.1   The "Monoaminergic Strategy"
2.2   *l*-Deprenyl as Monoamine-Enhancing Agent
3   Empirical Evidence
3.1   Case Series
3.2   Within Subject Design
3.3   Single-Blind, Parallel Group, Comparison Studies
3.4   Double-Blind, Placebo-Controlled, Parallel Group Studies
3.5   Summary of Empirical Data
3.6   Speculation Regarding Mechanism
4   Rationale for Chronic Administration
4.1   Endogenous Neurotoxins
4.2   Exogenous Neurotoxins
4.3   Longevity Studies
4.4   Summary
5   Conclusion
        References

1. Introduction

The purpose of this chapter is to summarize the theoretical and empirical bases for the administration of *l*-deprenyl (selegiline) to persons suffering from probable Alzheimer's disease (AD). Rationales exist for both *short-term* and *long-term* treatment: for the sake of clarity, these will be presented separately.

2. Rationale for Short-Term Administration

2.1. The "Monoaminergic" Strategy:

Dementia of the Alzheimer type (DAT) is a clinical syndrome characterized by progressive deterioration of intellectual functions and personality. The diagnosis of Alzheimer's *disease* (AD), an idiopathic degeneration of the brain, requires the syndrome of DAT and is confirmed by the coincident presence of neurofibrillary tangles and amyloid plaques in the cerebral cortex and hippocampus [1]. Neuropathological and neurochemical studies have demonstrated substantial deficits in ascending central cholinergic systems innervating the cortex [2]. Coupled with the known role of central cholinergic systems in different cognitive functions, especially memory and learning, the relative prominence of cholinergic deficits in AD has prompted empirical trials of a variety of cholinergic agents in this disorder [3–6]. In view of the widespread nature of the degenerative changes in the brains of persons dying with AD, it is perhaps not surprising that the behavioral and cognitive improvement resulting from selective cholinergic therapy has been modest at best. Other pharmacologic strategies are, therefore, in order.

Evidence has also accumulated which suggests that both structural and functional disturbances of central monoaminergic systems occur in AD. For example, reduced brain norepinephrine concentration has been reported in AD, which is associated with biochemical evidence of reduced norepinephrine turnover, decreased activity of the enzymatic marker for the epinephrine system, dopamine-β-hydroxylase, and loss of neurons of origin of noradrenergic innervation of the cortex in at least some subgroups of patients with AD. Similar disturbances have been described in dopaminergic and indoleaminergic systems [7–16].

Ascending monoamine pathways had previously been shown to play important roles in normal human and animal cognition, as well as in other behaviors [17–23]. This evidence is derived in part from neuropharmacologic studies demonstrating that drugs selectively affecting monoaminergic functions can influence a variety of brain-related behaviors and cognition.

Since monoaminergic neurotransmitter systems play important roles in the kinds of behaviors and cognitive functions disordered in patients with DAT, pharmacological manipulation of these systems offers a rational treatment approach. To the extent that functional monoaminergic deficits exist and contribute to the cognitive or behavioral dysfunction evident in patients with DAT, such drugs might enhance cognition, as well as improve our understanding of the relationship between neurochemical and behavioral changes.

Antidepressant medications as a class offer a readily-available pool of monoamine-enhancing drugs. Undesired effects limit the options, however. Central anticholinergic effects would have detrimental effects in view of the known central cholinergic deficits in AD and the demonstrated cognitive and behavioral sensitivity of these patients to anticholinergic administration [24]. Cardiovascular toxicity is also of particular concern in older patients. Other possible undesired effects include sedation, agitation, constipation, urinary retention, nausea, priapism, tardive dyskinesia, and seizures [25–27]. The dietary restrictions necessary for patients taking monoamine oxidase inhibitors pose a problem for patients with DAT. This array of relative contraindications for most commonly available antidepressants has likely contributed to the scarcity of studies of such medications in DAT without depression [28, 29].

2.2. l-Deprenyl as Monoamine-Enhancing Agent

l-Deprenyl is an irreversible monoamine oxidase B inhibitor with relatively specific effects on monoamine neurotransmitter systems [30–32]. Its neurochemical effects appear to vary in a dose-dependent fashion, with moderate selectivity for the monoamine oxidase (MAO) type-B isoenzyme at lower doses (e.g., 10 mg or less per day in humans) and nonselective MAO-A plus MAO-B inhibition, as well as other complex effects at higher doses [33]. At low doses it is less likely to produce a hypertensive reaction to tyramine, and has been reported to have significantly fewer undesired effects than other MAOI's, thus making it a relatively safe choice for study in DAT [34–36]. At lower doses it appears to have minimal antidepressant efficacy, while at higher doses increased antidepressant efficacy as well as amphetamine-like effects have been reported [32–40] (see Chapters 11, 17).

Further support for the study of *l*-deprenyl in DAT comes from its possible short-term "symptomatic" efficacy in Parkinson's disease (PD), which is also an idopathic degenerative brain disease with clinical, pathological, and neurochemical similarities to DAT [41–44]. *l*-Deprenyl administration resulted in at least short-term mood improvement and reduction of motor symptoms in one small study of patients with PD, some of whom received no other treatment [45]. These effects were associated with enhanced monoamine function. Studies in PD patients treated with dopaminergic agents have generally shown positive results [46]. The 800-subject DATATOP study of patients with untreated PD also showed improved motor and mental functioning within 1 month of receiving *l*-deprenyl 10 mg/day [47], which suggests a symptomatic benefit associated with short-term neurochemical effects. These findings, by analogy, suggest the possibility of short-term benefit of *l*-deprenyl administration to patients with DAT.

A final rationale for the study of the short-term effects of *l*-deprenyl administration relates to increased brain MAO-B activity in older persons, which is particularly prominent in patients with DAT [29, 48–51]. The functional significance of this is unclear, but it is possible that increase MAO-B activity *per se* might alter modulation of monoamines mediating the types of brain functions disordered in DAT. To the extent that this is so, short-term administration of *l*-deprenyl might ameliorate cognitive and/or behavioral symptoms associated with the illness.

3. Empirical Evidence

Based on the above-mentioned rationales, a surprisingly large number of trials of *l*-deprenyl in DAT have been performed. At this point there are at least 15 articles, abstracts, or manuscripts dealing with *l*-deprenyl in 636 patients with primary dementia; all but one have been published. There are several ongoing trials involving *l*-deprenyl in patients with probable AD. Published reports will be reviewed according to relevant design categories.

3.1. Case Series

Martini et al. [52] conducted an open trial of *l*-deprenyl in 11 patients (7 with DAT and 3 with multi-infarct dementia); patients were treated for 3 and 6 months, respectively. The authors reported qualitative findings indicating that 12 items on the Sandoz Clinical Geriatric Assessment Scale (SCAG) [53] improved, two worsened, and three were unchanged. All but one patient showed improved scores on a cognitive screening tool.

Schneider et al. reported a 4-week open pilot study of 14 patients with DAT treated with *l*-deprenyl 10 mg per day [54]. They found significant improvements in the agitation and depression factors of the brief Psychiatric Rating Scale (BPRS) [55], in the Cornell Scale for Depression in Dementia [56], and in spouses' blind ratings. Recall improved on the Buschke Selective Reminding Task [57], but intrusions also increased. Platelet MAO-B activity for all subjects was nearly completely suppressed after 4 weeks of treatment. Pretreatment and posttreatment EEG data showed reduction of amplitude in all five bands, and significant selective suppression of delta in the right frontal region. The results attested to the pharmacologic activity of *l*-deprenyl (as well as compliance), and to its effects on behavior (reduced agitation and mood-related symptoms), cognition, and CNS electrophysiology. The authors speculated that *l*-deprenyl might improve performance on the Selective Reminding Task by enhancing monoaminergic effects in mood and arousal systems with a possible disinhibiting effect (contributing to increased intrusions). There was no physiologic, electrocardiographic, or laboratory evidence of toxicity.

Goad et al. reported a single-blind study of 8 patients with DAT treated with 10 mg of *l*-deprenyl per day for 10 weeks [58]. Patients with behavioral problems were specifically selected for study. Five patients completed the study; two of the drop-outs had worsened behavior. No statistically significant effects on behavior assessed by the behave AD [59], cognitive function assessed by MMSE [60], or caregiver stress assessed by the Caregiver Burden Scale [61] were reported in the 5 subjects available for analysis. They reported, however, "mild clinical improvement" in cognitive function, caregiver stress, and "marked" clinical improvement in behavior symptoms. The trend in the data suggested improvement in areas of paranoia and delusions, hallucinosis, activity disturbances, anxiety, and phobias among patients completing the study. Blood pressure was unaffected, and no other adverse experiences were reported.

3.2. Within Subject Design

Tariot et al. administered *l*-deprenyl 10 mg per day and 40 mg per day in a serial crossover design to 17 patients with DAT in a double-blind, placebo-controlled trial [62]. Total BPRS scores [55] decreased significantly during the 10 mg per day treatment period (with decreases in measures of anxiety/depression, tension, and excitement). Approximately one-half of the patients were judged to have improved clinically, with evidence of increased activity and social interaction, along with reduced tension and retardation. Similar but smaller changes were observed during higher dose treatment. The behavioral changes were associated with improvement (in the same subjects) in performance on the Buschke Selective Reminding Task [57], particularly in late trials, although performance of other cognitive tasks did not change [63]. Significant and dose-dependent effects in hemodynamic state occurred, with slight decreases in standing systolic and diastolic blood pressure on the higher dose treatment which were consistent with monamine oxidase inhibition. Finally, dose-dependent effects on cerebrospinal fluid (CSF) on monoamine metabolites were observed, resulting in small but statistically significant reductions in HVA and 5-HIAA concentrations during 10 mg per day treatment vs. baseline, and larger reductions in HVAA and MHPG concentrations with still only slight reductions in 5-HIAA during 40 mg per day treatment [64].

Taken together the results of the study showed that there were dose-dependent behavioral, cognitive, and neurochemical effects in this sample. There were no adverse effects at the lower dose, two subjects experienced orthostatic hypotension at the higher dose, and there were no effects on observed sleep, laboratory tests, or weight. The authors speculated that the greater effect of low-dose therapy indicated that it might have been the inhibition of MAO-B, and not MAO-A, that was important in the clinical improvement noted, and they questioned the possible relationship between these findings and that of elevated MAO-B levels in AD (above).

Piccinin et al. treated 20 patients with DAT with *l*-deprenyl 10 mg/day in a placebo-controlled, crossover study with each treatment period being 3 months (total = 6 months) [65]. Significant effects in favor of drug were found in verbal fluency, digit span, visuospatial processing, letter cancellation, and constructional apraxia. No behavioral data were reported. Minimal side-effects (hyperexcitability in two cases, dizziness in two cases, and orthostatic hypotension in one case) were reported. The authors suggested that the results were consistent with a possible crucial role for disrupted dopaminergic innervation of frontal systems, pertaining to arousal and attention.

Sunderland et al. reported a two-period crossover study of 10 patients receiving *l*-deprenyl 10 mg per day who were also administered physostigmine [66]. There were essentially no significant effects reported in this abstract.

Schneider et al. examined the potential safety and efficacy of *l*-deprenyl 10 mg per day added to cholinesterase inhibitors such as tacrine or sustained release physostigmine [67]. This was a two-period crossover study in 10 patients. *l*-Deprenyl added to tacrine and sustained-release physostigmine was free of adverse effects and was associated with significant mean improvement on the Alzheimer Disease Assessment Scale, cognitive subscale [68]. No behavioral data were reported. The findings were interpreted to suggest that the use of this combination was possibly safe and effective.

3.3. Single-Blind, Parallel Group, Comparison Studies

Campi et al. reported the results of a single-blind, randomized, parallel study of *l*-deprenyl 10 mg per day vs. L-acetylcarnitine 1000 mg per day for 3 months in 40 patients with mild-to-moderate DAT [69]. A variety of cognitive measures was employed, all of which showed significant differences in favor of *l*-deprenyl. Changes were evident as early as the first visit, after 1 month of therapy. No behavioral effects were reported. There was no clinical or laboratory evidence of adverse reaction to either drug.

Monteverde et al. reported on the effects of *l*-deprenyl 10 mg per day vs. phosphatidylserine 200 mg per day in a 3-month parallel single-blind study in 40 patients with mild-to-moderate DAT [70]. The study design and findings were quite similar to that of Campi et al. [69]. All cognitive measures employed showed improvement with *l*-deprenyl, as did functional status in activities of daily living. No behavioral effects were noted; side-effects were minimal.

Falsaperla et al. administered *l*-deprenyl 10 mg per day and oxiracetam 1600 mg per day to a total of 40 patients in a single-blind, parallel 3-month study [71]. Activities of daily living performance improved in the *l*-deprenyl group, as did some cognitive measures. Tolerability was good.

3.4. Double-Blind, Placebo-Controlled, Parallel Group Studies

Martucci et al. reported the effect of *l*-deprenyl 10 mg/day vs. placebo in 20 patients with primary degenerative dementia [72]. The English abstract does not indicate what the findings were.

Agnoli et al. conducted a placebo-controlled, parallel study of *l*-deprenyl 10 mg/day for 90 days in 20 patients with mild-to-moderate DAT [73]. Patients underwent clinical, behavioral, and memory evaluations every 30 days. Subjects in the active treatment group, but not in the placebo group, showed improvement in several measures of attention and memory. One patient in each group dropped out of the study. There were no differences in type or number of side-effects or concomitant treatments. No changes in behavioral ratings were found in the treatment group, although the article indicated that the placebo group experienced "significant worsening" during the same period, which was consistent with "a positive sign of stabilization of gross behavioral variables" in the treatment group. The authors also pointed out the limited sensitivity reliability of behavioral scales available for use in studies of this nature, and urged caution in interpreting these behavioral findings.

Loeb and Albano reported, in abstract form, on 110 patients with mild to moderate DAT in a 3-month trial of *l*-deprenyl 10 mg per day [74]: "Improvement of some cognitive functions (mainly primary memory, declarative memory, and verbal fluency) was observed in the selegiline group." Improvement in functional performance was also reported. Side-effects were reported only in a few cases, none of which required cessation of treatment. No other information was provided.

Mangoni et al. reported on 119 patients with DAT randomized to *l*-deprenyl 10 mg per day vs. placebo for 3 months [75]. Virtually all cognitive measures showed effects in favor of *l*-deprenyl compared with placebo. Adverse reactions were roughly similar in both the placebo and *l*-deprenyl groups, and compounds were discontinued in three subjects in the *l*-deprenyl group and one subject in the placebo group. Performance in activities of daily living was better in the *l*-deprenyl group. No behavioral effects were reported.

Filip et al. reported in abstract form on a 6-month trial of *l*-deprenyl 10 mg per day in 173 inhabitants of residential homes who had met DSM III criteria for mild DAT [76]. Dropout rates in the placebo and *l*-deprenyl groups were 19 and 16%, respectively. *l*-Deprenyl was superior to placebo on a measure of personal neatness. A secondary analysis was performed according to whether patients had visuospatial abnormalities at baseline, suggesting a positive treatment effect on measures of cognition and behavior (irritability). There were no differences between the groups as to frequency and severity of adverse effects.

3.5. Summary of Empirical Data

The empirical evidence from these reports is summarized in the following. Three case series involving a total of 26 subjects with DAT (plus 4 with multi-infarct dementia) treated for 28 to 182 days suggested overall improvement of various behavioral ratings, generally good tolerability, and one trial showed suppression of EEG delta in the right frontal area. Some patients, especially three more severely impaired patients, developed side-effects.

Four studies of within-subjects design involving 57 patients have been reported. In two of these, *l*-deprenyl was the experimental medication in patients already being maintained on a cholinesterase inhibitor. Three of these studies showed significant or nearly significant improvement with *l*-deprenyl in a variety of ratings, both behavioral and cognitive. Obviously, one problem with crossover studies is that carryover effects may have mitigated or otherwise affected the results.

Three randomized parallel group studies involving 117 patients in which *l*-deprenyl was compared to acetylcarnitine, phosphatidylserine, or oxiracetam in 90-day trials have been reported. In all three studies, the Blessed Dementia Scale, Five-Item Recall, Short-Story Recall and, in some cases, other ratings showed significant improvement in the *l*-deprenyl group at the 0.01 level. The lack of double-blind treatment suggests that they should be considered as open clinical trials.

Finally, there are five published articles or abstracts which report results of randomized, parallel group, placebo-controlled, double-blind studies. These studies involved approximately 433 patients with generally mild to moderate dementia treated from 90 to 180 days. The parallel group studies generally showed improvement in measures of cognition with *l*-deprenyl treatment. Behavioral measures, where reported, showed improvement as well, as did functional performance in activities of daily living. Tolerability was good. In summary, there are only four placebo-controlled, parallel group, double-blind trials of *l*-deprenyl reported of sufficient sample size; one has been published in English. Tolerability was excellent in all studies.

The majority of studies indicates that beneficial effects of *l*-deprenyl are achieved in measures of cognition, usually within a few weeks. Positive effects on behavior and functional status are noted frequently as well.

Virtually all authors point toward the need for large, carefully controlled studies to address definitively the efficacy and tolerability of *l*-deprenyl in DAT. It is therefore surprising that there has been relatively little interest in further assessing the effects of short-term administration. In the United States, this may be related to the fact that the medication is now available by prescription (although approved by the Food and Drug administration only for use in PD), and that the proprietary license for its distribution will expire in 1995). The consequence of this is that a sponsor who supports definitive studies in patients with dementia of the Alzheimer type will not benefit financially from positive results.

3.6. Speculation Regarding Mechanism

It is possible to speculate regarding the mechanism of the apparent short-term beneficial effect of *l*-deprenyl in this population. Most studies used a dose of 10 mg per day; one study looked at 10 mg vs. 40 mg per day. One other report compared *l*-deprenyl with a nonspecific inhibitor, tranylcypromine, and found poor tolerability of tranylcypromine in a small group of patients with DAT who had previously received *l*-deprenyl [7]. The overall evidence suggests that the lower dose of *l*-deprenyl is more efficacious than the higher dose, and that nonspecific MAOI's may not be efficacious (or at least are not well tolerated).

As reviewed above, relatively selective inhibition of MAO-B is a major distinguishing feature of the lower dose of *l*-deprenyl. It is therefore possible that selective MAO-B inhibition plays a role in the effects of *l*-deprenyl in this population. This phenomenon, in turn, could be related to the known increase in MAO-B activity in the brains of patients with DAT. This elevation may be a marker of primary neuronal degeneration with secondary gliosis, in which case MAO-B inhibition might selectively result in improved modulation of monoaminergic neurotransmission and attendant reduction of symptoms.

The time-course of positive effects, generally within weeks, is consistent with this hypothesis. It is also possible that *l*-deprenyl achieves its effect via metabolism to *l*-amphetamine in the brain [37, 39]. It has been argued that this is unlikely to account for the cognitive and behavioral changes observed at the 10 mg dose, since minimal brain levels should be achieved with this dose; moreover, *l*-amphetamine is only weakly active, and the effects that were observed developed consistently over weeks and not over a span of days [62].

Finally, it is possible that patients with DAT experience improvement in subtle mood disturbance, and that this is the basis for the apparent beneficial effect of *l*-deprenyl. Some studies in patients with PD suggest that this might be the case [45, 47]. More generally, perhaps *l*-deprenyl has relatively nonspecific effects on mood and arousal. Indeed, the original reports in mixed psychiatric populations suggested a "psychic energizing" effect of the drug [78]. As previously suggested, it is possible that *l*-deprenyl's effects are quantitatively (occurring at very low doses) but not qualitatively unique in DAT [62]. Overall, it must be concluded that the precise mechanism of action of the drug in DAT is unclear, and that further studies with more selective MAO-B inhibitors would be useful in clarifying this issue (see Chapters 7, 8, 9, 15).

4. Rationale for Chronic Administration

All published studies of *l*-deprenyl have attempted to assess the effects of acute or subchronic administration. There are rationales to examine longer-term effects as well. The first is simply to learn the duration of the shorter-term effects, i.e., whether patients who experience any "symptomatic" relief (e.g. improvements in behavior, cognitive function, performance of daily living activities, or cooperation with caregivers, etc.) might experience this for prolonged periods of time. There are also theoretical grounds for examining possible longer-term benefits (regardless of whether short-term benefit occurs) aimed at reduction of levels of possible endogeneous neurotoxins and/or consequences of exposure to exogenous neurotoxins. This *highly speculative* rationale is summarized below. It is notable that there is more interest in long-term clinical trials, based on this theoretical foundation, than in shorter-term trials, which may have more empirical rationales.

4.1. Endogenous Neurotoxins

There is some evidence from animal and human studies suggesting a possible role for oxidative mechanisms (a common feature of many different neurotoxic events) in the loss of at least some neuronal systems in AD [79, 80]. The brain is known to be susceptible to oxidative stress, consequences of which can include disruption of DNA, damage to membranes, and neuronal death. Recent evidence suggests that oxidative injury may actually occur in AD. Smith et al. reported regional loss of glutamine synthetase activity (in essence, a measure of oxidative damage) in patients dying with AD, but not controls, which was confirmed by similar changes in another oxidized protein (carbonyl) [81]. As the authors indicate, possible explanations for this include excess generation of free radicals or other oxidant species, as well as deficits in free radical scavenging systems. There is some evidence to support both views [81]. In particular, oxidative deamination by MAO of endogenous monoamines results in the formation of hydrogen peroxide and other toxic byproducts such as hydroxyl radicals and superoxide [82] (see Chapters 8, 9, 18).

Additionally, the oxidation of some monoamines by MAO, including dopamine, can produce neurotoxins such as 6-hydroxydopamine and quinone [83–85]. Since brain MAO-B levels are known to be elevated in

AD, it is possible that one consequence is increased production of these endogenous neurotoxins. Such a cascade would be accelerated by other events causing reduction in surviving neuronal cells (age, trauma, illness), since these would likely compensate by providing excess neurotransmitters and thus toxic byproducts.

In sum, therefore, one rationale for chronic administration of *l*-deprenyl would be to reduce this chain of events by inhibition of MAO-B, leading to reduced free radicals and other neurotoxins. Indeed, some *in vitro* data indicate that *l*-deprenyl does indeed reduce the oxidant stress associated with catabolism of dopamine [86]. This theoretical rationale for the preventative use of *l*-deprenyl in DAT, aimed at reduction of "endogenous neurotoxins," has been proposed by Bowen et al. [87].

4.2. Exogenous Neurotoxins

The second line of evidence suggesting a *possible* toxic etiology for AD, and a rationale for the use of *l*-deprenyl on a preventative basis, is provided by analogy from studies of MPTP (1-methyl-4-phenyl-1,2,3,6-tetrahydropyridine) and its implications for PD. This rationale is developed further elsewhere in this volume (see Chapter 00), and will be only briefly reviewed. MPTP causes striatal dopaminergic neuronal degeneration and results in a clinical syndrome similar to idiopathic PD (see [88–90] for review). In experimental animals, depletion in striatal dopamine content similar to that found in patients dying with PD has been reported. In addition, neuropathological changes reminiscent of those found in humans with PD have also been reported in animals. The neurotoxic action of MPTP appears to be mediated by oxidative biotransformation (via MAO-B) to a charged species, 1-methyl-4-phenylpyridinium ion (MPP^+). This compound probably exerts neurotoxicity by disruption of mitochondrial functions, specifically, by blocking the reoxidation of NADH dehydrogenase by coenzyme Q10 leading to ADP depletion in a rotenone-like fashion [80]. Oxygen radicals themselves may also play a role in MPTP-induced neuronal damage [80]. Oxidative biotransformation of MPTP is blocked by administration of MAO-B inhibitors such as *l*-deprenyl at crucial junctures after exposure, thus preventing further MPTP-induced neurotoxicity as well as the development of parkinsonism in non-human primates and other experimental animals [91–93].

MPTP-induced parkinsonism represents a model of idiopathic PD that suggests the possible efficacy of preventative therapy with inhibition of MAO-B. There is some epidemiologic evidence in support of this. Barbeau et al. reported a high correlation between regional presence of agricultural pesticides and the prevalence of PD, suggesting a possible connection between the herbicide paraquat (similar structurally to MPP⁺) and the illness [94]. An earlier report by Rajput et al. suggested an association between early onset PD and rural living, raising the question of whether well water in particular was the responsible agent [95]. Perhaps environmental exposure to either toxic or nontoxic substances leads to the development of PD in vulnerable individuals via oxidative mechanisms.

The above rationales provided the foundation for preventatively oriented studies of the treatment of early PD with antioxidative strategies using *l*-deprenyl [47, 96]. These two studies indicated that early treatment with *l*-deprenyl in this population delayed the need, in the view of the treating neurologist, for treatment with L-dopa-carbidopa therapy. The basis for this is not known, nor has the duration of this effect been established.

4.3. Longevity Studies

The final strand of evidence suggesting a possible neuroprotective effect of *l*-deprenyl is based on longevity studies in animals and humans. Birkmayer reported a retrospective review of experience with patients with PD treated with *l*-deprenyl; he found increased longevity in this group of patients [97]. This has not yet been confirmed by other investigators. Additionally, Knoll et al. reported a significant increase in life span of rats treated with *l*-deprenyl, starting at 24 months of age [98]. Millgram et al. found a similar but less robust effect in a different strain of rats [99] (for details see Chapter 7).

4.4. Summary

The findings in PD are relevant to AD because it is also an idiopathic degenerative brain disease with clinical, pathological, and neurochemical similarities to AD [41–44]. These similarities suggest the theoretical possibility that oxidation of an exogenous toxin to reactive metabolites by MAO-B contributes to neuronal death in DAT and, therefore, that chronic administration of *l*-deprenyl might prevent or retard degeneration of vulnerable systems in at least a subgroup of patients with DAT.

5. Conclusion

A rationale exists for the short-term administration of *l*-deprenyl to patients with DAT, in the hope that restoration of functional neurotransmitter disturbances might improve some symptoms of the illness.

There is encouraging but not convincing empirical evidence that this is the case. Carefully controlled large clinical trials will be necessary to establish whether or not this is true, and to determine the nature and duration of the effect if it does indeed occur. The hope that *l*-deprenyl might exert a neuroprotective effect in AD is strictly theoretical and somewhat more tenuous. In view of the fact that the medication appears to be relatively safe, has potential short-term as well as long-term benefit, in view of the absence of other convincing treatment research strategies, and in view of the need to develop increased expertise in the conduct of trials in this population, large trials of the medication in patients with DAT are in order.

Acknowledgements

The authors are grateful to Maureen E. Herbstsommer for preparation of the manuscript. This work was supported by grants from the National Institute of Mental Health (00733, 40381, 19074), and by the NIA (05142), as well as the State of California Alzheimer's Disease Diagnosis and Treatment Center.

References

[1] Tomlinson BE, Blessed G, Roth M. Observations on the brains of demented old people. J Neurol Sci 1970; 11: 205–242.
[2] Coyle JT, Price DL, DeLong MR. Alzheimer's disease: a disorder of cortical cholinergic innervation. Science 1983; 219: 1184–1190.
[3] Thal LJ, Rosen W, Sharpless NS, Crystal H. Choline chloride fails to improve cognition in Alzheimer's disease. Neurobiol Aging 1981; 2: 205–208.
[4] Beller SA, Overall JE, Swann AC. Efficacy of oral physostigmine in primary degenerative dementia. Psychopharmacology 1985; 87: 147–151.
[5] Eagger SA, Levy R, Sahakian BJ. Tacrine in Alzheimer's Disease. Lancet 1991; 337: 989–992.
[6] Tariot PN, Cohen RM, Welkowitz JA, Sunderland T, Newhouse PA, Murphy DL, Weingartner H. Multiple-dose arecoline infusions in Alzheimer's disease. Arch Gen Psychiatry 1988; 45: 901–905.
[7] Adolfsson R, Gottfries CG, Roos BE, Winblad B. Changes in the brain catecholamines in patients with dementia of the Alzheimer type. Br J Psychiatry 1979; 135: 216–223.
[8] Gottfries CG, Adolfsson R, Aquilonius SM, Carlsson A, Eckernas S-A, Nordberg A, et al. Biochemical changes in dementia disorders of Alzheimer type. Neurobiol Aging 1983; 4: 261–271.
[9] Yates CM, Simpson J, Gordon A, Maloney AF, Allison Y, Ritchie IM, et al. Catecholamines and cholinergic enzymes in pre-senile and senile Alzheimer type dementia and Down's syndrome. Brain Res 1983; 280: 119–126.
[10] Rosser MN, Iversen LL, Reynolds GP, Mountjoy CQ, Roth M. Neurochemical characteristics of early and late onset types of Alzheimer's disease. Br Med J 1984; 288: 961–964.
[11] Arai H, Kosaka K, Iizuka R. Changes of biogenic amines and their metabolites in post-mortem brains from patients with Alzheimer type dementia. J Neurochem 1984; 43: 388–393.

[12] Crow TJ, Cross AJ, Cooper SJ, Deakin JW, Ferrier IN, Johnson JA, et al. Neuro-transmitter receptors and monamine metabolites in the brains of patients with Alzheimer's type dementia and depression, and suicides. Neuropharmacology 1984; 23: 1561–1569.

[13] Francis PT, Palmer AM, Sims NR, Bowen DM, Davison AN, Esiri MM, et al. Neurochemical studies of early onset Alzheimer's disease: possible influence on treatment. N Engl J Med 1985; 313: 7–11.

[14] Bondareff W, Mountjoy CQ, Roth M. Loss of neurons of origin of the adrenergic projection to cerebral cortex (nucleus locus coeruleus) in senile dementia. Neurology 1982; 32: 164–168.

[15] Mann DMA, Lincoln J, Yates PO, Stamp JE, Toper S. Changes in the monoamine-containing neurons of the human CNS in senile dementia. Br J Psychiatry 1980; 136: 533–541.

[16] Volicer L, Langlais PJ, Mattson WR, Mark KA, Gamache PH. Serotoninergic system in dementia of the Alzheimer type. Arch Neurol 1985; 42: 1158–1161.

[17] Kety SF. The biogenic amines in the central nervous system: their possible roles in arousal, emotion, and learning. In: Schmitt FO, editor. The neurosciences: second study program. New York: Rockefeller Press 1970; 324–336.

[18] Anzelark GM, Crow TJ, Greenway AP. Impaired learning and decreased cortical norepinephrine after bilateral locus coeruleus lesions. Science 1973; 181: 682–684.

[19] Gorelick DA, Bozewicz TR, Bridger WH. The role of catecholamines in animal learning and memory. In: Friedhoff AJ, editor. Catecholamines in behavior. New York: Plenum 1975; 1–30.

[20] Wise RA. Catecholamine theories of reward: a critical review. Brain Res 1978; 152: 215–247.

[21] Squire LR, Davis HP. The pharmacology of memory: a neurobiological perspective. Ann Rev Pharmacol Toxicol 1981; 21: 323–356.

[22] McGaugh JL. Hormonal influences on memory. Ann Rev Psychol 1983; 34: 297–323.

[23] Hopkins NF, Johnston D. Frequency-dependent noradrenergic modulation of long-term potentiation in the hippocampus. Science 1984; 226: 350–352.

[24] Sunderland T, Tariot PN, Cohen RM, Weingartner H, Mueller EA, Murphy DL. Anticholinergic sensitivity in Alzheimer patients and age-matched controls. Arch Gen Psychiatry 1987; 44: 418–426.

[25] Busse E, Simpson D. Depression and anti-depressants in the elderly. J Clin Psychiatry 1983; 44: 35–39.

[26] Neshkes RE, Gerner R, Jarvik LF, Mintz J, Joseph J, Linde S, et al. Orthostatic effect of imipramine and doxepin in depressed geriatric out-patients. J Clin Psychopharmacol 1985; 9: 102–106.

[27] Salzman C. Caution urged in using MAOI's with the elderly. Am J Psychiatry 1986; 143: 118–199.

[28] Cohen RM, Sunderland T, Aulakh CS. Antidepressants in states of cognitive dysfunction. Drug Dev Res 1984; 4: 517–532.

[29] Gottfries CG. Alzheimer's disease and senile dementia: biochemical characteristics and aspects of treatment. Psychopharmacology 1985; 86: 245–252.

[30] Knoll J, Ecseri Z, Kelemen K, Nievel J, Knoll B. Phenylisopropylmethyl-propinylamine (E-250), a new psychic energizer. Arch Int Pharmacodyn 1965; 155: 154–164.

[31] Knoll J. Deprenyl (selegiline): the history of its development and pharmacological action. Acta Neurol Scand 1983; (Supplement) 95: 57–80.

[32] Elsworth JD, Glover V, Reynolds GP, Sandler M, Lees AJ, Phuapradit P, et al. Deprenyl administration in man: a selective monoamine oxidase B inhibitor without the "cheese effect." Psychopharmacology 1978; 57: 33–38.

[33] Knoll J. Analysis of the pharmacological effects of selective monoamine oxidase inhibitors. CIBA Foundation Symposium 1976; 39: 135–161.

[34] Sunderland T, Mueller EA, Cohen RM, Jimerson DC, Pickar D, Murphy DL: Tyramine pressor sensitivity changes during deprenyl treatment. Psychopharmacology 1985; 86: 432–437.

[35] Quitkin FM, Liebowitz MR, Stewart JW, McGrath PJ, Harrison W, Rabkin JG, et al. l-Deprenyl in atypical depressives. Arch Gen Psychiatry 1984; 41: 777–781.

[36] Mann JJ, Aarons SF, Wilner PJ, Keilp JG, Sweeney JA, Perlstein T, Frances AJ, et al. A controlled study of the antidepressant efficacy and side-effects of (−)-deprenyl. Arch Gen Psychiatry 1989; 46: 45–50.

[37] Reynolds GP, Elsworth JD, Blau A, Sandler M, Lees AJ, Stern GM. Deprenyl is metabolized to amphetamine and methamphetamine in man. Br J Clin Pharmacol 1978; 6: 542–543.

[38] Mendis N, Pare CMB, Sandler M, Glover B, Stern GM. Is the failure of (−)-deprenyl a selective MAO-B inhibitor to alleviate the pressure related to freedom from cheese effect? Psychopharmacology 1981; 73: 87–90.

[39] Karoum F, Chuang LW, Isler T, Calne DB, Liebowitz MR, Quitkin MR, et al. Metabolism of (−)-deprenyl to amphetamine and methamphetamine. Neurology 1982; 32: 503–509.

[40] Mendlewicz J, Youdim MBH. *l*-Deprenyl, a selective monoamine oxidase-type B inhibitor, in the treatment of depression: a double-blind evaluation. Br J Psychiatry 1983; 142: 508–511.

[41] Rossor MN, Parkinson's disease and Alzheimer's disease as disorders of the isodendritic core. Br Med J 1981; 283: 1588–1590.

[42] Appel SH. A unified hypothesis for the cause of amyotrophic lateral sclerosis, parkinsonism, and Alzheimer disease. Ann Neurol 1981; 10: 499–505.

[43] Jellinger K. Neuropathological substrates of Alzheimer's disease and Parkinson's disease. J Neural Transm 1987; (Supplement) 24: 109–129.

[44] Ditter SM, Mirra SS. Neuropathologic and clinical features of Parkinson's disease in Alzheimer's disease patients. Neurology 1987; 37: 754–760.

[45] Eisler T, Teravainen H, Nelson R, Krebs H, Weise V, Lake CR, et al. Deprenyl in Parkinson disease. Neurology 1981; 31: 19–23.

[46] Golbe LI. Deprenyl as symptomatic therapy in Parkinson's disease. Clin Neuropharmacol 1988; 11: 387–400.

[47] The Parkinson Study Group. Effect of deprenyl on the progression of disability in early Parkinson's disease. N Engl J Med 1989; 321: 1364–1371.

[48] Robinson DS, Davis JM, Nies A, Colburn RW, Davis JN, Bourne HR, et al. Ageing, monoamines, and monoamine oxidase levels. Lancet 1972; i: 290–291.

[49] Adolfsson R, Gottfries CG, Oreland L, Wieberg A, Winblad B. Increased activity of brain and platelet monoamine oxidase in dementia of Alzheimer type. Life Sci 1988; 17: 1029–1034.

[50] Knoll J. Selective inhibition of B-type monoamine oxidase in the brain. A drug study to improve the quality of life in senescence. In: Weverling JA, editor. Strategy in drug research. Amsterdam: Elsevier Science Publishers 1982; 107–135.

[51] Reinikaninen KJ, Paljarvi L, Halonen T, Mallminen O, Kosma V, Laakso M, Riekkinen J. Dopaminergic system in monoamine oxidase B activity in Alzheimer's disease. Neurobiol Aging 1988; 9: 245–252.

[52] Martini E, Pataky I, Szilagyi K, Ventor V. Brief information on an early phase-II study with deprenyl in demented patients. Pharmacopsychiatry 1987; 20: 256–257.

[53] Shader RI, Harmatz JS, Salzman C. A new scale for clinical assessment (SCAG). J Amer Geriatr Soc 1969; 22: 107–113.

[54] Schneider LS, Pollack VE, Zemansky MF, Gleason RP, Palmer R, Sloane RB. A pilot study of low dose *l*-deprenyl in Alzheimer's disease. J Geriatr Psychiatry Neurol 1991; 4: 143–148.

[55] Overall JE, Beller SA. The brief psychiatric rating scale (BPRS) in geropsychiatric research: I. Factor structure on an in-patient unit. J Gerontol 1984; 39: 187–193.

[56] Alexopoulos GS, Abrams RC, Young RC, Shamoian CA. Cornell scale for depression in dementia. Biol Psychiatry 1988; 23: 271–284.

[57] Buschke H, Fuld PA. Evaluating storage, retention, and retrieval in disordered memory and learning. Neurology 1974; 24: 1019–1025.

[58] Goad DL, Davis CM, Liem P, Fuselier CC, McCormack JR, Olsen KM. The use of selegiline in Alzheimer's patients with behavior problems. J Clin Psychiatry 1991; 52: 342–345.

[59] Reisberg B, Borenstein J, Salob SP, Ferris SH, Franssen E, Georgotas A. Behavioral symptoms in Alzheimer's disease: phenomenology and treatment. J Clin Psychiatry 1987; 48 (Supplement): 9–15.

[60] Folstein MF, Folstein SE, McHugh PR. Mini-Mental State: A practical method for grading the cognitive state of patients for the clinician. J Psychiatr Res 1975; 12: 189–198.

[61] Zarit SH. Issues and directions in family intervention research. In: Light E, Lebowitz B, editors. Alzheimer's disease treatment and family stress: directions for research. Washington, D.C.: U.S. Government Printing Office. DHHS (ADM) 89-1569, 1989, Rockville, MD, USA, 458–486.

[62] Tariot PN, Cohen RM, Sunderland, T, Newhouse PA, Yount D, Mellow AM, et al. l-Deprenyl in Alzheimer's disease: preliminary evidence for behavioral change with monamine oxidase B inhibition. Arch Gen Psychiatry 1987; 44: 427–433.

[63] Tariot PN, Sunderland T, Weingartner H, Murphy DL, Welkowitz JA, Thompson K, Cohen RM. Cognitive effects of l-deprenyl in Alzheimer's disease. Psychopharmacology 1987; 91: 489–495.

[64] Sunderland T, Tariot PN, Cohen RM, Newhouse P, Mellow AM, Mueller EA, Murphy DLM. A multidose study of the effects of l-deprenyl on CSF monoamine metabolites in patients with Alzheimer's disease. Psychopharmacology 1987; 91: 293–296.

[65] Piccinin GL, Finali G, Piccirilli M. Neuropsychological effects of l-deprenyl on Alzheimer's type dementia. Clin Neuropharmacol 1990; 13: 147–163.

[66] Sunderland T, Molchan SE, LaLonde FM, Lawlor BA, Martinez RA, Martinson HF, Vitiello B. Combination pharmacotherapy in Alzheimer's disease: Deprenyl plus physostigmine (abstract). Am College Neuropsychopharmacol 1989.

[67] Schneider LS, Olin JT, Pawluczyk S. Combination of l-deprenyl and cholinesterase inhibitor in Alzheimer's disease: a double-blind, crossover, pilot study. Am J Psychiatry, 1992, in press.

[68] Rosen WG, Mohs RC, Davis KL. A new rating scale for Alzheimer's disease. Am J Psychiatry 1984; 141: 1356–1364.

[69] Campi N, Todeschini GP, Scarzella L. Selegiline vs. L-acetylcarnitine in the treatment of Alzheimer-type dementia. Clin Therap 1990; 12: 306–314.

[70] Monteverde A, Gnemmi P, Rossi F, Monteverde A. Selegiline in the treatment of mild to moderate Alzheimer-type dementia. Clin Therap 1990; 12: 315–332.

[71] Falsaperla A, Preti P, Oliani C. Selegiline vs. Oxiracetam in patients with Alzheimer-type dementia. Clin Therap 1990; 12: 376–384.

[72] Martucci N, Fabbrini G, Fioravanti M. Monoaminossidasi e demenza: trattamento con un inibitore dell'attivita MAO-B. Giornale D Neuropsicofarmacologia 1989; 11 (6): 265–269.

[73] Agnoli A, Martucci N, Fabbrini G, Buckley A, Fioravanti M. Monoamine oxidase in dementia: treatment with an inhibitor of MAO-B activity. Dementia 1990; 1: 109–114.

[74] Loeb C, Albano C. Selegiline: A new approach to DAT treatment. European conference on Parkinson's disease and extrapyramidal disorders 1990 (abstract).

[75] Mangoni A, Grassi MP, Fratolla L, Piolti R, Bassi S, Motta A, et al. Effects of a MAO-B inhibitor in the treatment of Alzheimer's disease. Eur Neurol 1991; 31: 100–107.

[76] Filip V, Kolibas E, Ceskova E, Hronek J, Novotna D, Novotny V, et al. Selegiline in mild SDAT: results of the multi-center, double-blind, placebo-controlled trial. Am Col Neuropsychopharm 1991 (abstract).

[77] Tariot PN, Sunderland T, Cohen RM, Newhouse PA, Mueller EA, Murphy DL. Tranylcypromine compared with l-deprenyl in Alzheimer's disease. J Clin Psychopharmacol 1988; 8: 23–27.

[78] Varga E, Tringer L. Clinical trial of a new type of promptly acting psychoenergetic agent. Acta Med Acad Sci Hung 1967; 23: 289–295.

[79] Volicer L, Crino PB. Review: Involvement of free radicals in dementia of the Alzheimer-type: a hypothesis. Neurobiol Aging 1990; 11: 567–571.

[80] LeBel CP, Bondy SC. Mini-review: oxygen radicals: common mediators of neurotoxicity. Neurotoxicol Teratol 1991; 13: 341–346.

[81] Smith CD, Carney JM, Starke-Reed PE, Oliver CN, Stadtman ER, Floyd RA, Markesbery WR. Excess brain protein oxidation and enzyme dysfunction in normal aging and in Alzheimer's disease. Proc Natl Acad Sci 1991; 88: 10540–10543.

[82] Cohen G. Oxidative Stress in the Nervous System. In: Sies H, editor. Oxidative stress. London: Academic Press 1985; 383–402.

[83] Jonsson G. Studies on the mechanisms of 6-hydroxydopamine cytotoxicity. Medical Biology 1976; 54: 406–420.

[84] Graham DG. Catecholamine toxicity: A proposal for the molecular pathogenesis of manganese neurotoxicity and Parkinson's disease. Neurotoxicol 1984; 5: 83–96.

[85] Heikkila R, Cohen G. Inhibition of biogenic amine uptake by hydrogen peroxide: a mechanism for toxic effects of 6-hydroxydopamine. Science 1971; 172: 1257–1258.

[86] Cohen G, Spina MB. Deprenyl suppresses the oxidant stress associated with increased dopamine turnover. Ann Neurol 1989; 26: 689–690.

[87] Bowen DM, Davison AN. Can the pathophysiology of dementia lead to rational therapy? In: Crook T, Bartus R, Ferris S, Gershon S, editors. Treatment development strategies for Alzheimer's disease. Madison, Conn.: Powley Assoc 1986; 35–66.

[88] Tetrud JW, Lansgton JW. R-(−)-deprenyl as a possible protective agent in Parkinson's disease. J Neurol Transm 1987; (Supplement) 25: 69–79.

[89] Shoulson I. Experimental therapeutics directed at the pathogenesis of Parkinson's disease. In: Handbook of experimental pharmacology: drugs for the treatment of Parkinson's disease. Calen DB, editor. Berlin: Springer-Verlag 1989; 289–305.

[90] Langston JW. The etiology of Parkinson's disease: new directions for research. In: Parkinson's disease and movement disorders. Jankovic J, Tolosa E, editors. Baltimore-Munich: Urban and Schwarzenberg 1988; 75–85.

[91] Langston JW, Irwin I, Langston EB. Pargyline prevents MPTP-induced parkinsonism in primates. Science 1984; 225: 1480–1482.

[92] Heikkila RF, Manzion L, Cabbat FS, Duvoisin RC. Protection against the dopaminergic neurotoxicity of MPTP by monoamine oxidase inhibitors. Nature 1984; 311: 467–469.

[93] Cohen G, Pasik P, Cohen B, Leist A, Mytilineou C, Yahr M. Pargyline and deprenyl prevent the neurotoxicity of MPTP in monkeys. Eur J Pharmacol 1984; 106: 209–219.

[94] Barbeau A, Roy M, Cloutier T, Plasse L, Paris S. Environmental and genetic factors in the etiology of Parkinson's disease. In: Yahr M, Bergmann K, editors. Advances in neurology. Vol 45: Parkinson's disease. New York: Raven Press 1987.

[95] Rajput AH, Stern W, Christ A, Laverty W. Etiology of Parkinson's disease: environmental factors. Neurology 1984; 34: 207.

[96] Tetrud JW, Langston JW. The effect of deprenyl (selegiline) on the natural history of Parkinson's disease. Science 1989; 245: 519–522.

[97] Birkmayer W, Knoll J, Riederer P, Youdim MBH, Hars V, Martin J. Increased life expectancy resulting from addition of *l*-deprenyl to Madopar treatment in Parkinson's disease: a long-term study. J Neurol Transm 1985; 64: 113–127.

[98] Knoll J. Striatal dopamine dependency of life span in male rats. Longevity study with (−)-deprenyl. Mechanisms of Aging and Development 1988; 46: 237–262.

[99] Milgram NW, Racine RJ, Nellis P, Mendonca I, Ivy GO. Maintenance on *l*-deprenyl prolongs life in aged male rats. Life Sci 1990; 47: 415–420.

Inhibitors of Monoamine Oxidase B
Pharmacology and Clinical Use in Neurodegenerative Disorders
ed. by I. Szelenyi
© 1993 Birkhäuser Verlag Basel/Switzerland

CHAPTER 17
Do MAO-B Inhibitors Have Any Role in the Treatment of Depression?

G. Laux

1 Introduction
2 Clinical Studies with Selegiline in Depressive Disorders
3 Pharmacotherapy of Depressive Disorders by Selegiline Combined with
  Phenylalanine or *l*-5-Hydroxytryptophan
4 Concluding Remarks
  Summary
  References

1. Introduction

Parkinson's disease (PD) is clearly associated with changes in affective state and a higher frequency of depression. Depressive symptoms have been found in about 70% of cases of PD [1], while depression that meets diagnostic criteria and significance is seen in about 40% of PD patients [2]. There is no single type of depression in PD, but rather there are several different depressive syndromes related to the nature of the PD. Mayeux et al. [3] described depressed PD patients with sleep disturbances, fatigue, psychomotor retardation, and difficulty in concentrating as dominant complaints. Schiffer et al. [4] reported atypical depression with anxiety and panic disorder to be found significantly more frequently among patients with PD. According to Starkstein et al. [5], depressed patients with PD reported a significantly higher frequency of worrying, loss of interest, hopelessness, loss of appetite and libido, as well as anxiety, i.e., they showed a predominance of autonomic and affective symptoms. Interestingly, these authors found anergia and motor retardation to be not significantly more frequent in PD patients with depression. In recent years controlled studies have provided evidence that monoamine oxidase inhibitors (MAOIs) are effective antidepressants and comparable to (tricyclic) reuptake inhibitors. They are very effective in the treatment of so-called therapy-resistant depressions (i.e., tricyclic-nonresponders), atypical depressions, phobias, panic disorders, and anxiety states [6]. Selective MAOIs are now available that offer greater safety (e.g., reduced risk of the "cheese effect"): moclobemide is a reversible, relatively selective MAO-A inhibitor with established antidepressant efficacy [7]. Inhibition of MAO-A is regarded as the decisive factor for the antidepressant effect, because, in man, noradrenaline and serotonin are almost exclusively catabolized by MAO-A, and disturbance and/or dysequilibrium of these neurotransmitters is considered as an important pathomechanism in depressive illnesses.

Selegiline is a selective MAO-B inhibitor that is effective as an antiparkinsonian drug due to dopaminergic activity [8]. And, there are some clinical observations and findings available from preliminary studies of the antidepressant efficacy and safety of selegiline [9]. The possible importance of the dopaminergic system, at least in some subtypes of depressive disorders, has been indicated by the antidepressant efficacy of nomifensine [10] or sulpiride [11]. According to pharmacological data, selegiline reduces the number of β-adrenoceptors after chronic treatment, as observed under treatment with typical antidepressants [12].

Recently, a significant relationship between Alzheimer's disease, major depression, PD, and low dopaminergic activity has been claimed [13].

2. Clinical Studies with Selegiline in Depressive Disorders

The antidepressant properties of selegiline have been assessed in several controlled clinical studies [14–20]; the results are summarized in Table 1. In most of the studies deprenyl had a statistically significant antidepressant effect compared with placebo. The dose seems to be the most critical issue: at doses under 10 mg/d selegiline is a selective MAO-B inhibitor, while higher doses result in non-selective MAO-inhibition including MAO-A inhibition and inhibition of dopamine reuptake (see Chapters 6, 9). This has been clinically shown by the study of Mann et al. [19] using two different doses of deprenyl in the treatment of depressed outpatients diagnosed as having a major depressive episode according to DSM-III-R criteria (Diagnostic and Statistical Manual of Mental Disorders (third ed., revised); American Psychiatric Association 1987). Only at higher doses did selegiline reveal an antidepressant effect superior to placebo. Additionally, no correlation has been found between inhibition of platelet MAO-B and clinical response [20].

Regarding undesired effects, the absence of many of the side-effects typical of nonselective MAOIs was impressive. Safety aspects ("cheese effect") can be a further argument in favor of selegiline compared with "classical" nonselective MAOIs. Regarding the clinical characteristics of the patients responding to selegiline, Mann et al. [9] found evidence in an open study for a better antidepressant efficacy in nonendogenous depressions (see Figure 1). However, the controlled study of Mann et al. [19] showed no significant difference between endogenous vs. nonen-

Table 1. Controlled studies with l-deprenyl in depressive disorders.

Authors	[Ref.]	N, patients	Study design	Dosage	Results	Side-effects
Mann and Gershon (1980)	[9]	10 (endogenous depression, outpatients)	open (Pl wash-out)	5–15 mg/day	HRSD reduction 68% Onset of action after 3 days	Sleep disturbances, anorexia
Mendis et al. (1981)	[14]	22		10–20 mg/day	No anitdepressant activity Improvement 50% of patients	
Mann et al. (1982)	[15]	25 (13 endogenous depressives, 12 nonendogenous depressives)	open (Pl wash-out)	5–20 mg/day	Response rate 64% (6 responders endogenous, 10 non-endogenous subgroup)	Insomnia, reduced appetite, increased energy, agitation
Mendlewicz and Youdim (1983)	[16]	14 (bipolars)	db vs. Pl (n = 13)	15 mg/day	10 Responders D 2 Responders Pl	D = Pl
Quitkin et al. (1984)	[17]	17 (atypical depressives)	open Pl (n = 24)	10–20 mg/day	Response rate 59% D > Pl (Response if $D \geqslant 30$ mg/d)	Insomnia (4×) Peripheral edema (1x)
Ceskova et al. (1986)	[18]	27 (endogenous depressives)	open	10–20 mg/day	10 Responders Stimulatory effect	Mild, no cheese effect (without diet)
Mann et al. (1989)	[19]	22 (outpatients, MDD)	db vs. Pl (n = 22)	10 mg/day 30 mg/day	No signif. antidepressant effect Response rate D 50% (HRSD reduction 41%) Pl 14% (HRSD reduction 10%)	D = Pl Insomnia, tremor, dry mouth, headache
McGrath et al. (1989)	[20]	30 (atypical depressives)	db vs. Pl (n = 50)	20–40 mg/day	Response rate D 50%, Pl 28% No correlation MAO inhibition/clinical response Ph > D	Dry mouth 1× hypertensive reaction after eating cheese

db = double-blind; D = l-deprenyl; HRSD = Hamilton Rating Scale of Depression; Pl = Placebo; MDD = Major Depressive Disorder; > = significantly better; = = equally frequent; ≥ = more than; Ph = Phenelzine

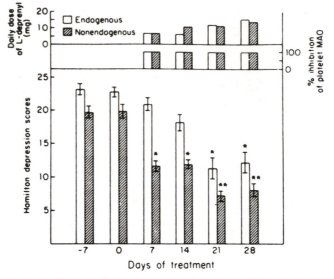

Figure 1. The effect of *l*-deprenyl upon endogenous and non-endogenous depression and platelet monoamine oxidase activity (from: [15]).

dogenous depressions. Some authors reported better results for selegiline in the treatment of so-called atypical depressions, which is in line with the prevailing view that MAOIs are the treatment of choice for atypical depressions [6]. Additionally, in recent years it has been shown that MAOIs constitute an effective drug treatment for phobias and panic disorders [6]. In direct contrast, the presence of panic attacks appeared to predict a nonresponse to selegiline [19]. This observation can give some evidence for a different therapeutic action compared to "classical" nonselective MAOIs, possibly based on dopamine-reuptake-inhibiting properties (see Chapters 6, 7). Other antidepressants acting on the dopaminergic system have also failed to show efficacy against panic attacks [24].

3. Pharmacotherapy of Depressive Disorders by Selegiline Combined with Phenylalanine or *l*-5-Hydroxytryptophan

The studies with selegiline combined with phenylalanine or *l*-5-hydroxytryptophan in the pharmacotherapy of depressive disorders are summarized in Table 2. The most striking results of these few studies are the rapid onset of action and the reported paucity of side-effects in both selegiline combination-treatment conditions.

Table 2. *l*-Deprenyl combination therapy of depressive disorders.

Authors	[Ref.]	N, patients	Study design	Drugs	Results
Mendlewicz and Youdim (1980)	[21]	14 (uni-/bipolars)	open	D (15 mg/d) + *l*-5-HTP (900 mg/d) plus benzerazide	10 Responders Correlation MAO inhibition/ clinical response Rapid onset of action
		58	db	D + *l*-5-HTP (n = 18) vs *l*-5-HTP (n = 21) vs placebo (n = 19)	D + *l*-5-HTP > Pl *l*-5-HTP = Pl Correlation MAO inhibition/ clinical response
Birkmayer et al. (1984)	[22]	155 (unipolars)	oral and i.v.	D (5–10 mg/d) plus phenylalanine (250 mg/d)	Potent antidepressive action
Sabelli (1991)	[23]	10 (drug resistant major depressions)	open oral	D (5 mg/d) plus phenylalanine (2–6 g/d) plus pyridoxine (100 mg/d)	9 Responders Rapid onset of mood elevation (within hours – 3 days) Lack of side-effects

db = double-blind; D = *l*-deprenyl; *l*-5-HTP = *l*-5-hydroxytryptophan; Pl = Placebo > = significantly better; = = equally effective

4. Concluding Remarks

Controlled studies in recent years have revealed that selegiline at higher doses (20–40 mg/d) has a statistically significant antidepressant effect compared with placebo. This seems to be based on the loss of selective MAO-B inhibition at higher doses with a predominance of MAO-A inhibition and inhibition of dopamine reuptake. The latter effect might be the reason why selegiline has a different profile from the new, reversible, selective MAO-A inhibitors like moclobemide, which are – in contrast to selegiline – also effective in panic disorders. Thus, it can be concluded that selegiline may hold a place in the pharmacotherapy of depressive disorders, especially of that in subgroups with reduced dopaminergic function, as hypothesized in organic and involutional depressions. Beside dopaminergic effects, pharmacokinetic and pharmacodynamic factors may contribute to the therapeutic benefits of selegiline: the conversion of selegiline to *l*-amphetamine and *l*-metamphetamine has been claimed as such a factor [25]. However, the concentrations of the *l*-enantiomers of amphetamine might be too low for induction of clinically relevant central effects. "Dirty drugs" (with effects on multiple, different neurotransmitters), from a clinical point of view, seem to be more effective than highly selective substances. Therefore, selegiline given as a "non-selective" MAOI could also become an antidepressant of interest because of its favorable profile with respect to side-effects. Controlled studies with adequate numbers of patients and carefully diagnosed subtypes and subgroups of affective disorders are necessary and recommended in order to establish the position of selegiline in the treatment of depressive illness.

Summary

In recent years controlled studies have provided evidence that monoamine oxidase inhibitors (MAOIs) are effective antidepressants especially in the treatment of so-called atypical and therapy-resistant depressions. Open and controlled clinical studies revealed that the MAO-B inhibitor selegiline (*l*-deprenyl) at higher doses (20–40 mg/d) has significant antidepressive efficacy. This seems to ground on the loss of selective MAO-B inhibition at higher dosage with predominance of MAO-A inhibition and inhibition of dopamine reuptake. Few studies are available with selegiline combined with phenylalanine or *l*-5-hydroxytryptophan showing a rapid onset of action and only few side effects. A special profile regarding the antidepressant action of selegiline is discussed.

References

[1] Brown RG, MacCarthy B. Psychiatric morbidity in patients with Parkinson's disease. Psychol Med 1990; 20: 77–87.
[2] Ring HA, Trimble MR. Affective disturbance in Parkinson's disease. Int J Geriatr Psychiatry 1991; 6: 385–393.
[3] Mayeux R, Stern Y, Williams JBW, Cote L, Frantz A, Dyrenfurth I. Clinical and biochemical features of depression in Parkinson's disease. Am J Psychiatry 1986; 143: 756–759.
[4] Schiffer RB, Kurlan R, Rubin A, Boer S. Evidence for atypical depression in Parkinson's disease. Am J Psychiatry 1988; 145: 1020–1024.
[5] Starkstein SE, Preziosi TJ, Forrester AW, Robinson RG. Specificity of affective and autonomic symptoms of depression in Parkinson's disease. J Neurol Neurosurg Psychiatry 1990; 53: 869–873.
[6] Pare CMB. The present status of monoamine oxidase inhibitors. Br J Psychiatry 1985; 146: 576–584.
[7] Laux G, Riederer P, editors. Clinical approaches to moclobemide, a new reversible inhibitor of MAO-A (RIMA). Psychiat Prax Suppl 1990; 17: 1–30.
[8] Riederer P, Przuntek H, editors. MAO-B-inhibitor selegiline (R-(−)-deprenyl). A new therapeutic concept in the treatment of Parkinson's disease. J Neural Transm 1987 (Supplement 25): 1–197.
[9] Mann JJ, Gershon S. l-Deprenyl: a selective monoamine oxidase type B inhibitor in endogenous depression. Life Sci 1980; 26: 877–882.
[10] Overall JE. Efficacy of nomifensine in different depressive syndromes. J Clin Psychiatry 1984; 45 (Sect. 2): 85–88.
[11] Aylward M, Maddock J, Dewland PM, Lewis PA. Sulpiride in depressive illness. Adv Biol Psychiat 1981; 7: 154–165.
[12] Zsilla G, Barbaccia ML, Gandolfi O, Knoll J, Costa E. (−)-Deprenyl, a selective MAO-B inhibitor increased 3H-imipramine binding and decreased beta-adrenergic receptor function. Eur J Pharmacol 1983; 11: 117.
[13] Wolfe N, Katz DI, Albert ML, Almozlino A, Durso R, Smith MC, Volicer L. Neuropsychological profile linked to low dopamine in Alzheimer's disease, major depression, and Parkinson's disease. J Neurol Neurosurg Psychiatry 1990; 53: 915–917.
[14] Mendis N, Pare CMB, Sandler M, Glover V, Stern M. Is the failure of (−)-deprenyl, a selective monoamine oxidase B inhibitor, to alleviate depression related to freedom from the cheese effect? Psychopharmacology 1981; 73: 87–90.
[15] Mann JJ, Frances A, Kaplan RD, Kocsis J, Peselow ED, Gershon S. The relative efficacy of l-deprenyl: a selective monoamine type B inhibitor, in endogenous and nonendogenous depression. J Clin Psychopharmacol 1982; 2: 54–57.
[16] Mendlewicz J, Youdim MBH. l-Deprenyl: a selective monoamine oxidase type B inhibitor, in the treatment of depression: a double-blind evaluation. Br J Psychiatry 1983; 142: 508–511.
[17] Quitkin FM, Liebowitz MR, Stewart JW, McGrath PJ, Harrison W, Rabkin JG, Markowitz J, Davies SO. l-Deprenyl in atypical depression. Arch Gen Psychiatry 1984; 41: 777–781.
[18] Ceskova E, Svestka J, Nahunek K, Rysanek R, Peska I, Novotna H. Clinical experience with l-deprenyl in endogenous depression. Activ Nerv Sup (Praha) 1986; 28: 47.
[19] Mann JJ, Aarons SF, Wilner PJ, Keilp JG, Sweeney JA, Pearlstein T et al. A controlled study of the antidepressant efficacy and side effects of (−)-deprenyl. Arch Gen Psychiatry 1989; 46: 45–50.
[20] McGrath PJ, Stewart JW, Harrison W, Wager S, Nunes EN, Quitkin FM. A placebo-controlled trial of l-deprenyl in atypical depression. Psychopharmacol Bull 1989; 25: 63–67.
[21] Mendlewicz J, Youdim MBH. Antidepressant potentiation of 5-hydroxytryptophan by l-Deprenyl in affective illness. J Affect Disord 1980; 2: 137–146.
[22] Birkmayer W, Riederer P, Linauer W, Knoll J. l-deprenyl plus l-phenylalanine in the treatment of depression. J Neural Transm 1984; 59: 81–87.

[23] Sabelli HC. Rapid treatment of depression with selegiline-phenylalanine combination. J Clin Psychiatry 1991; 52: 137.
[24] Sheehan DV, Davidson J, Manschreck T, Van Wyck Fleet J. Lack of efficacy of a new antidepressant (bupropion) in the treatment of panic disorder with phobias. J Clin Psychopharmacol 1983; 3: 28–31.
[25] Karoum F, Chuang LW, Eisler T. Metabolism of (−)-deprenyl to amphetamine and metamphetamine may be responsible for deprenyl's therapeutic benefit: a biochemical assessment. Neurology 1982; 32: 503–509.

Inhibitors of Monoamine Oxidase B
Pharmacology and Clinical Use in Neurodegenerative Disorders
ed. by I. Szelenyi
© 1993 Birkhäuser Verlag Basel/Switzerland

CHAPTER 18
The Therapeutic Place and Value of Present and Future MAO-B Inhibitors – *l*-Deprenyl as the Gold Standard

P. Riederer and M. B. H. Youdim

1   Introduction
2   Short-Term Action
2.1   Substrate Specificity in Humans
2.2   Symptomatic Effects
3   Long-Term Actions
3.1   MAO-B Activity and Neurotoxicity
3.2   Amphetamine-Like Action
3.3   Neuroprotective Action of *l*-Deprenyl after Chemical Intoxication
3.3.1   MPTP
3.3.2   6-Hydroxydopamine
3.3.3   DSP-4
3.4   Clinical Evidence for a Neuroprotective Role of *l*-Deprenyl
3.5   Inhibition of MAO-B and Possible Action on NMDA-Receptor-Associated Polyamine Binding Site
3.6   MAO-B Inhibition and Synthesis of Nerve Growth Factor
4   Concluding Remarks
          References

1. Introduction

The establishment of MAO inhibitors in the early 1960s failed, not because of the lack of intended efficacy but because of accompanying side-effects, e.g., hypotension and hypertension, psychic alteration, and hepatotoxicity. With Johnston's discovery in 1968 of the multiple forms (MAO-A, MAO-B), selective MAO inhibitors could be developed for the first time that considered substrate specificity. Thus, there was hope to reduce the initially observed side-effects. *l*-Deprenyl (selegiline), synthesized by Ecsery and developed as an antidepressant drug by Knoll, was such a substance. As an antidepressant *l*-deprenyl did not succeed, but as an anti-Parkinson drug it did [1]. Meanwhile, *l*-deprenyl has become the "gold standard" of MAO inhibitors. The clinical and theoretical innovations of the last decade have been decisively marked by *l*-deprenyl since it unites many synergistic biochemical and pharmacological properties. Any new MAO-B inhibitor must have comparable properties since they determine the therapeutic value. Some of these new inhibitors will be reviewed here in comparison to *l*-deprenyl.

Table 1. Biochemical Actions of *l*-Deprenyl.

Short-Term Action
- Inhibition of MAO-B
- Increase in PEA and DA (PEA ≫ DA)
- Inhibition of chemical neurotoxicity (MPTP, 6-OHDA, DSP-4)
- Metabolization to amphetamine and metamphetamine
- Amine-uptake-inhibiting properties
- Reduction of L-dopa dose
- Reduction of dopamine-related toxic metabolites

2. Short-term Action

2.1. Substrate Specificity in Humans

It is well known that dopamine is a relatively good MAO-B substrate [2]. As early as 1977, Birkmayer et al. [3] pointed out that *l*-deprenyl's clinical effect could also be due to the increased concentration of phenylethylamine (PEA) – an excellent and selective MAO-B substrate. In fact, it could later be demonstrated that, in the striatum of patients suffering from Parkinson's disease (PD), PEA increases up to 1190%. PEA releases dopamine and indirectly potentiates the dopaminergic function. Therefore, *l*-deprenyl increases the concentration of both amines and enhances the action of dopamine by increasing the rate of release via PEA at the same time [3]. Recent experiments confirm the significant increase of PEA (160–350%) in the striatum of rats after 0.5–4 mg/kg *l*-deprenyl i.p. without changing dopamine [4].

Electrophysiological studies also show that the neuronal response of the N. caudatus to dopamine agonists is potentiated after application of 2 mg/kg *l*-deprenyl. This effect is similar to PEA's in small doses [5]. Therefore, *l*-deprenyl is able to increase dopaminergic transmission without changing dopamine metabolism.

l-Deprenyl's mild effect on striatal dopamine is due to the fact that MAO-B cannot be identified intraneuronally in the substantia nigra [6–8]. Furthermore, dopamine is a relatively good MAO-B substrate. In contrast, noradrenaline and serotonin are exclusively MAO-A substrates. Thus, the modest dopamine increase after *l*-deprenyl administration compared to the very significant PEA increase can be explained. In addition, obviously, a part of dopamine is metabolized by MAO-A, even if MAO-B is completely inhibited. Additionally, most of the MAO-B activity can be demonstrated in the glia. Therefore, dopamine can also be enriched there after *l*-deprenyl induces MAO-B inhibition. However, a quick metabolization via MAO-A and COMT is likely. It is not known how much of the dopamine that is accumulated in the glia reaches the receptors under these particular circumstances in neurodegenerative diseases (hormone-like action). It would be important to clarify the meaning of MAO-A in this context. The investigation of selective MAO-A blockers in neurodegenerative diseases like PD and dementia of the Alzheimer type (DAT) would contribute to answering these questions. But, as long as there are no MAO-A blockers causing no hypertensive effects, appropriate studies (especially if chronic dopaminergic and (nor)adrenergic combination therapy is used) probably will not be conducted.

2.2. Symptomatic Effects

Recent clinical experiments demonstrate that L-dopa therapy, combined with a peripheral decarboxylase blocker, initially acts excellently. However, after about 5 years this therapy leads to an increase in side-effects such as motor fluctuations, the on-off-phenomenon, dyskinesia and dystonia, as well as susceptibility to pharmacotoxic psychosis. This is known as the L-dopa syndrome. Is it then accurate to label dopamine as a "neurotoxic" substance if it was possibly synthesized after L-dopa treatment in nonphysiological concentrations in degenerating neurons? The fact that L-dopa therapy yields excellent clinical effects is contrary to this hypothesis. Melamed [9] points out that the administration of L-dopa needs to be stopped if the threat of L-dopa syndrome is suspected or imminent. Since, for example, hyperkinesia is observed less often with bromocriptine and lisuride than with L-dopa combination therapy [9, 10] L-dopa syndrome cannot be correlated with the disease progression (neuronal cell death). On the other hand, *in vitro* experiments demonstrate possible neurotoxic effects of dopamine [11–13]. In our opinion, these experiments show that a reduction of the L-dopa dose is justified. Therefore, early combination with *l*-deprenyl has the following advantages:

1) Reduction of the L-dopa dose; therefore a more physiologic rate of dopamine synthesis;
2) Reduction of synthesis of dopamine-derived toxic metabolites like hydrogen peroxide, α,β-unsaturated aldehydes, 5-S-cysteinyl-dopamine, etc.;
3) Reduction of oxidative stress and, possibly, *l*-deprenyl-dependent neuroprotective action [14].

3. Long-term Actions

Long-term actions with adaptive changes in the brain which may account for some neuroprotective effects of *l*-deprenyl need further

Table 2. Biochemical Actions of *l*-Deprenyl.

Long-Term Action
• Reduction of "oxidative stress"
  – increase in SOD activity
  – increase in catalase activity
  – suppression of GSSG

• Neuroprotective action (?)
  – clinical evidence
  – morphological evidence
  – neurotrophic action
  – NMDA-receptor-associated polyamine binding site

---

examination. We should consider examining the long-term effects of this drug and other MAO-B inhibitors on such factors as hydrogen peroxide detoxicating enzymes, reduction of oxygen-free radicals, nerve growth factor and N-methyl-D-aspartate (NMDA) receptor-associated poly-amine binding sites.

3.1. MAO-B Activity and Neurotoxicity

By using PEA as substrate, MAO-B is increased by approximately 25% in the striatum of PD patients [2]. This result has been confirmed in thrombocytes [15]. Furthermore, *l*-deprenyl increases superoxide dismu-tase (SOD) activity in rats [16]. Clow et al. [17] demonstrate that it is mostly the soluble form of CuZnSOD which is induced by *l*-deprenyl. Ceballos et al. [18] show that the gene for CuZnSOD is mainly ex-pressed in neuromelanin-containing pigmented neurons. This neuron type degenerates especially in PD and it is likely that these cells in particular need protection against oxidation. Physiological aging implies an increase in the MAO-B activity in different brain regions. Knoll et al. [19] as well as Milgram et al. [20] have suggested that *l*-deprenyl prolongs the life of rats – an effect which could be due to the inhibition of MAO-B and reduction of oxidative stress, since MAO-B can generate toxic radicals. The highest MAO-B activity is observed in PD patients, and those with Alzheimer's disease (AD) or amyotrophic lateral sclero-sis [21] in comparison to matched healthy age groups. Therefore, an inhibition of the enzyme could have a neuroprotective effect, especially since hydrogen peroxide significantly increases MAO-B activity (but not MAO-A activity) [8].

3.2. Amphetamine-Like Action

l-Deprenyl seems to exert an endogenous "amphetamine-like" tonic effect. Because some monoamines, e.g., PEA, are not catabolized by

COMT, inhibition of MAO-B leads to an accumulation of these amines in the brain [2]. Since PEA acts as a DA-releasing agent [3, 22], and in this way stimulates dopaminergic neurons, an endogenous "amphetamine-like" activity of *l*-deprenyl could contribute to its overall tonic effect. In addition, *l*-deprenyl is metabolized to *l*-amphetamine and *l*-metamphetamine [23] (for details see Chapter 10).

However, recent preclinical studies clearly show that *l*-deprenyl lacks amphetamine-like abuse potential (see Chapter 11), a finding that confirms and supports the clinical experience [24, 25] that it neither has potential for drug abuse nor causes withdrawal symptoms.

Nevertheless, new attempts are aimed at synthesizing compounds which are not metabolized to *l*-amphetamine and *l*-metamphetamine. Such compounds are now available: Ro-19-6327 (lazabemide) and MDL 72974 are selective and reversible MAO-B inhibitors which are now being clinically tested.

In addition, it has recently been shown in post-mortem studies that the number of neurons in the medial portion of the substantia nigra was greater in PD patients who had been treated with *l*-deprenyl plus L-dopa in comparison to those on L-dopa treatment alone. Furthermore, in the same study the number of Lewy bodies was lower in the group receiving the combined treatment [26]. Although this report has been criticised (e.g., some patients were on *l*-deprenyl only for a few months, there were some statistical problems, a lower L-dopa dose was used in the *l*-deprenyl group, and it was a retrospective study) the principal design, i.e., counting of surviving neurons post-mortem after patients were treated for years with various drug strategies, seems to be the only plausible way to prove or disprove a drug's neuroprotective value. Animal experiments and long-term clinical studies may be valuable to screen substances with neuroprotective potency, but a final proof will not be possible in living humans as long as there is no further progress in the development of biochemical analysis or imaging techniques.

3.3. Neuroprotective Action of l-Deprenyl after Chemical Intoxication

3.3.1. MPTP: MPTP (1-methyl-4-phenyl-1,2,3,6-tetrahydropyridine) causes parkinsonism in man [27] and animals [28]. Selective inhibitors of MAO-B like *l*-deprenyl or AGN 1135 block MPTP-induced dopaminergic neurotoxicity [29–30]. MPTP does not mirror the complete symptoms of human PD, but can be regarded as a model of akinesia and rigidity [31]. Compounds with similar chemical structure include both natural and synthetic products that are used for a variety of applications (e.g., paraquat, etc.). Although Barbeau et al. [32], in an epidemiological study performed in various regions of Quebec, Canada, have proven a correlation between the use and amount of pesticides and the

occurrence of PD, there is no real clinical and experimental evidence that environmental compounds cause PD. On the other hand, it cannot be precluded that environmental toxins structurally similar to MPTP could cause the disease. Therefore, it is important and relevant to study the mechanism of intoxication and to regard MPTP as a model that mirrors motor symptoms of the disease. As *l*-deprenyl blocks this type of chemical intoxication, it has to be regarded as a useful adjuvant in the treatment of (chemical) parkinsonism.

It has to be considered, however, that *l*-deprenyl inhibits MPTP-induced neurotoxicity, and does so not only when given prior to the toxic compound [14]. Tatton and Greenwood [32] recently reported that *l*-deprenyl is also able to inhibit the neurotoxicity of MPTP when administered days after the dopaminergic neurons have been lesioned. This finding suggests that this type of neuroprotection is independent of MAO-B activity. Rather, it can be related to *l*-deprenyl's action to stimulate certain neurotrophic factors and to take part in processes of regeneration. This hypothesis, however, has to be substantiated by experiments designed to elucidate possible direct or indirect effects of *l*-deprenyl on the synthesis of certain nerve growth factors.

3.3.2. 6-Hydroxydopamine: 6-Hydroxydopamine (6-OHDA) is thought to induce nigro-striatal dopaminergic neuronal lesions via generation of hydrogen peroxide and oxygen free radicals derived from it, such as superoxide and hydroxyl radicals [34–36], presumably initiated by a transition metal [37]. There is evidence that *l*-deprenyl protects from 6-OHDA lesions [38]. A single intraperitoneal injection of a high dose of *l*-deprenyl (5 mg/kg), as well as pretreatment during 3 weeks with a low dose (0.25 mg/kg) led to normalization of acetylcholine-liberation in slices of striatum from rats which had been treated with 6-OHDA. Clorgyline did not show this effect [39, 40; for review 14]. It was concluded that the neuroprotective effects of *l*-deprenyl were due to the compound's increased scavenger function.

l-Deprenyl's ability to counteract this toxicity has been attributed to its facilitating action on SOD-dismutase activity [16, 40]. This effect has been confirmed recently [41, 42, for review 14]. In addition, *l*-deprenyl enhances catalase activity [41]. These effects of *l*-deprenyl are independent from its MAO-B-inactivating capacity, because clorgyline, even in high doses, is not able to stimulate either SOD or catalase.

3.3.3. DSP-4: However, *l*-deprenyl at rather high non-selective doses of more than 10 mg (that are not used in clinical practice), like with MPTP or 6-OHDA, also protects against DSP-4 in mice [43]. DSP-4 is a neurotoxin that selectively degenerates noradrenergic fibers. Because MDL 72974, another selective MAO-B inhibitor, failed to block this neurotoxicity, it has been assumed that the amine-uptake-inhibiting properties of *l*-deprenyl might be responsible for this effect. In fact, DSP-4 (as well as 6-OHDA) are monoamines and *l*-deprenyl might act by preventing access by the toxin to the neuron. On the other hand, *l*-deprenyl might act via stimulation of certain nerve growth factors. This effect, however, might not be specific for a certain neurodegenerative disease.

3.4. Clinical Evidence for a Neuroprotective Role of l-Deprenyl

"Symptomatic effects" of a drug have to be separated from "neuroprotective actions". It seems possible that a neuroprotective action is still operative even when no significant improvement in symptoms is noted. There is such clinical evidence for *l*-deprenyl's neuroprotective action [44–47].

The extended patient life-expectancy, and the ability to postpone the start of L-dopa therapy for PD patients who were initially treated with *l*-deprenyl is ascribed by the authors of the DATATOP study [46, 47] to a slowing of the progression of the disease (see Chapter 15).

A major argument against the DATATOP [47] evaluation has been the short, 1-month wash-out period employed. It has been suggested that the symptomatic effects of *l*-deprenyl may still have been apparent [48]. There are, however, two arguments against this criticism: First, an increase in the concentration of amines is seen only after MAO inhibition of about 80% [49]. Conversely, the symptomatic effect of an MAO inhibitor is lost relatively rapidly as the enzyme recovers from total blockade. New protein synthesis to about 30–40% enzyme protein (enough active enzyme to sufficiently metabolize the amine) appears within the first 2 weeks after cessation of an irreversible MAO inhibitor. Second, urinary PEA, which accumulates by 20–90 fold after *l*-deprenyl, drops to normal excretion concentration within a few days after *l*-deprenyl withdrawal [50]. Therefore, the design of the DATATOP study seems adequate to mirror the biochemical requirements for substantiating this interpretation of the clinical result.

Furthermore, a protective role of *l*-deprenyl has recently been shown in mice [12]. When oxidative stress associated with an increased turnover of DA was provoked by injection of haloperidol (1 mg/kg), the concentration of oxidized glutathione (GSSG), as an index of changes in the redox state in the striatum tripled. Treatment with *l*-deprenyl (2.5 mg/kg) 18 hours before the haloperiydol injection suppressed this rise in GSSG by 71.9%.

In addition, recent post-mortem studies show that the ratio of GSH and GSSG in the substantia nigra of PD is shifted towards GSSG. This finding supports the hypothesis of accelerated oxidative stress in this brain area [51].

3.5. Inhibition of MAO-B and Possible Action on NMDA-Receptor-Associated Polyamine Binding Site

The neuroprotective effect of *l*-deprenyl may, however, also receive a contribution from the antagonistic occupation of the polyamine binding site of the glutamatergic NMDA receptor by N-acetylated polyamines.

NMDA receptor antagonists have been proposed as anti-parkinson drugs [52–54]. It is hypothesized that *l*-deprenyl exerts antagonistic effects on this binding site by significantly increasing the concentration of the highly selective MAO-B substrates N-acetylputrescine, N-acetylspermidine, and N-acetylspermine. The K_m-value of these polyamine derivatives is in the range of the K_m-value for PEA [14, 55]. Therefore, *l*-deprenyl might act neuroprotectively by helping to reduce excessive calcium influx into the neuronal cell.

3.6. MAO-B Inhibition and Synthesis of Nerve Growth Factor

MAO-B is mainly localized in the glia [7, 8]. Therefore, *l*-deprenyl enhances, at least to some extent, extraneuronal dopamine concentration. Recent studies by Furukawa et al. [56] point to the assumption that methylated catecholamines stimulate synthesis of nerve growth factor. *l*-Deprenyl might facilitate this process via MAO-B inhibition, especially as COMT activity is not changed in the various brain regions in patients with PD and AD. However, selective MAO-A inhibitors should be even more potent in this respect. This hypothesis is now under experimental investigation.

4. Concluding Remarks

The biochemical as well as pharmacological properties of *l*-deprenyl share features that may be unique to this compound. Therefore, it cannot be precluded that MAO-B inhibition *per se* is independent of any neuroprotective action and may only be of palliative therapeutic value. In addition, it is not at all certain that MAO-A inhibitors do not show neuroprotective action. Therefore, a comparison with other selective MAO-B inhibitors such as AGN 1135 (N-propargylamino-indane) [57, 58], Ro 19-6327 (N-[2-aminoethyl]-5-chloro-2-pyridine carboxamide) [59], and MDL 72974 (2, 4-fluorophenethyl)-3-fluoroallylamine [60], etc. is required to establish whether there is some intrinsic property of *l*-deprenyl which is not shared by other MAO-B (or even MAO-A) inhibitors.

The beneficial effect of *l*-deprenyl as a symptomatic and neuroprotective agent in neuro-degenerative disorders like PD [44–47] and AD [61–67] is due to its pharmacological actions and its biochemical effects.

Therefore, the therapeutic place and value of present and future MAO-B inhibitors will be evaluated by comparing these drugs with the biochemical and pharmacological properties of the "gold standard" of MAO-B inhibitors, *l*-deprenyl. If, however, a neuroprotective action can be fully established, the early *l*-deprenyl treatment of patients with neurodegenerative disorders is advocated.

References

[1] Birkmayer W, Riederer P, Youdim MBH, Linauer W. The potentiation of the anti-aki-netic effect after L-dopa treatment by an inhibitor of MAO-B, Deprenyl. J Neural Transm, 1975; 36: 303–326.

[2] Riederer P, Jellinger K, Seemann D. Monoamine oxidase and parkinsonism. In: Tipton KF, Dostert P, Strolin-Benedetti M, editors. Monoamine Oxidase and Disease. London: Academic Press, 1984: 403–415.

[3] Birkmayer W, Riederer P, Ambrozi L, Youdim MBH. Implications of combined treatment with "Madopar" and *l*-deprenyl in Parkinson's disease – A long-term study. Lancet, 1977; i: 439–443.

[4] Paterson IA, Juorio AV, Boulton AA. Possible mechanism of action of deprenyl in parkinsonism. Lancet, 1992; i: 183.

[5] Paterson IA, Berry MD, Juorio AV. (−)Deprenyl and dopamine transmission: electrophysiological recordings in the rat caudate nucleus. Soc Neurosci Abstr. In press.

[6] Levitt P, Pintar JE, Breakfield XO. Immunocytochemical demonstration of monoamine oxidase B in brain astrocytes and serotoninergic neurons. Proc Natl Acad Sci USA, 1982; 79: 6385–6389.

[7] Konradi C, Kornhuber J, Frölich L, Fritze J, Heinsen H, Beckmann H, Schulz E, Riederer P. Demonstration of monoamine oxidase-A and -B in the human brainstem by a histochemical technique. Neurosci, 1989; 33: 383–400.

[8] Konradi C, Riederer P, Heinsen H. Histochemistry of MAO subtypes in the brainstem of humans: a relation to the radical hypothesis of Parkinson's disease? In: Przuntek H, Riederer P, editors. Early Diagnosis and Preventive Therapy in Parkinson's Disease. Key Topics in Brain Research. New York, Vienna: Springer-Verlag, 1989: 243–248.

[9] Melamed E. Chronic levodopa suppresses its own utilization in striatum. In: Rinne UK, Nagatsu T, Horowski R, editors. How to Proceed Today in Treatment. Proceedings International Workshop Berlin Parkinson's Disease. Medicom Europe, 1991: 206–215.

[10] Rinne UK. Early use of dopamine agonist in the treatment of Parkinson's disease. In: Rinne UK, Nagatsu T, Horowski R, editors. How to Proceed Today in Treatment. Proceedings International Workshop Berlin Parkinson's Disease. Medicom Europe, 1991: 326–336.

[11] Cohen G. Monoamine oxidase, hydrogen peroxide, and Parkinson's disease. In: Yahr MD, Bergmann KJ, editors. Advances in Neurology. New York: Raven Press, 1986: 119–125.

[12] Cohen G, Spina MB. Deprenyl suppresses the oxidant stress associated with increased dopamine turnover. Ann Neurol, 1989; 26: 689–690.

[13] Fornstedt B, Brun A, Rosengren E, Carlsson A. The apparent autoxidation rate of catechols in dopamine-rich regions of human brains increases with the degree of depigmentation of substantia nigra. J Neural Transm [PD Sect], 1989; 1: 279–295.

[14] Gerlach M, Riederer P, Youdim MBH. The molecular pharmacology of *l*-deprenyl. Europ J Pharmacol – Mol Pharmacol Sect, 1992; 226: 97–108.

[15] Jarman J, Glover V, Sandler M, Turjanski N, Stern G. Platelet monoamine oxidase B activity in Parkinson's disease: A re-evaluation. J Neural Transm [PDSect]. In press.

[16] Knoll J. The striatal dopamine dependency of life span in male rats. Longevity study with (−)deprenyl. Mech Ageing Devel, 1988; 46: 237–262.

[17] Clow A, Hussain T, Glover V, Sandler M, Dexter DT, Walker M. (−)-Deprenyl can induce soluble superoxide dismutase in rat striata. J Neural Transm, 1991; 86: 77–80.

[18] Ceballos I, Lafon M, Javoy Agid F, Hirsch E, Nicole A, Simet P, Agid Y. Superoxide dismutase and Parkinson's disease. Lancet, 1990; i: 1035–1036.

[19] Knoll J, Dallo J, Yen TT. Striatal dopamine, sexual activity and lifespan. Longevity of rats treated with (−)deprenyl. Life Sci, 1989; 45: 525–531.

[20] Milgram NW, Racine RJ, Nellis P, Mendonca A, Ivy GO. Maintenance on l-deprenyl prolongs life in aged male rats. Life Sci, 1990; 47: 415–420.

[21] Aquilonius SM, Jossan SS, Ekblom JG, Askmark H, Gillberg PG. Increased binding of l-deprenyl in spinal cords from patients with amyotrophic lateral sclerosis as demonstrated by autoradiography. J Neural Transm [Gen Sect]. 1992; 89: 111–122.

[22] Paterson IA, Juorio AV, Boulton AA. 2-Phenylethylamine: a modulator of catecholamine transmission in the mammalian central nervous system? J Neurochem, 1990; 55: 1827.

[23] Reynolds GP, Riederer P, Sandler M, Jellinger K, Seemann D. Amphetamine and 2-phenylethylamine in post-mortem parkinsonian brain after (−)deprenyl administration. J Neural Transm, 1978; 43: 271–277.

[24] Elsworth JD, Sandler M, Lees AJ, Ward C, Stern GM. The contribution of amphetamine metabolites of (−)-deprenyl to its antiparkinsonian properties. J Neural Transm, 1982; 54: 105–110.

[25] Birkmayer W, Riederer P. Die Parkinson-Krankheit. Biochemie, Klinik, Therapie, 2nd ed. Vienna, New York: Springer Verlag, 1985.

[26] Rinne JO, Röyttä M, Paljärvi L, Rummukainen J, Rinne UK. Selegiline (deprenyl) treatment and death of nigral neurons in Parkinson's disease. Neurol, 1991; 41: 859–861.

[27] Davis GC, Williams AC, Markey SP, Ebert MH, Calne ED, Reichert C, Kopin IJ. Chronic parkinsonism secondary to intravenous injection of meperidine analogues. Psychiat Res, 1979; 1: 249–254.

[28] Burns RS, Chiuen CC, Markey SP, Ebert MH, Jacobowitz D, Kopin I. A primate model of Parkinsonism: selective destruction of dopaminergic neurons in the pars compacta of the substantia nigra by N-methyl-4-phenyl-1,2,3,6-tetrahydropyridine. Proc Natl Acad Sci USA, 1983; 80: 4544–4551.

[29] Heikkila RE, Manzino L, Cabbat FS, Duvoisin RC. Protection against the dopaminergic neurotoxicity of 1-methyl-4-phenyl-1,2,3,6-tetrahydropyridine by monoamine oxidase inhibitors. Nature, 1984; 311: 467–469.

[30] Riederer P, Youdim MBH. Monoamine oxidase activity and monoamine metabolism in brains of parkinsonian patients treated with l-deprenyl. J Neurochem, 1986; 46: 1359–1365.

[31] Gerlach M, Riederer P, Przuntek H, Youdim MBH. MPTP mechanisms of neurotoxicity and their implications for Parkinson's disease. Europ J Pharmacol – Mol Pharmacol Sect, 1991; 208: 273–286.

[32] Barbeau A, Roy M, Cloutier T, Plasse L, Paris S. Environmental and genetic factors in the etiology of Parkinson's disease. In: Yahr MD, Bergmann KJ, editors. Advances in Neurology. New York: Raven Press, 1986: 299–306.

[33] Tatton WG, Greenwood CE. Rescue of dying neurons: a new action for deprenyl in MPTP parkinsonism. J Neurosci Res, 1991; 30: 666–672.

[34] Heikkila RE, Cohen G. Further studies on generation of hydrogen peroxide by 6-hydroxydopamine: potentiation by ascorbic acid. Mol Pharmacol, 1972; 8: 241.

[35] Sachs CH, Jonsson G. Mechanism of action of 6-hydroxydopamine. Pharmacol 1975; 24: 1.

[36] Graham DG. Oxidative pathways for catecholamines in the genesis of neuromelanin and cytotoxic quinones. Mol Pharmacol, 1978; 14: 333–343.

[37] Ben-Shachar D, Eshel G, Finberg JPM, Youdim MBH. The iron chelator desferrioxamine (Desferal) retards 6-hydroxydopamine-induced degeneration of nigrostriatal dopamine neurons. J Neurochem, 1991; 56: 1441–1447.

[38] Knoll J. The possible mechanism of action of (−)deprenyl in Parkinson's disease. J Neural Transm, 1978; 43: 177–198.

[39] Knoll J. Striatal dopamine, ageing and (−)deprenyl. Jugoslav Physiol Pharmacol Acta, 1986; 22: 261–273.

[40] Knoll J. R-(−)-deprenyl (selegiline, Movergan®) facilitates the activity of the nigrostriatal dopaminergic neuron. J Neural Transm [Suppl], 1987; 25: 45–66.

[41] Carillo MC, Kanai S, Nokubu M, Kitani K. (−)Deprenyl induces activities of both superoxide dismutase and catalase but not of glutathione peroxidase in the striatum of young male rats. Life Sci, 1991; 48: 517–521.

[42] Clow A, Hussain T, Glover V, Sandler M, Walker M, Dexter D. Pergolide can induce soluble superoxide dismutase in rat striata. J Neural Transm [Gen Sect]. 1991; 86: 77–80.

[43] Finnegan KT, Skratt JJ, Irwin I, DeLanney LE, Langston JW. Protection against DSP-4-induced neurotoxicity by deprenyl is not related to its inhibition of MAO B. Europ J Pharmacol, 1990; 184: 119–126.

[44] Birkmayer W, Knoll J, Riederer P, Youdim MBH. (−)Deprenyl leads to prolongation of L-dopa efficacy in Parkinson's disease. Modern Problems of Pharmacopsychiatry, Vol 19. Basel: Karger, 1983: 170–176.

[45] Birkmayer W, Knoll J, Riederer P, Youdim MBH, Hars V, Marton J. Increased life expectancy resulting from addition of l-deprenyl to Madopar® treatment in Parkinson's disease: a long-term study. J Neural Transm, 1985; 64: 113–117.

[46] Tetrud JW, Langston JW. The effect of deprenyl (selegiline) on the natural history of Parkinson's disease. Science, 1989; 245: 519–522.

[47] DATATOP (Parkinson Study Group). Effect of deprenyl on the progression of disability in early Parkinson's disease. N Engl J Med, 1989; 321: 1364–1371.

[48] Landau WM. Clinical neuromythology IX. Pyramid scale in the bucket shop: DATATOP bottoms out. Neurol, 1990; 40: 1337–1339.

[49] Green R, Youdim MBH. Use of a behavioral model to study the action of monoamine oxidase inhibition in vivo. In: Monoamine Oxidase and Its Inhibition (Ciba Foundation Symposium 39). Amsterdam: Elsevier, 1976: 231–246.

[50] Elsworth JD, Glover V, Reynolds GP, Sandler M, Lees AJ, Phuapradit P, et al. Deprenyl administration in man; a selective monoamine oxidase B inhibitor without the "cheese effect". Psychopharmacol, 1978; 57: 33–38.

[51] Sofic E, Lange KW, Jellinger K, Riederer P. Reduced and oxidized glutathione in the substantia nigra in Parkinson's disease. Neurosci Lett. 1992; 142: 128–130.

[52] Olney JW, Price MT, Labruyere J, Salles KS, Friedrich G, Mueller M, et al. Anti-parkinsonian agents are phencyclidine agonists and N-methyl-aspartate antagonists. Europ J Pharmacol, 1987; 142: 319–325.

[53] Kornhuber J, Bormann J, Retz W, Hübers M, Riederer P. Memantine displaces [^{3}H]MK-801 at therapeutic concentrations in postmortem human frontal cortex. Europ J Pharmacol, 1989; 166: 589–590.

[54] Kornhuber J, Bormann J, Hübers M, Rusche K, Riederer P. Effects of the 1-aminoadamantanes at the MK-801-binding site of the NMDA-receptor-gated ion channel: a human postmortem brain study. Europ J Pharmacol – Mol Pharmacol Sect, 1991; 206: 297–300.

[55] Youdim MBH, Ben-Shachar D, Riederer P. The role of monoamine oxidase, iron-melanin interaction and intracellular calcium in Parkinson's disease. J Neural Transm [Suppl], 1990; 32: 239.

[56] Furukawa S, Shinoda I, Furukawa Y. Regulatory mechanisms of nerve growth factor synthesis in vitro. Human Cell, 1989; 6 (2): 137–142.

[57] Finberg JPM, Sabbagh A, Youdim MBH. Pharmacology of selective propargyl "suicide" inhibitors of monoamine oxidase. In: Usdin E, Sourkes TL, Youdim MBH, editors. Enzymes and Neurotransmitters in Mental Disease. Chichester: Wiley, 1980: 205.

[58] Kalir A, Sabbagh A, Youdim MBH. Selective acetylenic "suicide" and reversible inhibitors of monoamine oxidase types A and B. Br J Pharmacol, 1981; 73: 55–62.

[59] Da Prada M, Kettler R, Keller HH, Cesura Am, Richard JG, Marti JS et al. From moclobemide to Ro 19-6327 and Ro 41-1049: the development of a new class of reversible, selective MAO-A and MAO-B inhibitors. J Neural Transm [Suppl], 1990; 29: 279–292.

[60] Zerika M, Fozard JR, Dudley MW, Bey P, McDonald IA, Palfreyman MG. MDL 72974: a potent and selective enzyme-activated irreversible inhibitor of monoamine oxidase type B with potential for use in Parkinson's disease. J Neural Transm (PD Sect.), 1989; 1: 243–254.

[61] Tariot PN, Cohen RM, Sunderland T, Newhouse PA, Yount D, Mellow AM et al. l-(−)Deprenyl in Alzheimer's disease. Arch Gen Psychiat, 1987a; 44: 427–433.

[62] Tariot PN, Sunderland T, Weingartner H, Murphy DL, Welkowitz JA, Thompson K et al. Cognitive effect of l-deprenyl in Alzheimer disease. Psychopharmacol, 1987b; 91: 489–495.

[63] Tariot PN, Sunderland T, Cohen RM, Newhouse PA, Mueller EA, Murphy DL. Tranylcypromine compared with *l*-deprenyl in Alzheimer disease. J Clin Psychopharmacol, 1988; 8: 23–27.
[64] Martini E, Pataky J, Szilagyi K, Venter V. Brief information on an early phase-II study with (−)deprenyl in demented patients. Pharmacopsychiat, 1987; 20: 256–257.
[65] Piccinin GL, Finali GC, Piccirilli M. Neuropsychological effects of *l*-deprenyl in Alzheimer's type dementia. Clin Neuropharmacol, 1990; 13: 147–163.
[66] Mangoni A, Grassi MP, Frattoli L, Piolti R, Bassi S, Motta A et al. Effects of a MAO-B inhibitor in the treatment of Alzheimer disease. Eur Neurol, 1991; 31: 100–107.
[67] Goad DL, Davis CM, Leim P, Fuselier CC, McCormack JR, Olsen KM. The use of selegiline in Alzheimer's patients with behavior problems. J Clin Psychiat, 1991; 52: 342–345.

Inhibitors of Monoamine Oxidase B
Pharmacology and Clinical Use in Neurodegenerative Disorders
ed. by I. Szelenyi
© 1993 Birkhäuser Verlag Basel/Switzerland

APPENDIX I
Chemical Structures and Pharmacological Features of MAO-B Inhibitors

W. Paul and I. Szelenyi

1	Irreversible Inhibitors
1.1	Acetylenic Inhibitors
1.2	Allylamine Derivatives
1.3	Cyclopropylamines
1.4	Oxazolidinones
1.5	Hydrazines
2	Reversible Inhibitors
2.1	Harmala Alkaloids
2.2	Endogenous Inhibitors
2.3	Phenylethylamines
2.4	Morpholinoethylamine Derivatives
3	Chemical and Pharmacological Data of Selected MAO-B Inhibitors
3.1	Irreversible Inhibitors
3.1.1	Acetylenic Inhibitors
3.1.1.1	Pargyline
3.1.1.2	Selegiline
3.1.1.3	Desmethyl-Selegiline
3.1.1.4	Chinoin-175 (Fludepryl)
3.1.1.5	TZ 650
3.1.1.6	U 1424
3.1.1.7	AGN-1133
3.1.1.8	AGN-1135
3.1.2	Allylamine Derivatives
3.1.2.1	MDL 72145
3.1.2.2	MDL 72638
3.1.2.3	MDL 72974
3.1.3	Cyclopropylamines
3.1.3.1	LY-54761
3.1.4	Oxazolidinones
3.1.4.1	MD 780236
3.1.4.2	Almoxatone
3.2	Reversible Inhibitors
3.2.1	Phenylethylamines
3.2.1.1	p-CMPEA
3.2.2	Morpholinoethylamine Derivatives
3.2.2.1	Ro 16-6491
3.2.2.2	Lazabemide (Ro 19-6327)
4	Tables
	References

The purpose of this appendix is to give the reader a short summary overview of the present state of some selected MAO-B inhibitors.

Although the number of MAO-B inhibitors is limited in comparison to other drug classes, we thought it beneficial to further reduce their number in this appendix; one of the selection criteria was the chemical structure. Our intention was to present at least one compound of a given chemical class. Beside relevant chemical information (e.g., international nonproprietory name (INN), synonyms, chemical name, structure, molecular weight), an effort was made to briefly describe the pharmacological properties of the compound. Chemical names have been given according to the 9th Collective Index (9CI) of Chemical Abstracts. Furthermore, we have included the readily available information about the development stages of the compounds. If a MAO-B inhibitor has already been released, the countries in which it is on the market have also been given (for a detailed description of the chemical and pharmacological properties of the particular compounds see also Chapters 4 and 6).

1. Irreversible Inhibitors

Four chemical types of so-called suicide inhibitors (see below in 1.1; 1.2; 1.3; 1.5) have been described for MAO-B thus far. Oxazolidinones are only partly irreversible inhibitors.

1.1. Acetylenic Inhibitors

Following an instantaneous reversible phase, the interaction between the FAD of the enzyme and the compound results in an irreversible inhibition. The classical representative of this class is selegiline. Some analogues are also described.

1.2. Allylamine Derivatives

Intensive structure-enzyme inhibitory activity studies led to interesting, potent, and selective inhibitors of MAO-B (see below in 3.1.2).

1.3. Cyclopropylamines

Tranylcypromine is another non-selective irreversible inhibitor that is unsuitable for parkinsonian therapy. Some cyclopropylamine analogues have been synthetized by E. Lilly (see LY 54761).

1.4. Oxazolidinones

Oxazolidinone derivatives such as MD 240931 and MD 780236 are reversible inhibitors in *vivo* and *ex vivo*. However, they inhibit the enzyme irreversibly under *in vitro* conditions. Almoxatone is apparently a fully reversible inhibitor *ex vivo*. Some pyrido-[1,2-alpha]pyrimidines containing 3-amino-2-oxazolidinone moiety display irreversible MAO-inhibitory activity [1].

1.5. Hydrazines

Iproniazid was the first MAO inhibitor to be used in the therapy of depression. Phenelzine and phenylhydrazine have some effects on MAO-B, but they cannot be used in the therapy of Parkinson's disease (PD) due to their nonspecificity, higher affinity to MAO-A, and their side-effects.

2. Reversible Inhibitors

2.1. Harmala Alkaloids

Banisterine (harmine) was the first MAO inhibitor used in the therapy of PD, although harmine and harmaline are selective and potent inhibitors of MAO-A and have a very low affinity to MAO-B. A hallucinogenic drink known in the western Amazon region contains these alkaloids. They have no therapeutic use today.

2.2. Endogenous Inhibitors

This group of inhibitors is described in Chapter 8.

2.3. Phenylethylamines

Structural changes to PEA, the preferential substrate of MAO-B, result not only in enzyme-inhibiting compounds, but also in substances with different effects on MAO-A and MAO-B. PEA with a methyl group in the alpha position is a selective MAO-A inhibitor. *p*-CMPEA has, however, higher affinity for MAO-B.

2.4. Morpholinoethylamine Derivatives

Two MAO-B inhibitors belong to this chemical class. Ro 16-6491 is chemically related to moclobemide, a potent MAO-A inhibitor, and is the latter's metabolite. A slight structural modification of Ro 16-6491 has led to lazabemide (Ro 19-6327), the most potent and selective MAO-B inhibitor developed so far.

3. Chemical and Pharmacological Data of Selected MAO-B inhibitors

In the following, we concisely present selected chemical, pharmacological and clinical results obtained with some MAO-B inhibitors. In addition, we summarize the enzyme inhibitory activity of some selected compounds evaluated *in vitro* and *in vivo* (Tables 1 and 2 at the end of the appendix).

It must be remembered that IC_{50}-values of irreversible MAO-B inhibitors are not really characteristic of the actual inhibitory activity of a given compound (for details see Chapters 4 and 6). Asterisks (∗) indicate chiral centers in the molecule. For abbreviations see the "List of Abbreviations."

3.1. Irreversible Inhibitors

3.1.1. Acetylenic Inhibitors

3.1.1.1. Pargyline *(INN)*

Benzenemethanamine, N-methyl-N-2-propynyl- (9CI)

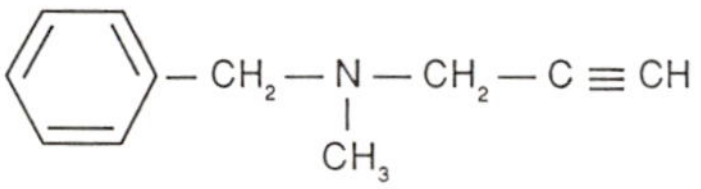

$$
\langle\!\!\langle \rangle\!\!\rangle - CH_2 - N - CH_2 - C \equiv CH
$$
$$
\qquad\qquad\qquad\;\; |
$$
$$
\qquad\qquad\qquad\; CH_3
$$

Synonyms

Pargylamine
NSC-43798
Eutonyl
A-19120

Derivative

Hydrochloride: $C_{11}H_{13}N \cdot HCl$ Mol. wt. 155.71

Pharmacology and therapy. Pargyline is a mixed-type inhibitor with relatively higher affinity to MAO-B (see Table 1) that inhibits metabolic changes induced by MPTP [2]. It is occasionally used in the treatment of moderate to severe hypertension, although less toxic compounds should be preferred.

Originator: Abbott (USA)

Development stage	Brand (Trade) name	Distributor	Country
Launched	Eudatine	Abbott (USA)	Belgium
Launched	Eutonyl	Abbott (USA)	UK
Launched	Eutonyl	Abbott (USA)	USA

3.1.1.2. Selegiline (INN)

Benzeneethanamine, N,α-dimethyl-N-2-propynyl-, (R)- (9CI)

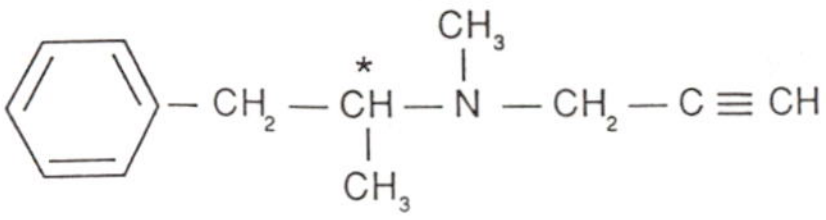

Synonyms

L-Deprenyl
L-Deprenalin
L-Deprenil
E 250

Derivative

Hydrochloride: $C_{13}H_{17}H \cdot HCl$ Mol. wt. 223.75

Pharmacology and therapy. Selective irreversible MAO-B inhibitor; selectivity (MAO-A/MAO-B) measured in rat brain: 400 [3]. Judged by its preclinical profile, selegiline is more than a simple MAO-B inhibitor; it has both MAO-B-dependent and MAO-B-independent properties. Inhibition of DA and PEA metabolism, reduction of ROS, NH_3 and aldehyde generation are typically MAO-B-dependent effects. On the other hand, effects such as enhancement of SOD and catalase activity, and reduction of neuromelanin synthesis are not dependent on the drug's MAO-B inhibitory activity (see Chapters 6–9, 13). Selegiline has been registered for the treatment of PD as an adjunct to L-Dopa (see Chapters 13–15) in many countries. Due to its multifaceted pharmacological profile, selegiline could also be used in the management of other neurological disorders (e.g., Alzheimer's disease, depression) (see Chapters 16, 17).

Originator: Chinoin Pharmaceuticals (Hungary)

Development stage	Brand (Trade) name	Distributor	Country
Launched	Eldepryl	Reckitt and Collman	Australia
Launched	Jumex	Splichal	Austria
Launched	Jumex	Armstrong	Argentina
Launched	Eldepryl	ASTA Medica	Belgium
Launched	Jumex	Chinoin	Bulgaria
Launched	Eldepryl	Deprenyl Research	Canada
Launched	Jumex	Chinoin	Cuba
Launched	Jumex	Chinoin	Czechoslovakia

Launched	Jumex	Star	Cyprus
Launched	Eldepryl	Ercopharm AS	Denmark
Launched	Jumex	Alpha-Chem	Egypt
Launched	Eldepryl	Farmos	Finland
Launched	Deprenyl	Shering Plough	France
Launched	Movergan	ASTA Medica	Germany
Launched	Pracythol	Sanofi Greece	Greece
Launched	Jumex	Star	Hong-Kong
Launched	Jumex	Chinoin	Hungary
Launched	Eldepryl	Themis	India
Launched	Eldepryl	Britannia	Ireland
Launched	Jumex	Dexxon	Israel
Launched	Jumex	Chiesi	Italy
Launched	Jumex	Medimpex West Indies	Jamaica
Launched	Jumex	Chinoin	Kenya
Launched	Eldepryl	ASTA Medica	Luxemburg
Launched	Jumex	Pahang Ph.	Malaysia
Launched	Jumex	Maurique Caprilles	Netherlands Antilles
Launched	Eldepryl	Pharm. Dagra	The Netherlands
Launched	Eldepryl	Reckitt and Collmann	New Zealand
Launched	Eldepryl	Hydropharma	Norway
Launched	Jumex	Sandoz	Portugal
Launched	Jumex	Shaheen	Pakistan
Launched	Jumex	Chinoin	Poland
Launched	Jumex	Sime Darby	Singapore
Launched	Eldepryl	Reckitt and Collmann	South Africa
Launched	Plurimen	Lab. Sarget	Spain
Launched	Eldepryl	Farmos Group AB	Sweden
Launched	Jumexal	Labatec	Switzerland
Launched	Jumex	Chinoin	Syria
Launched	Jumexal	Taiwan Major Chemical	Taiwan
Launched	Jumex	Medline	Thailand
Launched	Eldepryl	Britannia	UK
Launched	Jumex	Libra	Uruguay
Launched	Eldepryl	Sandoz	USA
Launched	Jumex	Chinoin	CIS*
Launched	Juprenyl	Zorka	Yugoslavia
under review	Jumex	Chinoin	Iran
under review	Jumex	Fujimoto	Japan
under review	Jumex	Imarsel	Nigeria
under review	Jumex	Cuvest	Philippines
under review	Jumex	Polinac	Venezuela

*Commonwealth of Independent States (the former Soviet Union)

3.1.1.3. Desmethyl-Selegiline

Benzeneethanamine, α-methyl-N-2-propynyl- (9CI)

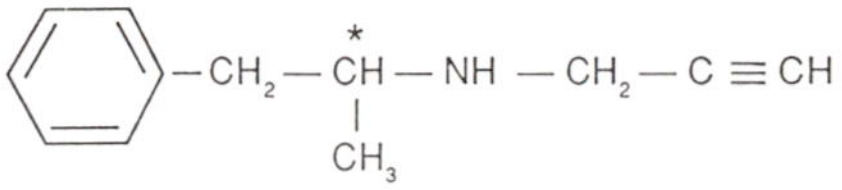

$$\text{—CH}_2\text{—}\overset{*}{\text{CH}}\text{—NH—CH}_2\text{—C}\equiv\text{CH}$$
$$\underset{\text{CH}_3}{|}$$

Synonyms

Nordeprenyl
Propargylamphetamine

Derivative

Hydrochloride: $C_{12}H_{15}N\cdot HCl$ Mol. wt. 209.74

Pharmacology and therapy. The desmethyl metabolite of selegiline is an irreversible inhibitor of MAO-B and nearly equipotent to the parent compound after multiple oral administration in rats [4]. Repeated oral administration of the desmethyl metabolite to conscious rats resulted in changes in the cortical electrical activity which were similar or even identical to those observed in animals treated with selegiline [5].

3.1.1.4. Chinoin-175

Benzeneethanamine, 4-fluoro-N,α-dimethyl-N-2-propynyl- (9CI)

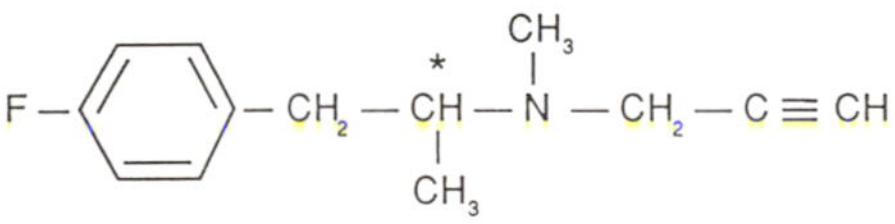

$$\text{F—}\quad\text{—CH}_2\text{—}\overset{*}{\text{CH}}\text{—}\overset{\overset{\text{CH}_3}{|}}{\text{N}}\text{—CH}_2\text{—C}\equiv\text{CH}$$
$$\underset{\text{CH}_3}{|}$$

Synonyms

Fludepryl
SR-96516 A

$C_{13}H_{16}FN$ Mol. wt. 206.54

Pharmacology and therapy. The *p*-fluoro-substituted derivative of selegiline shows about the same selectivity for MAO-B as selegiline [6]. Its pharmacological profile might be slightly different from that of selegiline (see Chapter 4). It has recently been demonstrated that fludepryl significantly decreased the number of neuromelanin granules in neurocytes of the SN in aged rats [7].

Originator: Chinoin Pharmaceuticals (Hungary)

3.1.1.5. TZ 650

Benzeneethanamine, N-Methyl-N-2-propynyl (9CI)

$$\text{Ph} - CH_2 - CH_2 - \underset{\underset{CH_3}{|}}{N} - CH_2 - C \equiv CH$$

$C_{12}H_{15}N$ Mol. wt. 173.28

Pharmacology and therapy. TZ 650 is a relatively selective MAO-B inhibitor [8], although it is structurally closely related to selegiline. The drug potentiates the response to tyramine ("cheese effect") [9].

3.1.1.6. U 1424

2-Furanethanamine, N,α-dimethyl-N-2-propynyl- (9CI)

$$\text{Furyl} - CH_2 - \overset{*}{C}H - \underset{\underset{CH_3}{|}}{N} - CH_2 - C \equiv CH$$
$$\underset{CH_3}{|}$$

Derivative

Hydrochloride: $C_{11}H_{15}NO \cdot HCl$ Mol. wt. 213.73

Pharmacology and therapy. U 1424 is a relatively selective MAO-B inhibitor [8], but it potentiates tyramine response *in vitro* [9].

3.1.1.7. AGN-1133

1H-Inden-1-amine, 2,3-dihydro-N-methyl-N-2-propynyl- (9CI)

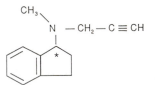

Synonym

Indanamin
SU-11739
J-508

Derivative

Hydrochloride: $C_{13}H_{15}N \cdot HCl$ Mol. wt. 221.58

Pharmacology and therapy. Although its MAO-B inhibitory activity is high, the drug's selectivity is very low (MAO-A/MAO-B: 0.4–1.0) [10, 11]. AGN-1133, given to mice prior to the administration of MPTP, protected against the neurotoxic effect of MPTP [12], thus again demonstrating its MAO-B inhibitory activity. It potentiates tyramine-induced hypertension [9].

Originator: Nicholas Kiwi (Australia)

3.1.1.8. AGN-1135

1H-Inden-1-amine, 2,3dihydro-N-2-propynyl- (9CI)

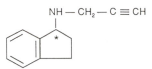

Derivative

Hydrochloride: $C_{12}H_{13}N \cdot HCl$ Mol. wt. 207.57

Pharmacology and therapy. The desmethyl analogue of AGN-1133 is a highly selective MAO-B inhibitor (MAO-A/MAO-B: 25–67 in the rat brain; 400 in the human frontal cortex) ([10]; Chapter 9). MCTP-induced neurotoxicity was prevented in mice [13]. At doses selective for MAO-B inhibition AGN-1135 did not potentiate tyramine response in the rat vas deferens *in vitro* [14]. AGN-1135 enhanced neither the potassium- nor the tyramine-induced catecholamine release from PC12 cells [15]. In contrast, potentiation of tyramine-induced response was observed using rabbit pulmonary artery strip [9]. In the cat, the pressure response to tyramine was not potentiated at the dose (1.0 mg/kg i.v.) which caused a near total inhibition of liver and brain MAO-B [16]. AGN-1135 could be a useful drug in potentiating the action of L-dopa in PD. The compound probably does not elicit the cheese effect; however this has not been clinically tested yet.

Originator: Nicholas Kiwi (Australia)

3.1.2. Allylamine Derivatives

3.1.2.1. MDL 72145

Benzeneethanamine, β-(fluoromethylene)-3,4-dimethoxy-, (E)- (9CI)

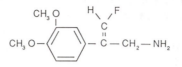

Derivative

Hydrochloride: $C_{11}H_{14}FNO_2 \cdot HCl$ Mol. wt. 247.70

Pharmacology and therapy. Selective, irreversible MAO-B inhibitor (MAO-A/MAO-B about 3 *in vitro* and *ex vivo*) [17, 18]. Higher selectivity (MAO-A/MAO-B: 43–133) was found by others ([19]; see Chapter 9). In contrast to selegiline (2.5–30 mg/kg, i.p.), MDL 72145 (0.5–10 mg/kg, i.p.) was inactive in the "behavioral despair" swim test in mice. It was also inactive in rats lesioned unilaterally in the ascending nigrostriatal bundle with 6-OHDA [19]. Inhibition of MPTP- but not MPP^+-induced neurotoxicity was observed [21, 22]. In humans, an oral dose of 16 mg totally inhibited MAO-B in platelets without potentiating the cardiovascular effects of oral tyramine (100 mg) [23]. Apparently, MDL 72145 is a pure MAO-B inhibitor without the additional effects of selegiline. Therefore, it can be considered a reliable tool for exploring the functional importance of MAO-B. Additionally, MDL 72145 is a potent inhibitor of SSAO. The physiological importance of SSAO and the significance of its inhibition by drugs is still unknown [18].

Originator: Marion Merrell Dow (USA)

Development stage: Clinical phase

3.1.2.2. MDL 72638

2-Propen-1-amine, 2-(2,4-dichlorophenoxy)methyl)-3-fluoro-, (Z)- (9CI)

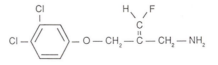

$C_{10}H_{10}Cl_2FNO$ Mol. wt. 250.11

Pharmacology and therapy. MDL 72638 is a clorgyline analogue which selectively inhibits MAO-B (MAO-A/MAO-B about 20) [24].

Originator: Marion Merrell Dow (USA)

3.1.2.3. *MDL 72974*

Benzenebutanamine, 4-fluoro-β-(fluoromethylene)-, (E)- (9CI)

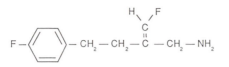

Synonyms
MDL 72974A (HCl)

Derivative

Hydrochloride: $C_{11}H_{13}F_2N \cdot HCl$ Mol. wt. 233.69

Pharmacology and therapy. MDL 72974A is the hydrochloride salt of MDL 72974. It is a highly selective irreversible inhibitor of MAO-B (MAO-A/MAO-B: 190) [25]. Its selectivity has been confirmed *in vivo*: after oral administration to rats, the brain MAO-B was inhibited by an ED_{50} of 0.18 mg/kg (MAO-A by an ED_{50} of 8.0 mg/kg) [25]. MAO-B selective doses protected mice and monkeys from neurodegeneration induced by MPTP [23, 25], but not against the neurotoxic effect of DSP-4 [26]. In contrast to selegiline, MDL 72974A has no amine-releasing or uptake inhibitory effects [27]. MDL 72974 did not significantly potentiate the cardiovascular effects of tyramine (given i.d.) in anesthetized rats [25]. In rats, it failed to generalize to *d*-amphetamine in high oral doses [28]. Judging from the preclinical data, MDL 72974A apparently is a selective MAO-B inhibitor without the additional, non-MAO-B-dependent actions of selegiline.

In a double-blind, randomized, placebo-controlled, healthy volunteer study, orally administered MDL 72974A was well tolerated in a range from 0.1 to 12 mg as a single dose (5 volunteers/dose [29, 30]. Only two cases of headache (one following the administration of 2 mg and one after giving 8 mg) were reported. There were no significant treatment-related changes in cardiovascular parameters [30]. Dose-dependent inhibition of platelet MAO-B activity was observed with a return to baseline values by day 14 [29]. Elimination half-life of the parent compound was 51 min.

MDL 72974A is a potent, irreversible inhibitor of MAO-B in man and can be useful as an adjuvant to L-dopa in the therapy of PD.

Interestingly, MDL 72974A is the most potent SSAO inhibitor that has been described thus far [31]. (See MDL 72145.)

Originator: Marion Merrell Dow (USA)

Development stage: Clinical phase

3.1.3. Cyclopropylamines

3.1.3.1. LY-54761

Ethanone, 2-(cyclopropylamino)-1-phenyl- (9CI)

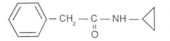

$C_{11}H_{13}NO$ Mol. wt. 175.22

Pharmacology and therapy. LY-54761 is a rather poorly selective MAO-B inhibitor, both *in vitro* (MAO-A/MAO-B: 1.0–1.6) and *in vivo* (MAO-A/MAO-B: 1.3) [32, 33]. Partial generalization was observed in rats trained on *d*-amphetamine [34].

Originator: E. Lilly (USA)

3.1.4. Oxazolidinones

3.1.4.1. MD 780236

2-Oxazolidinone, 3-(4-((3-chlorophenyl) methoxy) phenyl)-5-((methylamino)methyl)(+ −) (9CI)

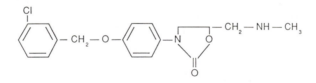

Derivative

Monomethanesulfonate: $C_{18}H_{19}ClN_2O_3 \cdot CH_4O_3S$ Mol. wt. 442.92

Pharmacology and therapy. MD 780236 is a highly selective MAO-B type inhibitor (MAO-A/MAO-B: 236–412) [34, 35]. The drug is a reversible inhibitor *in vivo* and *ex vivo*, but apparently not *in vitro*. It is likely that MD 780236 is oxidized by MAO-B, resulting in a reversible covalent bond. This would produce an irreversible inhibition *in vitro*. In the body, only small amounts of imine are formed. Major metabolites are alcohol and acid derivatives of the parent compound. The aldehyde formed could probably be further metabolized to a reversible inhibitor. Other enzyme systems may also be involved in the metabolism of MD 780236 [34, 35].

Originator: Delalande-Synthelabo (France)

3.1.4.2. Almoxatone (INN)

2-Oxazolidinone, 3-(4-((3-chlorophenyl) methoxy) phenyl)-
5-((methylamino)methyl)-, (R)- (9CI)

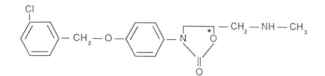

Synonym

MD 240928

Derivative

Monomethanesulfonate: $C_{18}H_{19}ClN_2O_3 \cdot CH_4O_3S$ Mol. wt. 442.91

Pharmacology and therapy. MD 780236 is a racemic compound. Its
R-configuration (Almoxatone, MD 240928) is fully reversible *ex vivo*,
whereas the S-enantiomer still possesses irreversible components observed with the racemic inhibitor [34]. Almoxatone is an extremely
specific inhibitor of MAO-B (MAO-A/MAO-B: 1667) [34]. In mice, the
drug protected against the neurotoxic effects (e.g., depletion of striatal
DA) of MPTP [37]. No generalization was observed in rats trained on
d-amphetamine [28, 38].

Originator: Delalande-Synthelabo (France)

3.2. Reversible Inhibitors

3.2.1. Phenylethylamines

3.2.1.1. p-CMPEA

Benzeneethanamine, 4-chloro-β-methyl- (9CI)

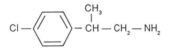

Synonym

4-chloro-β-methylphenethylamine

$C_9H_{12}ClN$ Mol. wt. 169.67

Pharmacology and therapy. p-Chloro-β-methylphenethylamine (*p*-CM-
PEA) is a competitive inhibitor with an approximately 620-fold higher
selectivity for MAO-B compared with MAO-A [39].

3.2.2. Morpholinoethylamine Derivatives

3.2.2.1. Ro 16-6491

Benzamide, N-(2-aminoethyl)-4-chloro- (9CI)

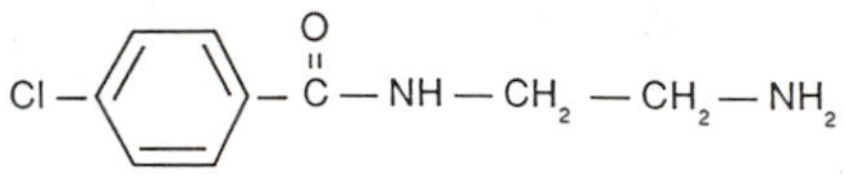

$$Cl - \langle \bigcirc \rangle - \overset{\overset{O}{\|}}{C} - NH - CH_2 - CH_2 - NH_2$$

Derivative

Hydrochloride: $C_9H_{11}ClN_2O\cdot HCl$ Mol. wt. 235.13

Pharmacology and therapy. Ro 16-6491 is a short-acting reversible MAO-B inhibitor in *in vitro* conditions [40]. Labeled Ro 16-6491 can be used as a selective probe for the affinity labeling of MAO-B [41]. Ro 16-6491 is a metabolite of moclobemide. This metabolic route is clearly dominant in rats, but not in humans [42]. Following oral administration of moclobemide, the concentration of Ro 16-6491 in human plasma is too low to produce relevant inhibition of MAO-B in platelets. Moclobemide can thus be considered as a selective MAO-A inhibitor in humans [42].

Originator: Hoffman-La Roche (Switzerland)

3.2.2.2. Lazabemide (INN)

2-Pyridinecarboxamide, N-(2-aminoethyl)-5-chloro- (9CI)

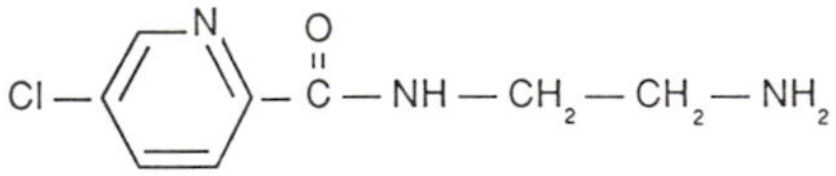

$$Cl - \langle \overset{N}{\bigcirc} \rangle - \overset{\overset{O}{\|}}{C} - NH - CH_2 - CH_2 - NH_2$$

Synonym

Ro 19-6327

Derivative

Hydrochloride: $C_8H_{10}ClN_3O\cdot HCl$ Mol. wt. 236.10

Pharmacology and therapy. Lazabemide is a highly selective reversible MAO-B inhibitor (IC_{50} for MAO-B 30–60 nmol/l, for MAO-A approx. 1 mmol/l or even higher; MAO-A/MAO-B > 20 000–30 000) [43, 44]. It prevents the toxicity of MPTP, but not that of MPP^+ [45]. Reversible MAO-B inhibitors such as Ro 19-6327 have virtually no effect on

DSP-4-induced neurotoxicity in rats [46]. In healthy volunteers, a dose of 0.685 mg/kg (50 mg) produces at least 90% inhibition of brain MAO-B for up to 12 h following oral administration [47].

Originator: Hoffman-La Roche (Switzerland)

Development stage: Clinical phase

Table 1. Effect of some selected MAO-B inhibitors on the brain MAO-A and MAO-B activity *in vitro*

Inhibitor	Tissue	IC_{50} (μmol/l) MAO-A (5-HT)	MAO-B (PEA)	Ratio of IC_{50}s MAO-A MAO-B	References
Pargyline	rat brain	1.6	0.022	73	10
	rat brain	1.8	0.850[1]	2	11
	mouse brain	2.85[1]	0.008[2]	356	48
IRREVERSIBLE					
Selegiline	rat brain	2.0	0.005	400	(Chapter 9)
(*l*-Deprenyl)	rat brain	0.8	0.05	16	10
	rat brain	180.0	0.73	247	49
	rat brain	180.0	0.50[1]	360	49
	mouse brain	70.5[1]	0.011[2]	6401	48
AGN-1133	rat brain	0.016	0.005	3	10
(J-508)	rat brain	0.180	0.126[1]	1.5	11
(Su-11739)	rat brain	—	0.1	—	8
	human brain	0.02	0.05	0.4	(Chapter 9)
AGN-1135	rat brain	2.0	0.08	25	10
	rat brain	2.0	0.03	67	(Chapter 9)
	rat brain	5.0	0.10	50	50
	mouse brain	339.0[1]	0.014	24200	48
	human brain	8.0	0.02	400	(Chapter 9)
TZ-650	rat brain	—	10.0	—	8
U-1424	rat brain	—	10.0	—	8
MDL-72145	rat brain	5.0	0.03	167	(Chapter 9)
	human brain	40.0	0.30	133	(Chapter 9)
MDL-72974	rat brain	0.68	0.004	170	25
LY 54761	rat brain	0.89	0.56	1.6	32
	rat brain	1.58	1.6	1.0	33
MD 780236	rat brain	14.0	0.034	412	34
	rat brain	13.0	0.055	236	35
MD 240931	rat brain	7.3	0.022	332	34
MD 240928 (Almoxatone)	rat brain	50.0	0.03	1667	34
REVERSIBLE					
Ro 19-6327 (Lazabemide)	rat brain	900.0	0.03	30000	44 (Chapter 9)

[1]tyramine was used;
[2]benzylamine was used;
5-HT = serotonin; PEA = β-phenylethylamine

Divergences (i.e., preincubation time) in the experimental design with the exception of the incubation temperature (mostly 37°C) were not taken into consideration.

Table 2. *Ex vivo* inhibition of MAO activity in different species after administration of some selected MAO-B inhibitors

Inhibitor	Species	Tissue	Route of Administration	Time[1]	Doses (mg/kg) and inhibition (%) MAO-A (5-HT)	MAO-B (PEA)	Ratio $\frac{\text{MAO-A}}{\text{MAO-B}}$	Ref.
IRREVERSIBLE								
Selegiline (*l*-Deprenyl)	rat[2]	brain	—[2]	—[2]	80.0: 50%	4.8: 50%	16.7	20
	rat (SPF-Fü)	brain	p.o.	2 h	>200.0: 50%	5.3: 50%	>37.7	35, 44
	rat (Sprague-Dawley)	brain	s.c.	1 h		1.0: 50%	—	51
	rat (CFY)	brain	i.v.	1 h	0.1: 10%	0.1: 56%	5.6	8
	mouse (C57BL/6)	brain	i.p.	1 h		10.0: 95%	—	26
	human volunteers	platelet	p.o.	4 h		0.074: 86%	—	18
AGN-1133 (J-508)	rat (Wistar)	brain	i.p.	2 h	0.5: ~35% 1.0: ~70%	0.5: ~75% 1.0: ~85%	~2.1 ~1.2	10, 50
(Sul1,739)	rat[2]	brain	s.c.	2 h	0.3: —[2]	0.3: —[2]	1.4	11
	rat (CFY)	brain	i.v.	1 h	1.0: 89%	1.0: 72%	0.8	8
AGN-1135	rat (Wistar)	brain	i.p	2 h	0.5: ~2% 1.0: ~8%	0.5: ~65% 1.0: ~75%	~33 ~9	10, 50
	rat[2]	brain	p.o.	2 h	5.3: 50%	0.4: 50%	13.3	51
MDL 72145	rat[2]	brain	—[2]	—[2]	8.5: 50%	0.35: 50%	24.3	20
	rat[2]	brain	i.p.	24 h	1.2: 50%	0.31: 50%[5]	—	18

Compound	Species	Tissue	Route	Time[1]			Value	Ref
MDL 72947	rat[2]	brain	—[2]	—[2]	8.0: 50%	0.18: 50%	44.4	20
	rat[2]	brain	p.o.	2 h	7.2: 50%	0.28: 50%	25.7	52
	mouse (C57BL/6)	brain	i.p.	1 h	—	1.25: 96%	—	26
	human volunteers	platelet	p.o.	1 h	—	0.007[4]: >95%	—	53
LY 54761	rat (Wistar)	brain	i.p.	1 h	7.6: 50%	5.8: 50%	1.3	32
MD 780236	rat (Sprague-Dawley)	brain	p.o.	2 h	5.0: 8%	5.0: 85%	10.6	34
MD 240928 (Almoxatone)	rat (Sprague-Dawley)	brain	p.o.	2 h	5.0: 0%	5.0: 77%	>70	34
MD 240931	rat (Sprague-Dawley)	brain	p.o.	2 h	5.0: 14	5.0: 87%	6.2	34
REVERSIBLE								
Ro 19-6327 (Lazabemide)	rat (SPF-Fü)	brain	p.o.	2 h	~300: 50%	0.07: 50%	>4000	44, 52
	human volunteers	brain	p.o.	—	—	0.7: ~90%	—	47
	human volunteers	platelet	p.o.	—	—	0.7: ~100%	—	47

[1]time prior to measurement of MAO activity;
[2]not mentioned
[3]tyramine was used;
[4]70 kg body weight;
[5]benzylamine was used;
PEA = β-phenylethylamine; 5-HT = serotonin

References

1. Hermecz I, Meszaros Z. Pyrido [1,2-alpha]pyrimidines], new chemical entities in medical chemistry. Med Res Rev 1988; 8: 203–20.
2. Cheeseman AJ, Clarke JB. Effects of 1-methyl-4-phenyl-1,2,5,6-tetrahydropyridine and its metabolite 1-methyl-4-phenylpyridine on acethylcholine synthesis in synaptosomes from rat forebrain. J Neurochem 1987; 48: 1209–14.
3. Riederer P, Youdim MBH. Monoamine oxidase activity and monamine metabolism in brains of parkinsonian patients treated with L-deprenyl. J Neurochem 1986; 46: 1359–65.
4. Borbe HO, Niebch G, Nickel B. Kinetic evaluation of MAO-B-activity following oral administration of selegline and desmethyl-selegiline in the rat. J Neural Transm 1990; 32 (Suppl): 131–7.
5. Nickel B, Borbe HO, Szelenyi I. Effect of selegiline and desmethyl-selegiline on cortical electric activity in rats. J Neural Transm 1990; 32 (Suppl): 139–44.
6. Ecsery Z, Knoll J, Somfai E, Török Z, Szinnyei E, Mozsolits K. Phenylisopropylamine derivative. PCY Int WO 8505617 (CA 105:78632).
7. Knoll J, Toth V, Kummert M, Sugar J. (−)-Deprenyl and (−)-parafluorodeprenyl-treatment prevents age-related pigment changes in the substantia nigra. A TV-image analysis of neuromelanin. Mech Aging Dev. 1992; 63: 157–63.
8. Knoll J, Ecsery Z, Magyar K, Satory E. Novel (−)deprenyl-derived selective inhibitors of B-type monoamine oxidase. The relation of structure to their action. Biochem Pharmacol 1978; 27: 1739–47.
9. Abdorubo A, Knoll J. The effect of various MAO-B inhibitors on rabbit arterial strip response to tyramine. Pol J Pharmacol Pharm 1988; 40: 673–83.
10. Kalir A, Sabbagh A, Youdim MBH. Selective acetylenic "suicide" and reversible inhibitors of monoamine oxidase types A and B. Br J Pharmac 1981; 73: 55–64.
11. Maitre L. Monoamine oxidase inhibiting properties of SU-11,739 in the rat. Comparison with pargyline, tranylcypromine and iproniazid. J Exp Pharm Therap 1967; 157: 81–8.
12. Heikkila RE, Davoison JP, Finberg M, Youdim MBH. Prevention of MPTP-induced neurotoxicity by AGN-1133 and AGN-1135, selective inhibitors of monoamine oxidase-B. Eur J Pharmacol 1985; 116: 313–7.
13. Youngster SK, Saari WS, Heikkila RE. 1-Methyl-4-cyclohexyl-1,2,3,6-tetrahydropyridine (MCTP): an alicyclic MPTP-like neurotoxin. Neurosci Lett 1987; 79: 151–6.
14. Finberg JPM, Tenne M, Youdim MBH. Tyramine antagonistic properties of AGN 1135, an irreversible inhibitor of monoamine oxidase type B. Br J Pharmac 1981; 73: 65–74.
15. Youdim MBH. Monoamine oxidase (MAO)-A but not MAO-B inhibitors potentiate tyramine-induced catecholamine release from PC12 cells. J Neurochem 1990; 54: 411–4.
16. Finberg JPM, Youdim MBH. Modification of blood pressure and nictating membrane response to sympathetic amines by selective monoamine oxidase inhibitors, types A and B, in the cat. Br J Pharmac 1985; 85: 541–46.
17. Zreika M, McDonald IA, Bey Ph, Palfreyman MG. MDL 72145, an enzyme-activated irreversible inhibitor with selectivity of monoamine oxidase type B. J Neurochem 1984; 43: 448–54.
18. Flucker CJR, Lyles GA, Marshall CMS. Ex vivo inhibition of amine oxidase activities in several rat tissues by MDL 72145. Br J Pharmac 1986; 87 (Suppl): 68P.
19. Fozard JR, Zreika M, Robin M, Palfreyman MG. The functional consequences of inhibition of monoamine oxidase type B: comparison of the pharmacological properties of L-deprenyl and MDL 72145. Naunyn-Schmiedeberg's Arch Pharmacol 1985; 331: 186–93.
20. Kabins D, Gershon S. Potential applications for monoamine oxidase B inhibitors. Dementia 1990; 1: 323–48.
21. Cheeseman AJ, Clark JB. Effects of 1-methyl-4-phenyl-1,2,5,6-tetrahydropyridine and its metabolite 1-methyl-4-phenylpyridine on acetylcholine synthesis in synaptosomes from rat forebrain. J Neurochem 1987; 48: 1209–14.
22. Bradbury AJ, Costall B, Jenner PG et al. The effect of 1-methyl-4-phenyl-1,2,3,6-tetrahydropyridine (MPTP) on striatal and limbic catecholamine neurones in white and black mice. Antagonism by monoamine oxidase inhibitors. Neuropharmacology 1986; 25: 897–904.
23. Palfreyman MG, Mcdonald IA, Bey P, Schechter PJ, Sjoerdsma A. Design and early clinical evaluation of selective inhibitors of monoamine oxidase. Prog Neuropsychopharmacol Biol Psychiatry 1988; 12: 967–87.

24. McDonald I, Palfreyman MG, Zreik M, Bey P. (Z)-2-(2,4-dichlorophenoxy)methyl-3-fluoroallylamine: a clorgyline analogue with surprising selectivity for monoamine oxidase type B. Biochem Pharmacol 1986; 35: 349–51.

25. Zreika M, Forzard JR, Dudley MW, Bey P, McDonald IA, Palfreyman MG. MDL 72,974: a potent and selective enzyme-activated irreversible inhibitor of monoamine oxidase type B with potential for use in Parkinson's disease. J Neural Trans Park Dis Dement Sect 1989; 1: 243–54.

26. Finnegan KT, Skratt JJ, Irwin I, DeLanney LE, Langston JW. Protection against DSP-4-induced neurotoxicity by deprenyl is not related to its inhibition of MAO B. Eur J Pharmacol 1990; 184: 119–26.

27. Dudley MW. The depletion of rat cortical norepinephrine and the inhibition of [^{3}H] norepinephrine uptake by xylamine does not require monoamine oxidase activity. Life Sci 1988; 43: 1871–7.

28. Moser PC. Generalization of l-deprenyl, but not MDL-72974, to the amphetamine stimulus in rats. Psychopharmacol 1990; 101: S240.

29. Hinze C, Harland D, Zreika M, Dulery B, Hardenberg J. A double-blind, placebo-controlled study of the tolerability and effects on platelet MAO-B activity of single oral doses of MDL 72,974A in normal volunteers. J Neural Trans 1990; 32 (Suppl): 203–9.

30. Harland D, Hinze C, Seppala A, Hardenberg J, Zreika M. A double-blind, placebo-controlled study of the tolerability and effects on platelet MAO-B activity of single oral doses of MDL 72,974A in normal volunteers. Eur J Pharmacol 1990; 183: 530.

31. Yu PH, Zuo DM. Inhibition of a type B monoamine oxidase inhibitor, (E)-2-(4-fluorophenethyl)-3-fluoroallylamine (MDL-72974A), on semicarbazide-sensitive amine oxidases isolated from vascular tissues and sera of different species. Biochem Pharmacol 1992; 43: 307–12.

32. Fuller RW, Hemrick SK, Mills J. Inhibition of monoamine oxidase by N-phenacylcyclopropylamine. Biochem Pharmacol 1978; 27: 2255–61.

33. Murphy DL, Donnelly CH, Richelson ET, Fuller RW. N substituted cyclo propylamines as inhibitors of monoamine oxidase B EC-1.4.3.4 forms. Biochem Pharmacol 1978; 27: 1767–72.

34. Dostert P, Strolin Benedetti M, Guffroy C. Different stereoselective inhibition of monoamine oxidase-B by the R- and S-enantiomers of MD 780236. J Pharm Pharmacol 1983; 35: 161–5.

35. Strolin Benedetti M, Dostert Ph, Boucher T, Guffroy Ch. A new reversible selective type B monoamine oxidase inhibitor: MD 780236. In: Kamijo K, Usdin E, Nagatsu T, editors. Monoamine oxidase. Basic and clinical frontiers. Amsterdam: Excerpta Medica, 1983; 209–20.

36. Strolin Benedetti M, Dow J. A monoamine oxidase-B inhibitor, MD 780236, metabolized essentially by the A form of the enzyme in the rat. J Pharm Pharmacol 1983; 35: 238–45.

37. Fuller RW, Hemrick-Luecke SK, Influence of selective, reversible inhibitors of monoamine oxidase on the prolonged depletion of striatal dopamine by 1-methyl-4-phenyl-1,2,3,6-tetrahydropyridine in mice. Life Sci 1985; 37: 1089–96.

38. Porsolt RD, Pawelec C, Roux S, Jalfre M. Discrimination of the amphetamine cue. Effects of A, B and mixed type inhibitors of monoamine oxidase. Neuropharmacology 1984; 23: 569–73.

39. Kinemuchi H, Arai Y, Toyoshima Y, Tadano T, Kisara K. Studies on 5-fluoro-alpha-methyltryptamine and p-chloro-beta-methylphenethylamine: determination of the MAO-A or MAO-B selective inhibition in vitro. Jpn J Pharmacol 1988; 46: 197–9.

40. Keller HH, Kettler R, Keller G, Da Prada M. Short-acting novel MAO inhibitors: In vitro evidence for the reversibility of MAO inhibition by moclobemide and Ro 16-6491. Naunyn-Schmiedeberg's Arch Pharmacol 1987; 335: 12–20.

41. Cesura AM, Imhof R, Takacs B, Galva MD, Picotti GB, Da Prada M. [^{3}H] Ro 16-6491, a selective probe for affinity labelling of monoamine oxidase type B in human brain and platelet membranes. J Neurochem 1988; 50: 1037–43.

42. Schoerlin M-P, Da Prada M. Species-specific biotransformation of moclobemide: a comparative study in rats and humans. Acta Psychiatr Scand 1990; 360 (Suppl): 108–10.

43. Da Prada M, Kettler R, Keller HH et al. From moclobemide to Ro 19-6327 and Ro 41-1049: the development of a new class of reversible, selective MAO-A and MAO-B inhibitors. J Neural Trans 1990; 29: 279–92.

44. Da Prada M, Kettler R, Cesura AM, Richards JG. Reversible, enzyme-activated monoamine oxidase inhibitors: new advances. Pharmacol Res Commun 1988; 20: 21–33.
45. Reinhard JF, Carmichael SW, Daniels AJ. Mechanisms of toxicity and cellular resistance to 1-methyl-4-phenyl-1,2,3,6-tetrahydropyridine and 1-methyl-4-phenylpyridinium in adrenomedullary chromaffin cell cultures. J Neurochem 1990; 55: 311–20.
46. Bertocci B, Gill G, Da Prada M. Prevention of the DSP_4-induced noradrenergic neurotoxicity by irreversible, not by reversible MAO-B inhibitors. Pharmacol Res Commun 1988; 20: 131–32.
47. Price CW, Bench CJ, Cremer JC et al. Inhibition of brain monoamine oxidase-B by Ro 19-6327—in vivo measurement using positron emission tomography. Eur J Pharmacol 1990; 183: 166.
48. Youdim MBH, Finberg JPM, Riederer P, Heikkila RE. Monoamine oxidase type B inhibitors in human and animal parkinsonism. In preparation.
49. Magyar K, Ecseri Z, Bernath G, Satory E, Knoll J. Structure activity relationship of selective inhibitors of MAO-B. In Magyar K, editor. Monoamine oxidases and their selective inhibition. Budapest: Akademia Kiado, 1980: 11–20.
50. Youdim MBH, Finberg JPM. MAO type B inhibitors as adjunct to L-dopa therapy. In: Yahr MD, Bergmann KJ, editors. Advances in Neurology. New York: Raven Press 1986; 45: 127–36.
51. Knoll J, Magyar K. Some puzzling pharmacological effects of monoamine oxidase inhibitors. Adv Biochem Psychopharmacol 1972; 5: 393–408.
52. Cesura AM, Pletscher A. The new generation of monoamine oxidase inhibitors. In: Jucker E, editor. Progress in Drug Research. Basel: Birkhäuser, 38: 171–296.
53. MDL 72,974A. Drugs of the Future 1991; 16: 428–31.

Inhibitors of Monoamine Oxidase B
Pharmacology and Clinical Use in Neurodegenerative Disorders
ed. by I. Szelenyi
© 1993 Birkhäuser Verlag Basel/Switzerland

APPENDIX II
Explanation of the Nomenclature for Optical Isomers

E. E. Polymeropoulos

The problem of distinguishing between enantiomers of optically active compounds is an old one. Many different prefixes are used in the current literature, a practice which often causes confusion. We shall try to give a historical account of this problem with the hope that the non-chemist reader may acquire a better understanding of the nomenclature.

To begin with, chemical compounds possessing an assymetric or chiral center (an atom with four different ligands lying in the middle of a tetrahedron) that rotate the electrical component of plane-polarized light clockwise (as the observer looks toward the beam of light) were specified as dextrorotatory or simply d-. On the other hand, compounds that rotate the electrical component of plane-polarized light counterclockwise were designated as levorotatory or l-. This assignment did not give any information about the spatial arrangement of the substituents on the assymetric atom. Later on, the configuration at the chiral center was assigned by taking glyceraldehyde as a standard. Dextrorotatory glyceraldehyde was arbitrarily assigned the d-configuration. The d- and l-prefixes now gave the relative configuration of the assymetric atom, while experimentally determined signs of rotation were added to the nomenclature. Thus, the two enantiomers of glyceraldehyde were known as d-($+$)- and l-($-$)-glyceraldehyde. The new assignment brought about confusion in the literature because of the multiple meaning of the d- and l-prefixes. It was then decided to characterize the absolute configuration of the chiral atom in dextrorotatory glyceraldehyde with a D- and in levorotatory glyceraldehyde with an L-. Experimental signs of rotation could also be added as ($+$) and ($-$). Thus, all compounds whose experimentally determined configuration corresponds to that of D-glyceraldehyde acquire the prefix D-, no matter what the sign of the optical rotation is; the same holds for the L-configuration. Soon, however, it became obvious that glyceraldehyde was not a sufficient standard according to which all compounds could be classified. Thus, the Cahn, Ingold, and Prelog (CIP) system evolved with which the absolute configuration of every chiral compound, hypothetical or real, can be determined unambiguously. According to a set of arbitrary but consistent rules based on atomic numbers, the ligands on the assymetric atom are given a priority. If we view the tetrahedral arrangement from the side remote from the substituent with the lowest priority, then the sequence of decreasing priority of the remaining three atoms can either be clockwise, in which case the configuration is R-(=Rectus), or counterclockwise, in which case the configuration is S-(=Sinister). Experimentally determined signs of rotation (+) or (−) may also be added to this nomenclature.

From these considerations it becomes evident that there is no necessary correspondence between the various prefixes, and that the unique CIP designation, together with experimentally determined signs of rotation, should be used whenever possible.

Subject Index

The subject index was compiled by B. Nickel, F. Stroman and U. Werner. It refers to keywords in Chapters 1 to 18. Tables and figures have been abbreviated as (T) and (F), respectively. For abbreviations see "List of Abbreviations".

Abuse liability
– amphetamine-like   215, 331
– assessments   215
– cocaine-like   215
– behavioral changes (rats)
 – d-amphetamine   216, 219, 220(T)
 – d,l-ampetamine   216, 219, 220(T)
 – l-amphetamine   216, 219, 220(T)
 – codeine   220 (T)
 – d-deprenyl   216, 219, 220(T)
 – l-deprenyl   216, 219, 220(T)
– description of methods   221, 222, 222(F), 223, 223(T), 224
– discriminative stimuli
 – amphetamine (d,l- or d-)   222
 – cocaine   224
 – l-deprenyl   225, 226
 – food-presentation schedule   225
 – reinforcement   221
– drug discrimination (rats)   221, 222, 222(F), 223, 223(T), 224
 – drug-effects
  – d-amphetamine   224, 225
  – clorgyline   202
  – d,l-deprenyl   224, 225
  – l-deprenyl   224, 225
  – MD 240928   224
  – MDL 72974   224
  – moclobemide   224
  – pargyline   224
– drug self-administration (monkeys) 226–230
 – methods   , 217(F), 218(F)226, 227, 228
 – drug-effects
  – cocaine   228, 229(F)
  – l-deprenyl   228, 229(F)
  – β-phenylethylamine   229(F), 230
– EEG changes (rats)
 – d-amphetamine   216, 217, 217(F), 218(F)
 – d,l-amphetamine   216, 217, 217(F), 218(F)
 – l-amphetamine   216, 217, 217(F), 218(F)
 – d-deprenyl   216, 217, 217(F), 218(F)
 – l-deprenyl   216, 217, 217(F), 218(F)
– physical dependency (rats)
 – d-amphetamine   218, 219, 220(F)

 – d,l-amphetamine   218, 219, 220(F)
 – l-amphetamine   218, 219, 220(F)
 – d-deprenyl   218, 219, 220(F)
 – l-deprenyl   218, 219, 220(F)
Accumbens nucleus   4, 5, 6(F), 9
L-Acetylcarnitine   332, 334
Acetylcholine (see cholinergic system)   5, 19, 26
– esterase   9
Acetylenic compounds   89, 90
N-Acetylputrescine   334
N-Acetylspermidine   334
N-Acetylspermine   334
Adenylate cyclase   29
Adenosine   19
Adrenaline (see Noradrenergic system)
Age
– chronological   147
– physiological   147, 330
Aging   176
– longevity by l-deprenyl   157, 164, 170
– morphological changes   160, 161, 162
– nigrostriatal neurons   160, 162
AGN 1133
– 95(F), 115, 115(F), 116(F), 117–119, 120(F), 121, 122
– selectivity of MAO-inhibition   186(T)
AGN 1135
– chemistry   95(F), 114, 115, 115(F), 118, 119, 120(F), 121, 122
– indane 116
– pharmacology   90, 130, 137, 186(T), 196, 334
– water/octanol partition coefficient (log/P) 117, 117(T)
Allenic amines   92
Allylamine derivatives   90, 91
Alzheimer Disease Assessment Scale   306
Alzheimer's disease (AD) (see also l-Deprenyl)   38, 61, 135, 147, 185, 255, 301–303, 329, 330, 334
treatment with l-deprenyl   303–309
AM1   116
Amantadine   60, 255
Aminal formation   119, 120, 121(F)
Amine oxidation
– mechanism   110, 110(F)
– nucleophilic attack   110, 112
– iminium cation   110, 112
– irreversible covalent bond   112
– steric hindrance   112
– flavin-adenosine-dinucleotide (FAD)   109
– 8a-carbon   109
– N5-nitrogen   110, 112
– flavin   109, 110(F), 111

Amitryptyline   87, 100(F)
Amphetamines   131
d-Amphetamine   112
–   dependence (see Abuse ability)
d,l-Amphetamine
–   dependence (see Abuse ability)
–   *l*-Amphetamine   112, 114(F), 118
–   dependence (see Abuse ability)
–   excretion   208(T)
–   metabolism   131, 206–209, 309, 324
–   pharmacokinetics   207(T)
–   pharmacological activity   133, 207, 324,
    331
Amygdala   3, 9, 11, 17, 19
Anterior cingulate areas   9
Anticholinergics   61
Antidepressants (see individual agents)
Anti-oxidant status   44
Apomorphine   59, 60
Area tegmenti ventralis (VTA)   27(T), 36
Atlantic Ocean Syndrome   250
Autoradiography; of *l*-deprenyl   131

Banisterine   255
Basal ganglia   3, 10(F), 12, 33
Basal forebrain
–   basal nucleus of Meynert   19, 38
–   magnocellular nuclei of the   4, 6(F), 18, 19
–   medial septal nucleus   19
–   nucleus of the diagonal band   19
Benserazide (see also *l*-Deprenyl, Parkinson's
    disease)   79–281
Benzodiazepine; improvement of rigidity   36
Benzylamine   85, 87
Benzylcyanide   87
Birkmayer, W.   245, 246(F), 251
Blaschko, H.   244
Blessed Dementia Scale   308
Bombesin   39
Brain
–   -derived neurotrophic factor (BDNF)   176
    –   injury   255
Brief Psychiatric Rating Scale (BPRS)   304,
    305
Britannia Pharmaceuticals   247
Brofaromine   136
Bromocriptine (see also DA agonists)   30, 33,
    59, 284
Buschke Selective Reminding Task   304, 305
Byske, D.   247, 250, 251

Calcium; influx   334
Carbidopa (see also *l*-Deprenyl, Parkinson's
    disease)   280, 281
β-Carbolines   175
Caregiver Burden Scale   304
Catalase   194(T)
–   in striatum   151, 152(T), 332
–   in tuberculum olfactorium   152(T), 153

Catechol-O-methyl transferase (COMT)   150,
    190, 332
–   activity in brain of PD patients   27, 29(T)
–   interaction with *l*-deprenyl   209
Caudate nucleus   5, 6(F), 18, 27
–   D$_2$-receptor binding   32(T)
Centromediano-parafascicular complex of the
    thalamus   9, 18
Cerebrospinal fluid; HVA   293
Cheese effect   62, 76, 90, 135–138, 150, 185,
    203, 243, 255, 262, 279, 320
Chinoin Pharmaceutical Company   241, 243,
    247
Chinoin-175 (Fludepryl)   90, 94(F)
p-Chloro-β-methylbenzeneethanamine
    (pCMPEA)   77, 98(F)
Chlorpromazine   87, 101(F)
Cholecystokinin (CCK-8)   39
Choline acetyltranferase; activity   8, 38
Cholinergic neurons; in the caudate   8, 149
Cholinergic system
–   degeneration of   31(F), 38
–   *l*-deprenyl   154
Cimoxatone   136
Clinical Geriatric Assessment Scala (SCAG)
    304
Clorgyline   76, 77, 79(F), 86, 110, 126, 137,
    151, 154, 176, 184, 243, 255, 278, 332
Cocaine; – like abuse liability (see Abuse
    ability)
"Complex loop"   37
Cornell Scale for Depression in Dementia   304
Cortex   31(F), 302
Covalent bond formation   111, 112
CQ-32084   30
Cyclopropylamine derivatives   91
Cytotoxic free radicals (see Radicals)

DDC (Dopa decarboxylase) (see also
    l-Deprenyl)   28, 284
DATATOP-study   159, 170, 172, 283,
    292–298, 303, 333
Dementia
–   Alzheimer type (DAT) (see Alzheimer's
    disease)
–   in PD   53
–   multi-infarct   304, 308
–   pathophysiology   38, 160, 163–165
–   subcortical (bradyphrenia)   52
–   *d*-Deprenyl
–   chemistry   112, 113(F)
–   conformational analysis   112
–   crystal structure   112
–   dependence (see Abuse liability)
–   structural comparison   112, 113(F), 114(F)
–   water-/octanol partition coefficient (logP)
    117, 117(T)
l-Deprenyl ((–)-deprenyl; selegiline)   129,
    169, 254

- chemical properties 110, 118–120
  - crystal structure 112
  - conformational analysis 112
  - structural comparison 112, 113(F), 114(F), 116(F)
  - structural formula 94(F), 115(F)
  - structure-activity relationship 130
  - water/octanol partition coefficient (logP) 117, 117(T)
- cheese effect (see Cheese effect)
- L-dopa sparing effect 132, 159, 256, 281, 328
- dopamine
  - release of 154(T), 155(T)
  - turnover 153, 188, 266, 296
  - uptake inhibition 133, 149, 150, 189, 190(F), 265, 320
- effect on
  - β-adrenoceptor 320
  - catalase 152(T)
  - SOD 152(T), 176
- history 237–243
- interaction with
  - COMT 209
  - L-dopa + DDC 209, 209(T), 210(F)
  - fluoxetine 209
  - non-selective MAO-inhibitors 209
  - pethidine 210
- long-term effects 155–164, 157(T), 158(F), 303, 310–312, 329, 330(T), 331
- MAO-B
  - dependent effects 268(T)
  - independent effects 268(T)
  - inhibition 132, 203, 204, 204(F), 327–330
  - PEA excretion 170, 205, 206(F)
  - recovery 204(F), 205
- multiple dose effects 150–155, 304–306
- neuromelanin (see Neuromelanin)
- neuroprotection (see also Neuroprotection) 133, 134, 172(T), 173(T), 193, 295–297, 310–312, 330, 333
- pharmacokinetics 132
  - absorption
    - labeled l-deprenyl 131, 201
  - distribution 201, 202
    - autoradiographic studies 131, 202
    - PET (see also Positron, emission tomography) 202
  - excretion 206–209
    - l-amphetamine 208(T)
    - desmethylselegiline 208(T)
    - l-methamphetamine 208(T)
  - metabolism 131, 206–209, 215, 324
    - metabolites in CSF 206, 207(T)
    - racemic transformation 206, 297
  - multiple dose kinetics 206, 207(T)
  - single dose kinetics 204, 206, 207(T)
- preventive medication 165

- side effects
  - monotherapy 263, 264(T)
  - combination therapy 263, 264(T)
- treatment of
  - AD (see also Alzheimer's disease) 160, 165
  - depression (see also Depression) 303, 319–324
  - PD (see also Parkinson's disease) 132, 190, 190(F), 256–261, 279–289, 291–295, 309, 327
    - combined with
      - DA-agonists 262, 284
      - L-dopa 56, 67, 256, 277, 278
      - L-dopa + DDC 56, 57, 67, 159, 160, 257(T), 258(T), 279–284
      - plus MAO-inhibitors 62, 63, 67, 278, 279
    - longevity (see also Life expectancy) 164(F), 165, 282, 292
    - long-term effects 292
    - monotherapy 62, 260(T), 261, 262, 283, 295
Deprenyl Research Ltd. 250, 251
Depression (see also l-Deprenyl)
- atypical 319
- in PD 52
- therapy-resistant 319
- therapy with
  - l-deprenyl 320, 320(F), 321(T), 324
    - + phenylalanine 322, 323(T)
    - + l-5-hydroxytryptophan 322, 323(T)
  - iproniazide 76, 240, 255
Desferrioxamine 193
Desmethylselegiline (desmethyldeprenyl) 131, 208(T)
Detoxification 194(T)
1,3-dimethyl-TIQ 176
Discrimination stimuli (see Abuse potential)
L-Dopa (see also l-Deprenyl) 26, 170, 175, 190, 277, 329
- treatment of PD (see l-Deprenyl)
- side effects 278, 329
- long-term use 278
- progression of PD 285
- substitution 43
Dopa-β-hydroxylase 302
DOPAC 27
- in various brain regions (PD patients) 28(T)
Dopamine (DA) 25–29, 31, 36, 37, 145, 146(F), 183, 191, 290, 328
- agonists (see also individual agents) 262
  - role in motor control 30
  - treatment of PD 59, 60, 284, 285
  - side effects 59, 60
- deficiency, nigrostriatal 25, 170, 278, 289

- distribution; in various brain regions of PD patients 27(T), 28(T)
- extraneural 191
- receptors 29–32
  - binding in PD 32(T)
  - classification 30(T)
  - in SN 31(F)
  - subtypes 8, 29, 30, 31, 31(F)
- turnover 153, 290
- uptake 134
Dopaminergic neurons 5, 9, 15, 19
- degeneration 280–285
- nigro-striatal system 25, 145, 153
Dopaminergic system; in AD 31(F), 302
"dopaminergic tone" 176, 177
Dopicar2 (see also l-Deprenyl) 284
Drug dependence (see Abuse liability)
Drug discrimination (see Abuse liability)
Drug-seeking 221
Drug self-administration behavior (see Abuse liability)
DSP-4 134, 171, 172, 191, 267, 332
Duvoisin, R. 248

E-250 240–245
Ecseri, Z. 241, 242(F)
EEG (electroencephalogram)
- drug effects on (see Abuse liability)
- in AD 308
- in parkinsonism 52
Ehringer, H. 245
Enantioselectivity 111
Entorhinal region 3, 9, 17
Epidermal growth factor (EGF) 171

Farmos 247
Fenton reaction 42, 290
Fire-Item Recall 308
Flavin 109, 110(F), 111
Flavin adenosine dinucleotide (FAD) (see also Amine oxidation) 109, 111, 117–119
- inhibitor complex 118, 120(F)
- 8a-carbon 109
- nucleophilic attack 110, 112, 114, 118
Flavin peptide 77, 78, 109, 110(F), 118
Fludepryl (CHINOIN-175) 90, 94(F)
Free radicals (see Radicals)
French Selegiline Multicenter Trial 295

GABA (γ-aminobutyric acid) 5, 26, 191
- receptors 39
GABA/enkephalin containing neuronal systems 5, 8, 9, 12, 12(F), 34, 34(F)
GABAergic systems 5, 8, 11, 17–19, 31(F)
- preservation of 39
- projections 5, 26
GABA/substance P-containing neuronal systems 5, 9, 11, 12, 12(F), 17, 34, 34(F), 35(F)

Galanine 19
Glia 188(T), 190(F), 328
- cell staining 189
- glial inhibition 132, 186
- role in PD 41
Glutamate 5, 31(F)
- receptor 195
Glutaminergic projection 13
Glutathione 193(F), 194
- oxidized 176(F), 193(F), 267, 333
- peroxidase 193(F), 194, 194(T)
- reduced 176(F), 193(F), 291

Haber-Weiss reaction 290
Heroin addicts 250
5-HIAA in CSF 305
Hippocampus 302
Hippocampal formation 3, 9, 17
- subiculum 9
Histamine 9, 19
Histochemistry
- antibody staining 188(T)
- histochemical staining 189, 189(T)
Hormone-like action 190
Hornykiewicz, O. 245
HVA
- in CSF 293, 305
- in various brain regions of PD patients 28(T)
Hydrogen peroxide (see Radicals)
- formation 41, 176(F), 266
- interaction with iron 42
Hydroxyl radical (see Radicals) 42, 290, 291
5-Hydroxytryptamine (5-HT) (see Serotonin)
l-5-Hydroxytryptophan 322
Hyperkinesia 329

Iminium cation 110, 119
Imipramine 87, 100(F)
Immunoreactivity
- somatostatin-like 40
- substance P-like 40
Indoleaminergic system 302
Intoxication; mechanism 332
Intraneural inhibition 127, 186
Iproniazid 76, 240, 255
Iron 42, 43, 291
- chelator 193
Isocortex 9, 17
- frontal association areas of 11, 19
- sensorimotor areas 9
Isoniazid 75

J-508 95(F), 114, 115, 115(F), 116(F), 117(T), 117–119, 120(F), 121, 122

Knoll, J. 241, 242(F), 343–345, 251
Kynuramine 84, 85

L 54761 (LY 54761) 98(F)
Langston, J.W. 249
Lazabemide (Ro 19-6327) 128, 131, 196, 297, 331, 334
– selectivity of MAO-inhibition 186(T)
Leucine-enkephaline (leu-enk) 39, 40
Levodopa (see L-dopa)
Lewy bodies 25, 164, 170
Liebermann, A. 251
Life expectancy; in PD 133, 164(F), 165, 256, 280, 282, 292, 333
Lipid peroxidation 42, 135, 267
Lipofuscin 17, 19, 148
Lisuride (see also Dopamine agonists) 30, 33, 59, 284
Locus coeruleus 9, 18

Madopar (see also l-Deprenyl) 150, 160, 169, 281
MAO-A and MAO-B (Monoamine oxidase of A and B type 154, 170, 243, 303, 305
– active sites 79, 109
– activity
  – in different brain regions 187(T)
  – in PD patients after l-deprenyl 187(T)
– distribution
  – in different organs 130
  – in tissues of different species 78, 328
  – in different brain regions 191(T), 188(T), 189(T)
– intraneural 27
– kinetic parameters 126, 127(T)
– lipophilic binding sites 110, 117
– selectivity 126, 127(T), 129
– substrates 81, 191
MAO-B (Monoamine oxidase B) 126, 148, 176, 184, 253, 289
– active centre 109, 186
– action 27, 111
– activity in SN 29(T)
– age 134, 135, 148, 149
– assays 85(T)
  – in vitro 84, 86
  – in vivo 86
– chemical properties (see also Amine oxidation, FAD) 77
– inhibitors
  – enzymatic reactions 77, 78, 82–84
  – irreversible 89–92, 114, 129
  – partly reversible 92, 93
  – reversible 86–88, 114, 130
– platelets 127, 204, 204(F)
– selectivity 186(T)
– stereoselectivity 116
Mazindol 134
MD 240928 97(F)
– drug discrimination 224
MD 780236 93, 97(F), 130
MDL 72145 91, 96(F), 114, 115, 115(F),

116(F), 117–119, 120, 121, 122, 130, 137, 186(T)
MDL 72392 90, 136
MDL 72394 90, 136
MDL 72638 90, 96(F)
MDL 72974 91, 97(F), 130, 134, 171, 178, 196, 331, 334
– drug discrimination 224
Meperidine 248
Mesostriatal dopaminergic system 36
l-Methamphematine 112, 131, 206–209, 309, 331
Methionine-enkephalin (Met-enk) 39, 40
MHPG; in CSF 203, 305
MPP+ 63, 87, 92, 93, 133, 173, 174(F), 175, 249(F), 254, 267, 297, 302
MPPP 248
MPTP 15, 35, 44, 63, 87, 133, 169, 171, 173, 174(F), 175, 183, 192, 248, 249(F), 289, 291, 311, 331, 332
MOLCAD computer program 113
Moclobemide 131, 136, 196, 319
– analogues 88
– drug discrimination 224
Monoamine metabolites; in CSF of AD patients 305
Monoamine oxidase (see MAO)
Monoaminergic system; in AD 302
Monoamines, exogenous 253
Monoclonal antibodies 128
Motor control 26
Motor loop (circuit) 4(F), 33–36
– "direct" pathway 12, 34, 34(F), 35, 35(F)
– "indirect" pathway 11, 12, 34, 34(F), 35, 35(F)
Muenter, M. 251

Nerve growth factor (NGF) 171, 332, 334
Neurodegenerative diseases 135, 329
Neuromelanin 15, 17, 178
– age related changes 147, 161, 162(T), 171
– area, number of granules 161
– effect of l-deprenyl 162, 163(T), 164, 171
– formation of 15, 147
Neuropeptides (see also individual peptides) 37, 39
Neuropeptide Y 7, 39
Neurotensin 39
Neuroprotection 129, 133, 170, 192, 196, 289, 290, 329, 330, 331, 334
Neurotoxins 174, 192, 193, 310–312
– endogenous 311, 312
– exogenous (see also MPTP, DSP-4) 310, 311
Neurotransmitter (see individual agents and systems)
Neurotrophic factors 332
Nigrostriatal system (see also Substantia nigra) 25

- degeneration of neurons 145, 278, 289
- D_1 and D_2 receptors 31(F)
- facilitation of 153–155
NMDA
- calcium influx 334
- polyamine binding site 195(F), 254, 268
- receptor 195, 195(F), 254, 268, 330, 334
NMIQ 175, 174(F)
NMTIQ 175, 174(F)
Noradrenaline 26, 183
- deficiency 37
- inhibition by l-deprenyl 149, 150
- uptake 133, 302
- turnover 151, 302
Noradrenergic system 9
- degeneration of 37, 302
Nucleus basalis of Meynert 19, 38

Octopamine 80
6-OHDA 44, 151, 171, 176, 192, 266, 267, 332
Optical isomerism 113
Oxazolidone derivatives 93
Oxidative stress 29, 41, 62, 63, 135, 193, 254, 261, 290, 291, 310, 329, 330, 333
- effect of l-deprenyl 193(F)
Oxiracetam 306, 308
Oxygen free radicals (see also Radicals) 290

Pallidum 3, 9, 10, 27
- connections 11
- external pallidal segment 6(F), 10–12
- internal pallidal segment 6(F), 10–12
- neuronal types 9
- ventral pallidum 3, 9–12
Panic disorders 322
Paranigral nucleus 4, 17, 18
Pargyline 94, 129, 240
- drug discrimination 224
Parkinson's disease (PD) 51, 145, 184, 277, 289, 303, 328
- antioxidative therapy 292
- course of disease 54, 55
- history 54
- life expectancy (see also Life expectancy) 54–56, 292
- pathobiochemistry 29(T), 42(T)
- pathophysiology 25
  - degeneration of NAergic system 37
  - degeneration of serotonergic system 37
  - degeneration of SN 42(T), 55, 145
  - extrastriatal dopaminergic system 36
  - non-dopaminergic system 37
  - receptor-effector coupling 33
  - role of glia 41
- prevalence 146
- side effects
  - anticholinergics 61
  - DA-agonists 59, 60

- L-dopa 56, 58
- L-dopa + DDC-inhibitors 57–59
- L-dopa + DDC-inhibitors + l-deprenyl 62
- symptoms
  - motor symptoms 51, 52
  - mental disorders 52, 53
  - disorders of the autonomic nervous system 53
- treatment with (see also l-Deprenyl and DA-agonists)
  - anticholinergics 61
  - DA-agonists 60
    - plus L-dopa 59, 60, 67
  - long-term pharmacotherapy 65, 66
  - MAO-B inhibitors 278, 279
  - physiotherapy 64, 65
  - surgical methods 63, 64
  - sustained release L-dopa 56, 57
  - "triple" combination 284, 286
- vulnerability of substantia nigra 42(T)
"Parkinson plus" 66, 67
Peptidergic system; dysfunction in PD 39, 40, 41
Pergolide 30, 59, 172, 284
Phenylalanine 322
PEA 77, 79(F), 81(T), 88, 126, 149, 183, 188, 190, 266, 327, 331
- release of catecholamines 266, 331
- urinary excretion 205, 206(F)
Pigmented parabranchial nucleus 4, 17, 18
Phosphatidylserine (PS) 100(F), 306, 308
Physical dependence (see Abuse liability)
Physostygmine 306
Polyamines 191, 195, 254, 334
Positron emission tomography (PET) 32, 88, 128, 131, 202
Progabide 35
Putamen 4, 5, 6(F), 9, 18
- D_2-receptor binding 32(T)
Pyridopyrimidine derivatives 91

Quinones 178, 310

Radicals 41, 42, 148, 177, 193, 266, 290, 330, 332, 336
- cytotoxic free radicals 62, 193, 310
- hydrogen peroxide (H_2O_2) 62, 77, 330
- formation 176(F), 191(F)
- hydroxyl radicals 77, 193(F)
- scavenger function; facilitation 150–153
- superoxide anions 176(F), 193(F)
Raphe nuclei, anterior 9, 18
Respiratory chain (Complex I)
- activity in the brain of PD patients 28, 29(T), 267
Retrosplenial region 9
Riederer, P. 245, 246(F), 251

Ro 16-6491   98(F), 114, 115, 115(F), 116(F),
    117–119, 120(F), 121, 122, 131, 137
Ro 19-6327 (see Lazabemide)
Ro 41-1049   88, 128

Salsolinol   87
Sandler, M.   247, 251
Scavenger function (see Radicals)
SDZ-201-678   30
Selegiline (see also l-Deprenyl)   110, 112
Serotonergic system   9
– degeneration of   26
Serotonin (5-Hydroxytryptamin; 5-HT)   26,
    76, 79(F), 80, 81(T), 126, 128, 183, 243
– turnover   153
Short-Story Recall   308
Shulmann, M.   250
Silyl compounds   92
Somatostatin   39, 40
– somatostatin-containing cells   7, 9
Somerset Pharmaceuticals   248, 250, 251
Stern, G.   247
Substantia innominata   19
Substance P (SP)   39, 40
Subthalamic nucleus   4, 11, 13
Substantia nigra (see also Nigrostriatal
    system)   4, 9, 11, 13, 14(F), 25, 31(F), 266
– age-related changes   160
– connection   17
– loss of projections in PD   53, 291
– neuronal types   15, 16(F)
– vulnerability in PD   42(T)
Suicide inhibitors   89, 129
Superoxide anion (see also Radicals)
– formation   41, 176(F), 193(F), 249, 266,
    290
Superoxide dismutase (SOD)   130, 151, 176,
    177, 194(T)
– activity   330, 332
    – in the striatum   151, 152(T)
    – in the tuberculum olfactorium   152(T),
        153
Su-11,739 (see also AGN-1133)   130
Striatum   4, 5, 12, 12(F), 31(F)
– connections   8

– dorsal striatum   4, 5, 8, 9, 10(F), 18
– matrix   9
– neuronal types   4, 7(F)
– proto-striosomes   8
– striosomes   8
– ventral striatum   4, 6(F), 8, 18
Sympathomimetic amines
– indirectly acting   128
– potentiation   137

Tacrine   306
Tetrahydroisoquinoline (TIQ)   174(F), 175
Thalamus
– centromediano-parafascicular complex   9,
    18
– intralaminar nuclei   9
– mediodorsal nuclei   3, 19
– reticular nucleus   18, 19
– ventrolateral nuclei   3
Thyreotropin releasing hormone (TRH)   39
Tocopherol   290
Tranylcypromine   91, 129, 309
Tryptamine   80
Tuberomamillary nucleus (hypothalamic)   4,
    9, 18
TV-image analyzer   160
Tyramine (TA)   76, 80, 81
– potentiation   133
– containing foodstuffs   135, 262
– hypertensive reaction to   303
Tyrosine hydroxylase (TH)   28
– activity in the brain of PD patients   29(T)
– antibody staining in the brain   188(T)
TZ-650   95(F), 137

U-1424   96(F), 114, 115, 115(F), 117–119,
    120(F), 121, 122, 130, 137

Vasoactive intestinal peptide (VIP)   39
Vasopressin   39
Vinca alkaloids   87, 101

Water/octanol partition coefficient   117(T)

Youdim, M.   244, 246, 246(F), 251